Cases on Communication Disorders in Culturally Diverse Populations

Diane M. Scott
North Carolina Central University, USA

A volume in the Advances in Linguistics and Communication Studies (ALCS) Book Series

IGI Global
DISSEMINATOR OF KNOWLEDGE

Published in the United States of America by
IGI Global
Information Science Reference (an imprint of IGI Global)
701 E. Chocolate Avenue
Hershey PA, USA 17033
Tel: 717-533-8845
Fax: 717-533-8661
E-mail: cust@igi-global.com
Web site: http://www.igi-global.com

Library of Congress Cataloging-in-Publication Data

Names: Scott, Diane M., 1956- editor.
Title: Cases on communication disorders in culturally diverse populations / Diane M. Scott, editor.
Description: Hershey PA : Information Science Reference, [2020] | Includes bibliographical references and index. | Summary: "This book explores how to provide culturally competent hearing, language, and speech services to culturally diverse populations"-- Provided by publisher.
Identifiers: LCCN 2019037789 (print) | LCCN 2019037790 (ebook) | ISBN 9781799822615 (hardcover) | ISBN 9781799822622 (paperback) | ISBN 9781799822639 (ebook)
Subjects: LCSH: Communicative disorders--Case studies. | Transcultural medical care--Case studies. | Cultural competence--Case studies.
Classification: LCC RC423 .C297 2020 (print) | LCC RC423 (ebook) | DDC 362.19685/5--dc23
LC record available at https://lccn.loc.gov/2019037789
LC ebook record available at https://lccn.loc.gov/2019037790

This book is published in the IGI Global book series Advances in Linguistics and Communication Studies (ALCS) (ISSN: 2372-109X; eISSN: 2372-1111)

British Cataloguing in Publication Data
A Cataloguing in Publication record for this book is available from the British Library.

Advances in Linguistics and Communication Studies (ALCS) Book Series

Abigail G. Scheg
Western Governors University, USA

ISSN:2372-109X
EISSN:2372-1111

Mission

The scope of language and communication is constantly changing as society evolves, new modes of communication are developed through technological advancement, and novel words enter our lexicon as the result of cultural change. Understanding how we communicate and use language is crucial in all industries and updated research is necessary in order to promote further knowledge in this field.

The **Advances in Linguistics and Communication Studies (ALCS)** book series presents the latest research in diverse topics relating to language and communication. Interdisciplinary in its coverage, ALCS presents comprehensive research on the use of language and communication in various industries including business, education, government, and healthcare.

Coverage

- Sociolinguistics
- Non-Verbal Communication
- Language and Identity
- Media and Public Communications
- Language Acquisition
- Computer-Mediated Communication
- Cross-Cultural Communication
- Language in the Media
- Discourse Analysis
- Dialectology

IGI Global is currently accepting manuscripts for publication within this series. To submit a proposal for a volume in this series, please contact our Acquisition Editors at Acquisitions@igi-global.com or visit: http://www.igi-global.com/publish/.

The Advances in Linguistics and Communication Studies (ALCS) Book Series (ISSN 2372-109X) is published by IGI Global, 701 E. Chocolate Avenue, Hershey, PA 17033-1240, USA, www.igi-global.com. This series is composed of titles available for purchase individually; each title is edited to be contextually exclusive from any other title within the series. For pricing and ordering information please visit http://www.igi-global.com/book-series/advances-linguistics-communication-studies/78950. Postmaster: Send all address changes to above address.

Titles in this Series

https://www.igi-global.com/book-series/advances-linguistics-communication-studies/78950

Internal and External Narrative Generation Based on Post-Narratology Emerging Research and Opportunities
Takashi Ogata (Iwate Prefectural University, Japan)
Information Science Reference • © 2020 • 300pp • H/C (ISBN: 9781522599432) • US $175.00

Enhancements and Limitations to ICT-Based Informal Language Learning Emerging Research and Opportunities
Rashad Ahmed (Miami University, USA) Abdu Al-kadi (Ibb University, Yemen) and Trenton Hagar (Utrecht University, The Netherlands)
Information Science Reference • © 2020 • 201pp • H/C (ISBN: 9781799821168) • US $175.00

Redefining the Role of Language in a Globalized World
Ai-Ling Wang (Tamkang University, Taiwan)
Information Science Reference • © 2020 • 300pp • H/C (ISBN: 9781799828310) • US $195.00

International Approaches to Bridging the Language Gap
Cristina-Aránzazu Huertas-Abril (University of Córdoba, Spain) and María Elena Gómez-Parra (University of Córdoba, Spain)
Information Science Reference • © 2020 • 317pp • H/C (ISBN: 9781799812197) • US $195.00

Toward an Integrated Approach to Narrative Generation Emerging Research and Opportunities
Takashi Ogata (Iwate Prefectural University, Japan)
Information Science Reference • © 2020 • 432pp • H/C (ISBN: 9781522596936) • US $215.00

Code-Switching for Equitable STEM Pedagogy Emerging Research and Opportunities
Miriam Chitiga (Fayetteville State University, USA)
Information Science Reference • © 2020 • 135pp • H/C (ISBN: 9781799809654) • US $125.00

Applied Linguistics for Teachers of Culturally and Linguistically Diverse Learners
Nabat Erdogan (University of Central Missouri, USA) and Michael Wei (University of Missouri-Kansas City, USA)
Information Science Reference • © 2019 • 504pp • H/C (ISBN: 9781522584674) • US $195.00

Language, Power, and Ideology in Political Writing Emerging Research and Opportunities
Önder Çakırtaş (Bingöl University, Turkey)
Information Science Reference • © 2019 • 206pp • H/C (ISBN: 9781522594444) • US $185.00

Deep Semantics and the Evolution of New Scientific Theories and Discoveries

IGI Global
DISSEMINATOR OF KNOWLEDGE

701 East Chocolate Avenue, Hershey, PA 17033, USA
Tel: 717-533-8845 x100 • Fax: 717-533-8661
E-Mail: cust@igi-global.com • www.igi-global.com

Editorial Advisory Board

Table of Contents

Detailed Table of Contents

This chapter will focus on providing intervention services for an eight-year-old African-American female, Dawn, with multiple disabilities. Dawn has been diagnosed with Down syndrome, a comorbid diagnosis of an intellectual disability, and exhibits behavior problems at home and school. In this scenario, she has been evaluated within the school system to determine eligibility for services, and the speech-language pathologist needs to develop intervention goals and select therapy strategies to provide appropriate services. While both parents are involved in the child's care, the family does not have permanent housing and moves frequently. Information from actual cases has been incorporated into this chapter.

This case focuses on the effects of trauma on the language and social pragmatic communication of a 10-year-old girl who was one of the many children separated from familial caregivers between 2016 and 2019 when she and her parents came to the U.S. from Central America seeking asylum due to gang violence and economic reasons. The child spent 8 months in the detention center without her parents and then was transferred to a foster home where she suffered neglect as well as physical and psychological abuse. This case study focuses on the long-term effects of structural violence and maltreatment on child development, and specifically on language and social pragmatic communication.

Silvia and Antonio Juarez described their 4-year-old son Emanuel as often happy. Emanuel came from a bilingual home and spoke both Spanish and English. His favorite activities were reading and playing with his iPad over-and-over again. Reading was a favorite pasttime and something that the Juarez's felt he did well. While he was described as "loving to engage people," it was not clear that his efforts were successful nor was it clear that they were reciprocated. Briefly observing Emanuel's interaction with his parents, it was noted Emanuel used echolalic phrases and engaged in repetitive and restricted behaviors, toe walking, and finger flicking. These behaviors were noted to be unusual and warranted further evaluation. The Juarez's primary concern was regarding Emanuel's "talking and being able to hold a conversation." Through speech and language therapy, the family expected that Emanuel's communication skills would improve, and he would be able to participate in conversations and talk in sentences.

This chapter will provide readers with an overview of how a systems-based approach can be used to understand the relationship between culture, environment, language, and disability. It will identify a useful model of ecology, culture, and development that can and should be considered in conjunction with the WHO-ICF framework to guide service delivery in school-based settings. This chapter will also provide an overview of systems-based approaches that can be used when working with children from traditionally marginalized backgrounds. Finally, a case study example will be used to provide guidance on the application of systems-based approaches to service delivery for children in school-based settings.

With the constantly rising multilingualism in the United States, cultural and linguistic diversity is gradually becoming more and more present at schools throughout the country. Therefore, there is a critical need for resources to support speech-language pathologists (SLPs) to work with culturally and linguistically diverse (CLD) clients. This case study examines a CLD client with a diagnosis of specific learning disability (SLD). SLD is a disorder characterized by one or more significant impairments in reading, spelling, writing, or arithmetical skills, which are not the direct result of other disorders or inadequate schooling. This chapter discusses approaches to appropriately assess the client's language skills and provides intervention suggestions to account for the CLD nature of the client and her SLD.

An increasing number of deaf and hard-of-hearing (D/HH) children live in homes where languages other than English or American Sign Language (ASL) are used. This chapter reviews issues of culture and linguistic diversity when working with D/HH multilingual learners (DMLs) from identification and early intervention through school entry. The authors will provide two case studies to explore the issues of service delivery to DMLs and their families: 1) Ji-Hun, who appears to use several spoken languages, including Korean, Japanese, and English, and 2) Ana, who is a recent immigrant to the USA and appears to use ASL, spoken Spanish, and spoken English. The discussion of these two case studies will encompass some cultural differences, including 1) openness to engagement with providers, 2) cultural beliefs about hearing loss, 3) community systems and familiar support, 4) perceptions of systems and authorities. The case studies presented are not based on actual clients but are drawn from the clinical experiences of the authors.

Sickle cell disease (SCD) is an autosomal recessively inherited group of red blood cell disorders. It is more commonly found in African Americans and Hispanics in the United States. The sickle-shaped cells characteristic of the disease cause physiological problems, including hemolytic anemia and vaso-occlusion. Research has linked hearing loss to sickle cell disease. Studies have shown that children and adults with sickle cell disease may have higher rates of sensorineural and central auditory hearing impairment. This case study examines hidden hearing loss in an African American boy with SCD who presents with normal hearing thresholds. It also discusses the role of audiologists in the care of individuals with sickle cell disease and hearing loss.

This chapter provides a brief overview of stroke, aphasia, and aphasia assessment. Additionally, it considers various issues associated with the standardized assessment of aphasia, including problems related to cultural and linguistic biases. The chapter also includes information on working with people who are bilingual, as well as working with interpreters. A hypothetical case study is presented as a teaching avenue to discuss these topics in greater length. This section contains details regarding how both cultural and linguistic barriers associated with the assessment of the patient's aphasia may have influenced the intervention provided by the speech-language pathologist (SLP). Medical terminology and procedures related to stroke intervention are also discussed as it relates to the SLP's plan of care.

Culturally competent management of adults with swallowing disorders involves more than simply including ethnically appropriate foods in dysphagia therapy. It requires an understanding of the client's health beliefs, challenges, and unique cultural perspective regarding all aspects of food to ensure unbiased and culturally appropriate services are provided. This chapter begins with an overview of dysphagia management followed by a closer look at cultural beliefs regarding food and ethical conflicts that may arise. The strategies for shared decision-making presented help create a culturally sensitive dynamic between the clinician and the patient/family that positively influence therapy outcomes. The chapter concludes with a case study that highlights the importance of ethnographic interviewing needed to establish understanding and trust between the clinician and an elderly Mexican woman and her family. The strategies and techniques presented here can be applied across all cultures to achieve successful management of dysphagia.

The Hispanic community has both positive and negative health indicators related to their Hispanic culture. This chapter details aspects of the Hispanic culture that can influence healthcare prevention, diagnosis, and intervention, including traditional healthcare beliefs and practices. Additionally, various health disparities associated with the Hispanic population are discussed, particularly related to neurological disorders. The chapter concludes with a case study presentation based loosely upon an actual event from a young man with neurocysticercosis. This section details how the patient's Hispanic culture influenced lifestyle choices, which increased risk for this disease, while also detailing how his culture impacted certain aspects of his medical intervention.

This chapter highlights traumatic brain injury (TBI) and various health disparities within this population, particularly gaps related to patients from culturally diverse backgrounds. A review of three main health disparities is included, related to increased risk for sustaining a TBI, intervention barriers related to TBI, and long-term outcome after TBI. This chapter also evaluates how culture influences aspects of TBI intervention by exploring cultural considerations apparent in diverse populations. The chapter concludes with an examination of a case study based on an actual patient who sustained a TBI and details how his Native American culture impacted his healthcare choices and how his healthcare providers adapted intervention strategies given cultural influences unique to his clinical presentation.

Research has linked hearing loss to other medical conditions such as diabetes. Studies have shown that hearing loss is more common in individuals who have diabetes than in those who do not. Hyperglycemia, or raised blood sugar, is a common effect of uncontrolled diabetes and over time leads to serious damage to many of the body's systems, especially the nerves and the blood vessels. Consequently, diabetes can affect the blood vessels of the inner ear and the vestibulocochlear (VIII cranial) nerve fibers. This case study examines the interrelationship between diabetes and hearing loss in an African American adult while examining the issues of the higher prevalence of diabetes in African Americans and the role of audiologists in the care of individuals with hearing loss and diabetes.

This chapter addresses the cultural diversity of supervisees encountered by supervisors. This case study addresses the cultural dynamics of a clinical fellow from Saudi Arabia who is completing her clinical fellowship in the United States. Aneshia is a clinical fellow who received her Bachelor of Science degree from King Saud University in Saudi Arabia and then earned her Master's degree from an American university. As a Muslim woman such topics as dress, religion, and culture are described and addressed as it relates to Aneshia and her interaction with patients, coworkers, and caregivers. Areas such as appropriate communication distance, appropriate greetings, and physical interactions (oral motor examination, etc.) are discussed along with strategies for addressing these challenges. Areas including documentation as it relates to Arabic syntax and morphology versus standard American English are described. Strategies for working with professionals from Middle Eastern and Arabic countries are also discussed.

Foreword

I have found that the case-study format is an excellent way to provide clinical information that is evidence based. This textbook does just that through the work of an excellent group of experienced professionals in the field of speech-language pathology and audiology. These authors are all veterans of both clinical practice and clinical teaching. They now provide us their expertise through selected cases that address the questions we have today. We continue to see an increase in the diversity of our caseloads, culturally and linguistically, and at the same time we search for authentic resources that can help us meet the needs of these individuals.

The uniqueness of this textbook is the ease in which you will find the answers to your questions. The information is well-laid out, thoroughly researched and presented in a way that is easy to read. The presentation of cases will lead you to engage in the "story" of these individuals and draw you into taking a personal interest in these cases. The authors do an excellent job of providing the answers to the problems they identify, or at least food-for-thought regarding the concerns and issues that these cases represent.

This textbook will be that book you will return to often to guide your clinical work. The information provided in the book can be adapted to your cases in ways you do not see initially. On further reading you will learn that questions you have had from other cases can be answered through a case presented here. The descriptions of cases are so rich with information that one case can provide answers to a broad range of questions you have been pondering.

Another excellent use of this case format will be for teaching graduate students. The cases are current and can parallel the class lectures. They can give students the "all important" complete look at a casc from beginning to end. As professors we are always looking for good clinical examples to expand the textbook narrative readings. This case-based book will do just that for you.

The authors that have been gathered for this textbook are experts across many areas in speech-language pathology and audiology, but most importantly, they have all had a long-standing interest in connecting the clinical and academics worlds. This is to be commended. Many times these two worlds are disjointed or simply not integrated as well as they could be. This book feels like a bridge has been made not only across clinical and academic pedagogy, but also across diversity issues which so often remain unattended. We see in this book the evidence-based practice principles that are critical to meet the needs of our diverse clients, students and patients.

As I read through the chapters I found myself thinking how important this book would be for the classroom teacher, the psychologist, the occupational therapist and other professionals. In this day of interprofessional practice and education this is the type of book that is needed. I will be sure to pass this book on to my professional colleagues from across a wide spectrum and feel confident their understanding of our field will be increased.

This book will be an excellent addition to the professional libraries of students, clinicians, academicians and other educators and healthcare providers. We are fortunate to have this excellent work to help us address our clinical challenges with individuals from culturally and linguistically diverse populations across settings. I know this book will be up front and center in my professional library.

Marlene B. Salas-Provance
A. T. Still University, USA

Preface

In the field of communication sciences and disorders, the demographic and caseload changes related to culturally and linguistically diverse (CLD) populations require *cultural competence* in order to provide *clinically competent services*. What is cultural competence? Cultural competence involves both understanding and appropriately responding to the combination of cultural variables and range of diversity that professionals and families bring to clinical interactions. Cultural diversity can incorporate a variety of factors, including but not limited to age, disability, ethnicity, gender identity, national origin, race, religion, sex, and sexual orientation. Linguistic diversity can go together with cultural diversity. Developing cultural competence is a dynamic and multifaceted process that requires ongoing and continuous self-assessment and expansion of one's cultural knowledge, which includes interactions with individuals from various cultures. It evolves over time and is a lifelong process.

This book addresses serving CLD populations with communication disorders by using case studies. Case studies offer a practical and detailed means for assisting students in communication sciences and disorders programs as well as faculty instructors and practitioners in appropriately applying assessment and intervention techniques to CLD populations. It is a pathway to expanding one's cultural knowledge.

The case studies begin with Tanveer, a first grader in the public schools who is an Urdu-speaking immigrant from Pakistan. Chapter 1, "The Preassessment Process for English Language Learners With Potential Language Impairment: Best Practices for Public School Professionals," asks the question, "Does Tanveer have a language impairment?" In order to accurately differentiate a language difference from a language impairment in this student, SLPs must demonstrate cultural competence by departing from "typical" testing procedures and using nonbiased assessment methods based on the principles of evidence-based practice.

Once again, the importance of culturally and linguistically appropriate assessment is illustrated in Chapter 2, "Navajo Speech and Language Evaluation: Difference vs. Disorder." The chapter highlights Carl, a five-year old Navajo boy who lives on the reservation in New Mexico with his Navajo-speaking family members. Carl speaks English primarily with exposure to Navajo and English in his home and community. He has been referred for an evaluation by his kindergarten teacher for speech and language concerns. The case illustrates systemic issues that result in lack of coordinated care and appropriate diagnosis, along with the lack of American Indian speech-language pathologists who understand linguistic and cultural differences.

In Chapter 3, "Intervention Services for a Child With Multiple Disabilities," intervention services for Dawn, an eight-year-old African-American female with multiple disabilities, are described. Dawn has been diagnosed with Down syndrome, a comorbid diagnosis of an intellectual disability, a congenital heart problem, and exhibits behavior problems at home and school. While both parents are involved in the child's care, the family does not have permanent housing and moves frequently. Children from transient home environments are at higher risk for poor academic and emotional outcomes. This case illustrates that intervention services should consider the support systems needed by both the child and the family.

The focus of Chapter 4, "Language, Social Pragmatic Communication, and Childhood Trauma," is on the effects of trauma on the language and social pragmatic communication of a 10-year-old girl who is separated from her family at the U.S. border and then spends 8 months in a detention center without her parents. Isidra is then transferred to a foster home where she suffers neglect, as well as physical and psychological abuse. Her biological parents are from Guatemala. Isidra and her family identify as Latinx and Garifuna, and racially identify as of African descent or Black. Isidra's parents are proficient speakers of Garifuna (language derived from African, Indian and European languages), Spanish, and English. Isidra frequently misinterprets facial expressions and the intentions of her peers. She is currently going to school within a residential center and is receiving psychological counseling. Isidra has been brought to a transdisciplinary clinic for further assessment.

In Chapter 5, "A Bilingual Child Diagnosed With Autism Spectrum Disorder," the case of 4-year-old Emanuel is described. He is from a bilingual home where both Spanish and English are spoken. While briefly observing him, it is noted that Emanuel uses echolalic phrases and engages in repetitive and restricted behaviors, toe walking, and finger flicking. Through speech and language therapy the family expects that Emanuel's communication skills will improve and he will be able to participate in conversations and talk in sentences.

Chapter 6, "Systems-Based Approaches to Speech-Language Pathology Service Delivery in School Age Children," provides readers with an overview of how a systems-based approach can be used to understand the relationship between culture, environment, language, and disability. It identifies a model of ecology, culture, and development that can be considered in conjunction with the WHO-ICF framework to guide service delivery in school-based settings, which in turn is applied to the case of Jeff. Jeff is 5-year-old boy from Jamaica. Jeff's family migrated to Tampa, FL. Jeff and his 10-year-old sister speak English, but their mother usually speaks to them using English or her native Jamaican Patois. Jeff's father is not in the U.S. The family lives with extended family while the mother looks for permanent employment and housing. Jeff's kindergarten class is staffed by three long-term substitutes and one parent volunteer. The SLP is trying to determine if Jeff has any significant communication issues that are impacting his learning.

The next case study, Chapter 7, "Working With a Culturally and Linguistically Diverse Individual With Specific Learning Disability," examines a CLD student, Nancy, who shows some signs of specific learning disability (SLD). Nancy is 10 years old and lives with her biological family. They emigrated from China when Nancy was 8 years old. Nancy spoke only Mandarin when she was in China and the dominant language used at home is Mandarin. She began to learn English after moving to the United States. The case study focuses on approaches to appropriately assess her language skills and provides intervention strategies to account for Nancy's SLD and her CLD background.

Deaf and hard-of-hearing (D/HH) children in the U.S. live in homes where languages other than English or American Sign Language (ASL) are used. Chapter 8, "Working With Deaf and Hard-of-Hearing Children From Linguistically Diverse Backgrounds," reviews issues of culture and linguistic diversity when working with D/HH multilingual learners (DMLs) from identification of the hearing impairment and implementation of early intervention services through school entry. Two case studies explore the issues of service delivery to DMLs and their families: 1) Ji-Hun, who appears to use several spoken languages, including Korean, Japanese, and English, and 2) Ana, who is a recent immigrant to the USA and appears to use ASL, spoken Spanish, and spoken English.

Chapter 9, "Sickle Cell Disease and Hidden Hearing Loss," examines the case of Brian, a 12-year-old African American male with sickle cell disease (SCD). SCD is an autosomal recessively inherited group of red blood cell disorders. The sickle-shaped cells characteristic of the disease cause physiological problems, including hemolytic anemia and vaso-occlusion. Research has linked hearing loss to sickle cell disease. This case study examines hidden hearing loss in Brian who presents with normal hearing thresholds.

Karl is a 68-year-old male who speaks only German. Karl is admitted to the hospital with a sudden onset of difficulties communicating, slurred speech, and right sided weakness. Chapter 10, "Factors Influencing Aphasia Assessment for Bilingual Adults," considers various issues associated with the standardized assessment of aphasia, including problems related to cultural and linguistic biases. The chapter includes information on working with people who are bilingual, as well as working with interpreters. It details how both cultural and linguistic barriers associated with the assessment of the patient's aphasia may have influenced the intervention provided by the speech-language pathologist (SLP).

Culturally competent management of adults with swallowing disorders involves more than including ethnically appropriate foods during intervention services. It requires an understanding of the client's health beliefs and cultural perspectives regarding food. Chapter 11, "Dysphagia Management in Culturally-Linguistically Diverse Populations," describes strategies for shared decision making that help create a culturally sensitive dynamic between the SLP and the patient/family. HL is an 84-year-old Hispanic woman with dysphagia following a left hemisphere subcortical stroke receiving services from a monolingual (English) SLP in a skilled nursing facility. The chapter highlights the importance of utilizing ethnographic interviewing to establish understanding and trust between an SLP and an elderly Mexican woman and her family.

Chapter 12, "Healthcare Considerations for the Hispanic Population," details aspects of the Hispanic culture which can influence healthcare prevention, diagnosis, and intervention, including traditional healthcare beliefs and practices. Additionally, various health disparities associated with the Hispanic population are discussed, particularly related to neurological disorders. Antonio is a 27-year-old Hispanic male whose neurological examination revealed mild cognitive, motor, and sensory impairments. Combined with the results from Antonio's head CT, a neurology team diagnoses him with neurocysticercosis. Antonio's Hispanic culture influenced his lifestyle choices which increased his risk for this disease; his culture also impacts certain aspects of his medical intervention.

Chapter 13, "Traumatic Brain Injury in Culturally Diverse Populations: Navigating Healthcare Intervention for Adults," highlights traumatic brain injury (TBI) and various health disparities within this population, particularly gaps related to patients from culturally diverse backgrounds. Jonas is 53 years old when he is in a severe motor vehicle collision. Jonas and his family are Native American and members of the Lumbee tribe. The chapter details how his Native American culture impacts his healthcare choices and how his healthcare providers modify their intervention strategies given unique cultural influences on his clinical presentation.

Research has linked hearing loss to other medical conditions such as diabetes. Studies have shown that hearing loss is more common in individuals who have diabetes than in those who do not. Research has shown that diabetes can affect the blood vessels of the inner ear and the vestibulocochlear (VIII cranial) nerve fibers. Chapter 14, "Hearing Loss and Diabetes in an African American Adult," examines the interrelationship between diabetes and hearing loss in an African American female, ST, in her mid-

50s. The case study examines the issues of hearing loss and the higher prevalence of diabetes in African Americans, along with the role of audiologists in the care of individuals with hearing loss and diabetes.

Chapter 15, "Supervision: The Other Side of Cultural Diversity," addresses the cultural diversity of supervisees encountered by supervisors. This case study addresses the cultural dynamics of a clinical fellow, Aneshia, from Saudi Arabia who is completing her clinical fellowship in the United States. As a Muslim woman such topics as dress, religion, and culture are addressed as it relates to Aneshia and her interaction with patients, coworkers and caregivers, including her interactions with male coworkers, patients and caregivers. Appropriate communication distance, physical interactions, and use of her native language versus standard American English are among the other challenges examined.

Speech-language pathologists and audiologists are expected to provide clinically and culturally competent services. This book describing clinical cases involving culturally and linguistically diverse populations across age groups and communication disorders will assist in meeting the need for more cultural knowledge. It provides practical information on serving CLD populations with communication disorders.

The underlying foundation for this casebook and all its chapters is the following: all clinical interactions should be approached from a cultural competence perspective. All clinical interactions are influenced by linguistic, cultural, ethnic, and societal intricacies along with healthcare beliefs brought to the interactions by clients/patients/families and practitioners.

Diane M. Scott

Section 1
Pediatric Populations

Chapter 1
The Preassessment Process for English Learners With Potential Language Impairment:
Best Practices for Public School Professionals

Celeste Roseberry-McKibbin
California State University, Sacramento, USA

EXECUTIVE SUMMARY

This chapter presents the case of Tanveer, a first-grade boy from an Urdu-speaking immigrant family from Pakistan. He is in the public schools and has been struggling academically since kindergarten. This chapter discusses the preassessment process and interventions that took place before Tanveer underwent a full special education evaluation, including testing by a speech-language pathologist for the possible presence of an underlying language impairment. (Note: this author personally worked with this child, and this is a true story with some details changed for confidentiality.) This chapter shows how even before formal special education testing commenced, conducting an extensive preassessment process helped to greatly increase the accuracy of the formal evaluation, eventual diagnosis, and intervention provided for Tanveer.

INTRODUCTORY KEY POINTS

ASHA (2019b) reminds us that best practices with clients are evidence-based. These practices must incorporate three major components: client perspectives, clinical experience, and external scientific evidence. Accordingly, the following four tasks are put forth as preassessment best practices for differentiating a language impairment from a language difference in an EL student: (Karanth, Roseberry-McKibbin, & James, 2017; Paradis, Schneider, & Duncan, 2013; Pua, Lee, & Liow, 2017; Roseberry-McKibbin, 2018):

DOI: 10.4018/978-1-7998-2261-5.ch001

1. Determine a child's proficiency in both the first language (L1) and English
2. Gather a case history of the child's speech and language development in L1 from the child's parents or other primary caregivers (e.g., a grandparent)
3. Interview individuals who have observed the child's linguistic performance in multiple settings (e.g., classroom teacher, interpreter/bilingual associate)
4. Conduct dynamic assessment of a child's ability to learn through using a response-to-intervention (RtI) model

These tasks are consistent with ASHA's (2019a; 2019b) mandates to provide culturally competent services that reflect principles of evidence-based practice.

INTRODUCTION

The United States has more immigrants than any other country in the world. Today, more than 40 million people living in the U.S. were born in another country. The population of immigrants is very diverse, representing almost every country in the world (Pew Research Center, 2019). At this time, there are more than 350 languages spoken in the U.S. Speakers of Russian have increased by 391%; speakers of Korean and Arabic have quadrupled (Accredited Language Services, 2019). Consequently, the number of English Learner (EL) students in the public schools is increasing dramatically. According to the National Center for Education Statistics (2019), in fall of 2016, the percentage of U.S. public school students who were English Learners (ELs) ranged from 0.9% in West Virginia to 20.2% in California.

When EL students struggle in the classroom, teachers often refer them to speech-language pathologists (SLPs) and other special education personnel for assessment for suspected language impairment and other special education diagnoses (e.g., autism spectrum disorder, reading disability). Many SLPs, having heavy caseloads and very little time, assess these EL students through a "business-as-usual" approach. Specifically, the SLPs conduct a brief screener and, if the child fails it, obtain signed permission from parents for a full evaluation. For this full evaluation, the SLPs frequently bring the child into their speech-language room and carry out formal standardized testing in English, even if the child is not fluent in English (Arias & Friberg, 2017). In approximately 1-1.5 hours, the SLP obtains formal scores (e.g., percentile ranks and standard scores) and then makes a diagnosis of "language impairment" or "no language impairment" based upon the findings from this static testing process, which measures the child's given knowledge at one point in time. The SLP then writes a report. If the child is diagnosed with a language impairment, the SLP holds an IEP meeting, obtains parent signatures, and places the student onto the speech-language caseload for intervention.

Numerous sources have documented the fact that assessment of the language skills of EL children is often biased, and that the typical procedures described above are not ideal. Use of such procedures over-identifies EL students as having language impairments (Barragan, Castilla-Earls, Martinez-Kieto, Restrepo, & Gray, 2018; Benavides, Kapantzoglou, & Murata, 2018; Lazewnik et al., 2019; Moore & Montgomery, 2018; Roseberry-McKibbin, Hegde, & Tellis, 2019). Use of standardized tests in English with ELs is fraught with problems (Arias & Friberg, 2017; Kraemer & Fabiano-Smith, 2017). Many of these tests contain potentially unfamiliar items that EL students have not been previously exposed to. For example, EL students from countries near the equator would not recognize test items that assumed exposure to ice and snow. Many EL students have been taught, in their cultures, to respectfully remain silent in the presence of an unfamiliar adult. Thus, they will not speak openly with an SLP who they do not know. This can definitely negatively impact their expressive language performance in an assessment, and lead to inaccurate conclusions like "this child has an expressive language delay" or "this child has clinically significant difficulties with pragmatics." In addition, use of formal test scores is psychometrically invalid for ELs because they have not been represented in the norming sample. Unfortunately, SLPs continue to use standardized tests in English anyway because school districts demand quantitative data such as standardized scores. In addition, many SLPs have not had the benefit of coursework or continuing education training in less-biased, culturally appropriate assessment practices.

In order to accurately differentiate a language difference from a language impairment in an EL student, SLPs must demonstrate cultural competence by departing from "typical" testing procedures and using legally sound, nonbiased assessment methods that represent principles of evidence-based practice. ASHA (2019a) states that cultural competence involves understanding and appropriately responding to the unique combination of cultural variables that clients and families bring to interactions. Use of scientifically-supported strategies for assessing the language skills of ELs demonstrates adherence to ASHA's mandate to use culturally competent strategies.

One such strategy is the implementation of an extensive preassessment process when differentiating a language difference from a language impairment in an EL student. The purpose of this process is to gather as much information as possible about the student's performance and language learning ability before a full, formal evaluation of his or her language skills takes place.

This chapter describes the case of Tanveer and discusses the preassessment process used before formal special education testing was initiated. The chapter discusses interventions that were used before Tanveer was formally assessed for a language impairment or other special education diagnosis (e.g., reading disability). The chapter emphasizes that a thorough preassessment process helps school teams examine closely whether or not the EL student's performance is primarily impacted by environmental variables (e.g., poverty, lack of home literacy) and therefore amenable to added non-special education supports, or whether the student truly has an underlying language impairment and will need special education in the form of speech-language services and possibly other services as well.

BACKGROUND INFORMATION/CLINICAL HISTORY

Tanveer D. and his family moved to California from Pakistan when Tanveer was three years old. At that time, he spoke only Urdu, the language of his immigrant family. Tanveer's mother worked full time inside the home caring for her children; Mr. D. was a postal worker. Both parents spoke fluent Urdu to their children at home; the parents' English skills were limited. The family was experiencing poverty and struggled to make ends meet. They did not speak, read, or write in English and did not read with their children in either Urdu or English. Research has documented the fact that in the homes of some culturally diverse families, reading with children is not a common practice (Guiberson & Ferris, 2019; Kummerer, 2012; Owens, 2020; Palafox, 2017; Simon-Cereijido, 2015). Tanveer's family fit this profile. However, his parents worked hard to provide the best life that they could for themselves and their two sons.

Tanveer had a brother, Abdul, who was two years younger than he was. The D. family did not put Tanveer into preschool, believing that staying home full time with his mother would provide the most secure, stable environment for their young son. They did attend the local Muslim mosque where Tanveer was exposed to other children; however, this only occurred once a week for 2-3 hours.

Tanveer began kindergarten when he was 5;7 years old. He spoke only Urdu; kindergarten was his first exposure to English or to any kind of structured school setting. His kindergarten teacher, Ms. Povey, had had many ELs in her classroom for the last 15 years, as the school district was home to a great many immigrant families. Ms. Povey estimated that in her 15 years with the school district, she had personally taught more than 500 EL students from a wide range of linguistic backgrounds including Urdu, Telegu, Farsi, Tagalog, Vietnamese, Spanish, Afrikaans, Mandarin, Dari, Maay, Arabic, and others. The elementary school itself had 1,000 students; 91% were culturally and linguistically diverse, and 9% were White. Most of the children's families received Aid to Families with Dependent Children.

When Tanveer first entered Ms. Povey's classroom in the fall of kindergarten, he was very quiet and had few friends. He had difficulty with classroom routines (e.g., lining up for recess, sitting in circle time). He often appeared confused. As an experienced teacher, Ms. Povey knew she should give Tanveer plenty of time to adjust to the school setting and learn English.

Ms. Povey was hesitant to refer him to the special education team because she thought that his difficulties might be due primarily to his EL status and his background of poverty, no preschool exposure, and lack of literacy in the home. She hoped that more time in school might help spontaneously resolve Tanveer's issues. She talked with Ms. Jimenez, the site SLP, about her concerns. Ms. Jimenez said she would help Ms. Povey informally monitor Tanveer's progress, agreeing that his difficulties might be entirely traceable to environmental and linguistic differences, not an underlying language impairment. Both Ms. Jimenez and Ms. Povey were aware that EL students are often overidentified for special education, and they did not want to do this to Tanveer.

In the spring of Tanveer's kindergarten year, Ms. Povey noticed that the other EL students in her class were reciting the alphabet accurately and writing spelling words accurately as well. They could read very simple English sight words and tell stories (although grammatically imperfect) in English. They had friends. Tanveer, on the other hand, struggled with all these tasks. He stood out noticeably among the other ELs as having inordinate difficulty with reading and writing especially. He only had 1-2 friends, and had difficulty interacting appropriately with other children. Upon Ms. Jimenez' advice, Ms. Povey introduced Tier 1 interventions through a Response to Intervention (RtI) model.

CLINICAL EVALUATIONS

RtI incorporates a dynamic assessment model whose purpose is to evaluate a student's ability to learn over time when provided with instruction. RtI emphasizes a process that attempts to provide additional, increasingly intensified support to students over time before labeling them as having disabilities (Moore & Montgomery, 2018). If the student shows treatment resistance, or limited ability to learn when provided with additional support and instruction, usually the student has a language impairment or other diagnosis that requires special education services (Roseberry-McKibbin, 2018).

Basic principles of RtI include: (Moore & Montgomery, 2018; Roseberry-McKibbin, 2018; Roth, Dixon, Paul, & Bellini, 2013)

- Intervening early
- Using a multi-tier model of service delivery
- Monitoring student progress to adapt instruction
- Using research-based, scientifically supported interventions as much as possible
- Making decisions based upon data
- Monitoring progress to determine if academic and/or behavioral interventions are producing the desired result

Usually, there are three tiers of instruction in the RtI model. Tier 1 activities provide high quality scientifically based instruction to whole classrooms of children; this can be tailored to meet the learning needs of individual students (Roth et al., 2013). Tier 2 activities are usually provided in small groups (e.g., 4-6 students) and are more differentiated. Tier 2 activities are intended for students who need additional support to successfully access the classroom curriculum. Students who participate in Tier 2 RtI often work on reading accuracy, fluency, and comprehension. They engage in additional activities focused on their needs, giving them more exposure to develop those skills (Edutopia, 2019). Tier 3 activities provide further, more highly specialized and differentiated support for smaller groups and even for students on an individualized basis. Thus, in Tier 3, students receive 1:1 instruction with the teacher or work in groups of 2-3 students. Tier 3 activities are usually provided more intensively and more frequently than those activities provided in Tiers 1 and 2 (Roth et al., 2013). For example, students receiving Tier 2 RtI might be seen in a group of 5 twice a week for 30 minutes. Students receiving Tier 3 RtI might be seen individually 3-4 days a week for 45 minutes.

With Ms. Jimenez' support, Ms. Povey began the preassessment process through implementation of an RtI model to ascertain whether or not Tanveer had a language difference that would resolve with time, or an underlying language impairment that would require special education services. In spring semester of kindergarten, Ms. Povey began implementing Tier 1 RtI methods. Ms. Jimenez provided Ms. Povey with strategies for helping Tanveer develop literacy-based skills, vocabulary, and increase his overall academic performance. Ms. Povey moved Tanveer to the front row of the classroom and seated him beside a peer buddy who was instructed to support him with following directions for classroom tasks. Ms. Povey kept careful data on Tanveer's progress.

Questions for the Reader

1. Was Tanveer a was a typically-developing student who simply needed more time to learn English, or did he have an underlying language impairment that impacted both Urdu and English and would require an IEP and formal special education services, including speech-language therapy?
2. What are best practices for nonbiased assessment of an EL to differentiate language difference from language impairment?
3. What is the role of a preassessment process that occurs before formal special education testing is carried out?
4. What is the role of RtI in the preassessment process?
5. Would implementation of RtI be sufficient to meet Tanveer's needs, or would he ultimately need special education?

Discussion of Questions for the Reader

1. It can be very difficult to differentiate a language impairment from a language difference that is impacted by linguistic and environmental variables such as lack of English proficiency, poverty, and lack of literacy in the home. This was a major challenge faced by Tanveer's school team.
2. This team realized that one of the best practices for nonbiased assessment of an EL to differentiate language difference from language impairment was to carry out a thorough preassessment process.
3. The preassessment process included parent interview and dynamic assessment of Tanveer's underlying language learning ability through a response-to-intervention (RtI) model.
4. The role of RtI in the preassessment process was to evaluate Tanveer's ability to learn when provided with increasingly intense amounts of instruction. Tanveer came from a home where parents' English was very limited. He had never been to preschool. The family was experiencing poverty, and Tanveer was not exposed to literacy practices within the home. Thus, increasing amounts of support were provided at school through an RtI model to ascertain if this support was sufficient to help him perform adequately in the classroom without special education intervention.
5. The school team hoped that provision of RtI would be sufficient for meeting Tanveer's academic needs without special education.

Implementing RtI

At the end of kindergarten, Ms. Povey and Ms. Jimenez examined data gathered to document Tanveer's response to Tier 1 RtI modifications. They discovered that despite these modifications, Tanveer had made minimal progress. At the beginning of fall of Tanveer's first grade year, Ms. Jimenez met with his teacher, Mr. Jarecki, and the school team. They decided that Mr. Jarecki would implement Tier 2 RtI methods to ascertain whether or not Tanveer would respond positively to more intensive support.

These Tier 2 methods provided Tanveer with more focused directed instruction for diagnostic and therapeutic instructional purposes. The team utilized the services of an Urdu-speaking tutor, Ms. Bukhari. Ms. Bukhari was an interpreter who the district hired and trained to assist with service delivery to Urdu-speaking children as well as meet with parents and explain school policies, district procedures, and relevant state and federal laws pertaining to their and their children's rights. Ms. Bukhari came to the classroom three times a week for an hour to help Tanveer and two other Urdu-speaking students with their school work. She saw them in a small group at the back of the classroom. She explained tasks in Urdu and helped the students with class assignments. The two other Urdu-speaking students in Tanveer's small group progressed quickly. Mr. Jarecki noticed that after several months of in-class support during the fall semester (September-December), they were performing better academically. Tanveer, on the other hand, showed minimal gains after four months of additional support.

In December of first grade, Mr. Jarecki met with the school team and reported on Tanveer's progress given Tier 2 RtI. Mr. Jarecki shared that unfortunately, Tanveer's progress was minimal. Tanveer showed very low reading fluency, even in comparison with other ELs, and appeared to have difficulty retaining information. He was struggling academically in every area. Mr. Jarecki also shared that Tanveer had difficulty maintaining a simple conversation, telling a story sequentially, and interacting appropriately with other children. The team decided that in January of first grade, more intensive Tier 3 RtI interventions would be implemented (Roseberry-McKibbin, 2018).

In January, these more intensive interventions began. They included:

1. A peer tutor for classroom support
2. Individual tutoring for ½ hour five days a week with Ms. Bukhari to help support Tanveer in Urdu
3. After-school homework club where Tanveer could receive individualized homework help from a classroom teacher
4. Support from the school's Reading Clinic, a non-special education pullout program where struggling students received one hour a week of small group instruction in reading and writing

Mr. Jarecki and the school team agreed to take a "watch-and-wait" approach to see if these extra, increased supports would help Tanveer to achieve grade-level skills. In April of Tanveer's first grade year, he had made minimal gains in his skills and was noticeably lower (academically) than all his EL classmates.

Gathering Case History

At that point, Ms. Jimenez decided to interview Tanveer's mother, Ms. D., to find out more about his language development and skills in Urdu. Ms. Jimenez reviewed ASHA's (2019b) evidence-based practice portal and was reminded that evidence-based practice focuses on including client perspectives as well as clinical experience and external scientific evidence. She wanted to obtain Ms. D's perspective on Tanveer's language development.

Remembering that evidence-based practice also involves the use of external scientific evidence, Ms. Jimenez found research showing that parent report is valid and reliable in terms of helping identify language impairment in bilingual children. She had read the research of Paradis, Emmerzael, and Duncan (2010) and Paradis et al. (2013), who found that use of parent reports on first language development was an accurate way to predict language impairment in children. She also read that Bedore, Pena, Joyner, & Macken (2011) found that parent and teacher reports correlate with children's language performance.

Ms. Jimenez read the research of Guiberson, Rodriguez, and Dale (2011) which showed that parent report was accurate and helpful in evaluating the language of young bilingual children. Continuing her research, Ms. Jimenez read that Benavides, Kapantzoglou, and Murata (2018) reported, based on their study's findings, that parent concerns plus low grammaticality scores on language samples yielded very high diagnostic accuracy in the assessment of monolingual Spanish-speaking children at risk for specific language impairment.

Ms. Jimenez reviewed information from child language development books and remembered that it is especially important to ascertain, from parents, the child's language development milestones in L1. Children from across all cultures should say their first word at around 12 months of age, speak 50 words expressively and put two words together around 18 months of age, and have an expressive vocabulary of 200-300 words at 24 months of age. In cultures where children's expressive language is not a high priority for caregivers, there may be minor variations in this timeline (e.g., speaking the first word at 13-14 months of age).

However, children's language across cultures should generally follow a similar timeline for the development of language milestones; this timeline does not appear to be negatively impacted by differences in interaction patterns between mothers and their babies in various cultures (Owens, 2020). Delving further, Ms. Jimenez read the research of Dar, Anwaar, Vihman, and Keren-Portnoy (2015), who conducted a cross linguistic comparison of Pakistani Urdu-speaking children and those learning other languages. Dar et al. found that there were similarities between the vocabulary growth of the Pakistani children in their study and children learning other languages.

With the help of Ms. Bukhari, the SLP discovered the following through interviewing Tanveer's mother (see Appendix for questions):

Tanveer spoke his first word in Urdu slightly before he turned two. He did not combine words into phrases in Urdu until after three years old. Ms. D. said that she began to suspect that "something was wrong" with Tanveer when his younger brother Abdul started surpassing him in Urdu language production. At age two, Abdul was speaking "lots of words" in Urdu and speaking mostly in short phrases. Abdul enjoyed conversing with others, and he used his words to communicate. Tanveer, on the other hand, often pointed and gestured but "didn't talk much." While Abdul had many friends in the neighborhood and at their temple, Tanveer had very few friends and seemed to be "a loner."

Ms. D. shared that at home, when she gave Tanveer multiple-step directions in Urdu, he would only carry out one of them and forget the others. Abdul, on the other hand, followed multiple step directions with no problem. Tanveer's mother said "Tanveer has always been a little slow, but he is a boy; we thought he'd outgrow his problems. Now we are starting to worry because at home, Tanveer cries and says that his school work is" too hard.'"

Ms. Jimenez felt concerned while interviewing Tanveer's mother. She had read a study by Morgan et al. (2016), who analyzed data from the Early Childhood Longitudinal Study -Birth Cohort, a nationally representative data set that is maintained by the U.S. Department of Education. Analyses were performed for a population-based sample of 9600 participating children and families. It was found that expressive vocabulary delays at 24 months of age were strongly associated with and predictive of children's receiving speech/language intervention at later ages. It was sounding to Ms. Jimenez like Tanveer might indeed have an underlying language impairment, not just a language difference that would resolve with time.

Ms. Jimenez shared with Tanveer's mother that she (Ms. Jimenez) had observed Tanveer in the classroom, on the playground, and at crosswalk duty as well. Ms. Jimenez had noticed that Tanveer seemed to need many repeats of directions, even when the other EL students had comprehended them the first or second time. Tanveer had difficulty telling a simple story sequentially in English and was slow to follow basic classroom directions and routines. He required a high degree of structure to learn new information, even when compared with EL peers.

Tanveer's mother said that these sounded like accurate observations that she herself had made based on Tanveer's behavior at home. For example, at home, Tanveer had difficulty following more than one simple direction given in Urdu. When he told her (in Urdu) about his school day, he seemed "disorganized" and she had difficulty following his story line. He was not able to complete homework independently, and always required a parent (usually her) to be by his side for extra structure and support. His younger brother Abdul, on the other hand, communicated effectively in Urdu and followed simple 2-3 step directions with no problems. Abdul worked well independently.

After Ms. Jimenez interviewed Tanveer's mother, she asked the Student Study Team (SST) to meet with Tanveer's parents. Mr. Jarecki was at the meeting, as was the school principal, Ms. Jimenez, and the school psychologist and resource specialist. The SST summarized these points:

1. Tanveer was slow to achieve basic language milestones in Urdu.
2. His younger brother Abdul had surpassed him in Urdu language skills.
3. Despite multiple and increasingly intensive school interventions in a dynamic assessment model utilizing RtI, Tanveer showed treatment resistance; he was benefitting very minimally from extra supports in both English and Urdu.
4. Tanveer's parents were concerned about his language development in Urdu, and believed that their son had difficulties that went beyond a language difference.

The SST decided that a formal special education evaluation was necessary, and his parents signed papers to have Tanveer evaluated by the SLP, psychologist, and resource specialist. The team reviewed the provisions of the Individuals with Disabilities Education Act (2004). According to the IDEA, when bilingual children are evaluated for special education needs:

1. There must be procedures to ensure that testing and evaluation materials and methods are provided and administered in the child's native language or mode of communication, unless it is not clearly feasible to do so.
2. Those who assess students must use a variety of data-gathering strategies and tools and may not rely upon a single procedure.
3. Alternative, research-based procedures may be used in evaluating students if standardized tests are not appropriate.
4. States must permit the use of a process based on the child's response to scientific, research-based intervention (RtI) to minimize overidentification and prevent unnecessary referrals to special education.

The special education team had Tanveer's language proficiency evaluated in both Urdu and English. It was found that he had lost some of his Urdu skills and that English was now his dominant language. Despite this, the special education team members had Ms. Bukhari present during all evaluations to provide support and scaffolding in Urdu if needed.

When the team assessed Tanveer for a possible underlying language impairment and/or other special education needs, they used informal evaluation measures supported by research. For example, they utilized language samples in Urdu and English; the use of language samples to evaluate the skills of ELs is supported by multiple studies (Arias & Friberg, 2017; Ebert & Pham, 2017; Lazewnik et al., 2019; Wood, Diehm, & Callender, 2016). The team also utilized narrative re-tells in both Urdu and English, knowing that ample research supports the use of analysis of narratives in differentiating a language difference from a language impairment in EL students (Ebert & Pham, 2017; Fiestas & Pena, 2004; Rezzonico et al., 2016). The team evaluated Tanveer's working memory, as difficulties with working memory are highly correlated with language impairment in both bilingual and monolingual children (Dispaldro, Leonard, & Deevy, 2013; Guiberson & Rodriguez, 2013; Kapantzoglou, Restrepo, Gray, & Thompson, 2015; Paradis, 2016; Thordardottir & Brandeker, 2013).

Each team member observed Tanveer in daily settings such as the classroom, playground, cafeteria, and bus duty line. The team observed that Tanveer often played alone and seemed to have very few friends. Other children did not approach him, and he did not initiate conversations with them. When Tanveer did converse with other children, he had difficulty staying on topic. In the classroom, Tanveer was slow to respond to directions. He appeared disorganized and confused, even as EL classmates appeared to understand directions and assignments. He was frequently off task and sometimes bothered other students.

In class, Tanveer appeared to have great difficulty paying attention, and often asked the teacher to repeat information that other students seemed to understand. It was noted that Tanveer's writing appeared large, awkward, and immature for his age. He had difficulty spacing his words appropriately, and his writing was noticeably less legible than that of other ELs in his class. His pencil grasp was awkward. Tanveer read out loud very slowly and laboriously, and appeared to have difficulty copying from the whiteboard to his paper.

Outcomes

At the conclusion of this multidisciplinary evaluation, it was discovered that Tanveer indeed had an underlying language impairment that affected verbal and written language skills. He was placed on an IEP and received weekly small group support from both the resource specialist and SLP. He made good gains after that, and his grades in the classroom improved. Ms. Bukhari ensured that Tanveer's parents were always kept apprised of his progress, and she helped them with home assignments to increase Tanveer's language skills.

ASHA (2019a) encourages SLPs to utilize culturally competent practices such as appropriately responding to the unique combination of variables that the family brings to interactions. Based upon this information, Ms. Jimenez and Ms. Bukhari met several times with Tanveer's parents and modeled literacy strategies that they could use at home with Tanveer. Because they were not literate in English or Urdu, Tanveer's parents were encouraged to discuss picture books with him in Urdu and talk about the stories. Ms. Bukhari and Ms. Jimenez modeled how to ask comprehension and prediction questions, for example, and showed Tanveer's parents how to help him tell stories sequentially based upon the pictures in the books. It was explained that this would help increase Tanveer's overall literacy skills, especially his ability to comprehend and produce narratives. Ms. Bukhari and Ms. Jimenez strongly encouraged Tanveer's parents to continue to build his skills in Urdu, as a plethora of research supports the finding that building skills in the first language contributes to greater skill in the second language (Genesee, 2016; Guiberson & Ferris, 2019; Pham, Ebert, & Kohnert, 2015; Roseberry-McKibbin, 2018; Simon-Cereijido, 2015). In addition, Ms. Jimenez knew that culturally competent service delivery to Tanveer and his family would include building on their unique needs and strengths (ASHA, 2019a).

The special education team, especially Ms. Jimenez, was very impressed at the accuracy of the preassessment process in pinpointing an underlying language impairment before a direct, formal evaluation occurred. Tanveer's case reinforced to them that for EL children, it is extremely important to not "jump the gun" and go directly from teacher referral to formal assessment with standardized tests. Doing so can result in overidentification of EL students for special education and mislabel them as "language impaired." The team resolved that in the future, when struggling EL students were referred for academic problems, a thorough preassessment process would be undertaken first in order to help rule out environmental and linguistic influences such as poverty, limited English skills, lack of literacy in the home, and others.

The RtI model, combined with parent and team interviews and observations, provided a comprehensive triangulation of data that was completely accurate in identifying an underlying language impairment in an EL student with linguistic and environmental differences. The team made plans to share this information with specialists all over the district so that evaluation procedures for EL students could improve district-wide.

Additional Questions for the Reader

1. Why was the preassessment process so important in Tanveer's case?
2. What information did Tanveer's mother share that served as a "red flag" that Tanveer might have a language impairment, not just a language difference?
3. Why was it a red flag that RtI was minimally successful in helping Tanveer improve his academic skills?
4. Why were environmental observations of Tanveer's interaction with other children helpful?
5. When Tanveer was finally formally evaluated by the special education team, did their findings corroborate with the results of preassessment procedures?

Discussion of Questions for the Reader

1. The preassessment process was so important in Tanveer's case because his initial difficulties in school could have been caused by his EL status (not speaking English) and environmental variables. These variables included coming from a background of poverty, not having any preschool experience, and not being exposed to literacy practices in the home such as reading with caregivers. The only way to differentiate language difference (due to linguistic and environmental variables) and language impairment is to use extensive preassessment methods to evaluate a student's ability to learn over time when provided with instruction.
2. Tanveer's mother shared "red flags" that were very helpful when Ms. Jimenez gathered Tanveer's case history information. His slowness in developing Urdu language milestones, especially compared to his younger brother, was key. His preference for gestures and pointing over verbalizing was revealing, as was his inability to follow instructions given in his primary language of Urdu. His frustration with school was indicative of potential clinically significant language difficulties.
3. It was a red flag that RtI—provided in increasingly intensive doses over time—was minimally effective for Tanveer. His treatment resistance, or inability to learn when provided with additional instruction, indicated that his difficulties and challenges in school could not be accounted for solely by linguistic and environmental variables. Clearly, Tanveer had an underlying language impairment that impacted both of his languages; he needed special education support that included speech-language services.
4. Environmental observations of Tanveer's classroom performance and interactions with other children were helpful because these observations were ecologically valid—they were made in naturalistic settings where Tanveer could be compared with peers of similar backgrounds. When EL students are showing inordinate difficulty in school, it is always best practice to compare them with peers from a similar cultural and linguistic background. If the students in question are showing a great deal more difficulty than these similar peers, usually there is an underlying language impairment or other type of special need.
5. The special education team obtained parental permission and formally evaluated Tanveer's language skills using research-supported practices such as language samples, narrative assessment, and evaluation of working memory. The team's results were completely congruent with the findings obtained in the preassessment process. The team could be assured that they had not "jumped the gun" and mislabeled Tanveer as having a language impairment when his struggles were due solely to linguistic and environmental differences that would have resolved with more time in school.

KEY POINTS

In the case of Tanveer D., an Urdu-speaking student from a Pakistani immigrant family, the following four preassessment tasks were successful in differentiating a language impairment from a language difference due to linguistic and environmental variables. These tasks were consistent with ASHA's (2019a; 2019b) mandates to provide culturally competent services that reflect principles of evidence-based practice:

1. Determine a child's proficiency in both the first language (L1) and English
2. Gather a case history of the child's speech and language development milestones in L1 from the child's parents or other primary caregivers (e.g., a grandparent)
3. Interview individuals who have observed the child's linguistic performance in multiple settings (e.g., classroom teacher, interpreter/bilingual associate)
4. Conduct dynamic assessment of a child's ability to learn when provided with instruction through using a multi-tiered approach where increasing amounts of support are provided over time.

REFERENCES

Accredited Language Services. (2019). *The 10 most popular languages in the U.S.* Retrieved from https://www.accreditedlanguage.com/languages/the-10-most-popular-languages-in-the-us/

American Speech-Language-Hearing Association (2019a). *Cultural competence*. Retrieved from asha.org/Practice-Portal/Professional Issues/Cultural-Competence/.

American Speech-Language-Hearing Association (2019b). *Evidence-based practice*. Retrieved from asha.org/Research/EBP/Evidence-Based-Practice.

Arias, G., & Friberg, J. (2017). Bilingual language assessment: Contemporary versus recommended practice in American schools. *Language, Speech, and Hearing Services in Schools*, *48*(1), 1–15. doi:10.1044/2016_LSHSS-15-0090 PMID:27788525

Barragan, B., Castilla-Earls, A., Martinez-Nieto, M., Restrepo, A., & Gray, S. (2018). Performance of low-income dual language learners attending English-only schools on the Clinical Evaluation of Language Fundamentals-4th edition, Spanish. *Language, Speech, and Hearing Services in Schools*, *49*(2), 292–305. doi:10.1044/2017_LSHSS-17-0013 PMID:29330555

Bedore, L. M., Pena, E. D., Joyner, D., & Macken, C. (2011). Parent and teacher rating of bilingual language proficiency and language development concerns. *International Journal of Bilingual Education and Bilingualism*, *14*(5), 489–511. doi:10.1080/13670050.2010.529102 PMID:29910668

Benavides, A., Kapantzoglou, M., & Murata, C. (2018). Two grammatical tasks for screening language abilities in Spanish-speaking children. *American Journal of Speech-Language Pathology*, *27*(2), 690–705. doi:10.1044/2017_AJSLP-17-0052 PMID:29554217

Dar, M., Anwaar, H., Vihman, M., & Keren-Portnoy, T. (2015). Developing an Urdu CDI for early language acquisition in Pakistan. *Journal of Child Speech and Language Studies*, *16*, 12–27.

Dispaldro, M., Leonard, L. B., & Deevy, P. (2013). Real-word and nonword repetition in Italian-speaking children with specific language impairment: A study of diagnostic accuracy. *Journal of Speech, Language, and Hearing Research: JSLHR*, *56*(1), 232–336. doi:10.1044/1092-4388(2012/11-0304) PMID:22761319

Ebert, K., & Pham, G. (2017). Synthesizing information from language samples and standardized tests in school-age bilingual assessment. *Language, Speech, and Hearing Services in Schools*, *48*(1), 42–65. doi:10.1044/2016_LSHSS-16-0007 PMID:28055056

Edutopia. (2019). *Response to intervention*. Retrieved from https://www.edutopia.org/topic/response-to-intervention

Fiestas, C. E., & Pena, E. D. (2004). Narrative discourse in bilingual children: Language and task effects. *Language, Speech, and Hearing Services in Schools*, *35*(2), 155–168. doi:10.1044/0161-1461(2004/016)

Genesee, F. (2016). *At-risk learners and bilingualism: Is it a good idea?* Retrieved from http://www.colorincolorado.org/article/at-risk-learners-and-bilingualism-is-it-a-good

GeneseeF.idea.

Guiberson, M., & Ferris, K. P. (2019). Early language interventions for young dual language learners: A scoping review. *American Journal of Speech-Language Pathology*, *28*(3), 945–963. doi:10.1044/2019_AJSLP-IDLL-18-0251 PMID:31398304

Guiberson, M. M., & Rodriguez, B. L. (2013). Classification accuracy of nonword repetition when used with preschool-age Spanish-speaking children. *Language, Speech, and Hearing Services in Schools*, *44*(2), 121–132. doi:10.1044/0161-1461(2012/12-0009) PMID:23188260

Guiberson, M. M., Rodriguez, B. L., & Dale, P. S. (2011). Classification accuracy of brief parent report measures of language development in Spanish-speaking toddlers. *Language, Speech, and Hearing Services in Schools*, *42*(4), 536–549. doi:10.1044/0161-1461(2011/10-0076) PMID:21844403

Individuals with Disabilities Education Improvement Act of 2004 (IDEA). (2004). *Public Law 108-446, 108th Congress*. Retrieved from https://sites.ed.gov/idea/

Kapantzoglou, M., Restrepo, M. A., Gray, S., & Thompson, H. (2015). Language ability groups in bilingual children: A latent profile analysis. *Journal of Speech, Language, and Hearing Research: JSLHR*, *58*(5), 1549–1562. doi:10.1044/2015_JSLHR-L-14-0290 PMID:26200211

Karanth, P., Roseberry-McKibbin, C., & James, P. (2017). *Intervention for preschoolers with communication delays: Practical strategies*. San Diego, CA: Plural Publishing, Inc.

Kraemer, R., & Fabiano-Smith, L. (2017). Language assessment of Latino English learning children: A records abstraction study. *Journal of Latinos and Education*, *16*(4), 349–358. doi:10.1080/15348431.2016.1257429

Kummerer, S. E. (2012). Promising strategies for collaborating with Hispanic parents during family-centered speech-language intervention. *Communication Disorders Quarterly*, *33*(2), 84–95. doi:10.1177/1525740109358453

Lazewnik, R., Creaghead, N. A., Smith, A. B., Prendeville, J., Raisor-Becker, L., & Silbert, N. (2019). Identifiers of language impairment for Spanish-English dual learners. *Language, Speech, and Hearing Services in Schools*, *50*(1), 126–137. doi:10.1044/2018_LSHSS-17-0046 PMID:30521665

Moore, B., & Montgomery, J. K. (2018). *Making a difference for America's children: Speech-language pathologists in public schools* (3rd ed.). Austin, TX: Pro-Ed.

Morgan, P. L., Hammer, C. S., Farkas, G., Hillemeier, M. M., Maczuga, S., Cook, M., & Morano, S. (2016). Who receives speech/language services by 5 years of age in the United States? *American Journal of Speech-Language Pathology*, *25*(2), 183–199. doi:10.1044/2015_AJSLP-14-0201 PMID:26579989

National Center for Education Statistics. (2019). *English language learners in public schools.* Retrieved from https://nces.ed.gov/programs/coe/indicator_cgf.asp

Owens, R. E. (2020). *Language development: An introduction* (10th ed.). New York: Pearson Education.

Palafox, P. L. (2017). The unique speech needs of children in poverty. *ASHA Leader*, *22*(3), 30–31. doi:10.1044/leader.SCM.22032017.30

Paradis, J. (2016). The development of English as a second language with and without specific language impairment: Clinical implications. *Journal of Speech, Language, and Hearing Research: JSLHR*, *59*(1), 171–182. doi:10.1044/2015_JSLHR-L-15-0008 PMID:26501845

Paradis, J., Emmerzael, K., & Duncan, T. (2010). Assessment of English learners: Using parent reports on first language development. *Journal of Communication Disorders*, *43*(6), 474–497. doi:10.1016/j.jcomdis.2010.01.002 PMID:20304411

Paradis, J., Schneider, P., & Duncan, T. S. (2013). Discriminating children with language impairment among English-language learners from diverse first language backgrounds. *Journal of Speech, Language, and Hearing Research: JSLHR*, *56*(3), 971–981. doi:10.1044/1092-4388(2012/12-0050) PMID:23275391

Pew Research Center. (2019). *Key findings about U.S. immigrants.* Retrieved from https://www.pewresearch.org/fact-tank/2019/06/03/key-findings-about-u-s-immigrants/

Pham, G., Ebert, K., & Kohnert, K. (2015). Bilingual children with primary language impairment: Three months after treatment. *Journal of Language and Communication Disorders*, *50*(1), 94–105. doi:10.1111/1460-6984.12123 PMID:25134887

Pua, E. P. K., Lee, M. L. C., & Liow, S. J. R. (2017). Screening bilingual preschoolers for language difficulties: Utility of teacher and parent reports. *Journal of Speech, Language, and Hearing Research: JSLHR*, *60*(4), 950–968. doi:10.1044/2016_JSLHR-L-16-0122 PMID:28297001

Rezzonico, S., Goldberg, A., Mak, K. K., Yap, S., Milburn, T., Belletti, A., & Girolametto, L. (2016). Narratives in two languages: Storytelling of Bilingual Cantonese-English Preschoolers. *Journal of Speech, Language, and Hearing Research: JSLHR*, *59*(3), 521–532. doi:10.1044/2015_JSLHR-L-15-0052 PMID:27253078

Roseberry-McKibbin, C. (2018). *Multicultural students with special language needs: Practical strategies for assessment and intervention* (5th ed.). Oceanside, CA: Academic Communication Associates.

Roseberry-McKibbin, C., Hegde, M. N., & Tellis, G. E. (2019). *An advanced review of speech-language pathology: Preparation for the Praxis SLP and comprehensive examination* (5th ed.). Austin, TX: Pro-Ed. Inc.

Roth, F. P., Dixon, D. A., Paul, D. R., & Bellini, P. I. (2013). RtI grades 3-5 in action: Oral and written language activities for the Common Core State Standards. Rockville, MD: American Speech and Hearing Association.

Simon-Cereijido, G. (2015). Preschool language interventions for Latino dual language learners with language disorders: What, in what language, and how. *Seminars in Speech and Language*, *36*(2), 154–164. doi:10.1055-0035-1549110 PMID:25923000

Thordardottir, E., & Brandeker, M. (2013). The effect of bilingual exposure versus language impairment on nonword repetition and sentence imitation scores. *Journal of Communication Disorders*, *46*(1), 1–16. doi:10.1016/j.jcomdis.2012.08.002 PMID:23021785

Wood, C., Diehm, E. A., & Callender, M. E. (2016). An investigation of language environment analysis measures for Spanish-English bilingual preschoolers from migrant low-socioeconomic status backgrounds. *Language, Speech, and Hearing Services in Schools*, *47*(2), 123–124. doi:10.1044/2015_LSHSS-14-0115 PMID:27019230

Wood, C., Wolford, M. C., & Schatschneider, C. (2018). Relationship between performance on oral narrative retells and vocabulary assessments of Spanish-speaking children. *Communication Disorders Quarterly*, *39*(3), 402–414. doi:10.1177/1525740117722507

KEY TERMS AND DEFINITIONS

Culturally Diverse: Cultural diversity refers to diverse or different cultures, as opposed to monoculture (a situation where everyone holds and practices the same cultural values). The term cultural diversity also refers to having different cultures respect each other's differences.

English Learner: Person who learns English as another language. This person speaks a first or primary language other than English and learns English sequentially (after they learn their first or primary language). The English learner may speak more than two languages: their primary language, English, and others.

Informal Testing: Testing of language learning ability that does not involve the use of standardized tests that are norm-referenced. Informal testing can involve use of strategies such as gathering and analyzing language samples, dynamic assessment of a child's ability to learn when provided with instruction, and others.

Language Impairment: Also known as Developmental Language Disorder (DLD), is a label used by professionals to explain difficulties with language development that are not due to physical abnormality, hearing loss, acquired brain damage, or lack of language experience. These difficulties are not part of a general developmental delay that affects other skills.

Linguistically Diverse: This term refers to the situation where persons from different backgrounds speak languages that differ from the mainstream language of the geographic region. For example, in the

U.S., English is the mainstream language. Linguistically diverse individuals speak languages such as Spanish, Dari, Mandarin, Arabic, and others.

Nonbiased Assessment: Assessment of the language-learning ability of a child whose first language is one other than English. The purpose is to differentiate language difference from language impairment. Nonbiased assessment involves using materials and methods of testing that are not linguistically or culturally biased against the child.

Parent Report: Information provided by parents about their children's development, communication skills, and progress in multiple areas such as academic, linguistic, social, and others.

Prereferral: Period before a child is formally referred for special education testing, including that provided by the speech-language pathologist, psychologist, and resource specialist.

Response to Intervention: RtI incorporates a dynamic assessment model whose purpose is to evaluate a student's ability to learn over time when provided with instruction. RtI emphasizes a process that attempts to provide additional, increasingly intensified support to students over time before labeling them as having disabilities.

Teacher Report: Information provided by teachers about children's development, communication skills, and progress in multiple areas such as academic, linguistic, social, and others.

APPENDIX

Case History Questions for Culturally and Linguistically Diverse Students

(adapted from Roseberry-McKibbin, C. (2018). *Multicultural students with special language needs: Practical strategies for assessment and intervention* (5th ed.). Oceanside, CA: Academic Communication Associates)

Language Development Background

1. What was the first language your child learned?
2. What languages is your child currently exposed to in the home?
3. When and under what circumstances was your child exposed to English?
4. What language(s) is/are spoken by the adults in the home?
5. At this time, what do you perceive to be your child's strongest and most fluent language?
6. How old was your child when she spoke her first word? (should be around 12 months)
7. How old was your child when she first began putting two words together? (should be around 18 months)
8. When your child turned two, how many words was she using expressively? (should be 200-300)
9. Does your child have normal vision and hearing? Are there any medical concerns?

Language Use

Can your child: (in the first language, English, or both)
__Answer simple questions
__Communicate basic needs
__Follow 2- and 3-step directions
__Tell a simple story sequentially
__Describe familiar events and objects

School Social Interaction

Does your child:
___Communicate effectively with peers
___Often play alone
___Get teased or bullied by others
___Get excluded from activities by peers
___Rarely initiate with peers

Does Your Child Exhibit any of the Following Challenges?

___Has difficulty communicating in our primary language
___Has a family history of learning difficulties

___Learns language more slowly than siblings
___Prefers gestures to talking
___Is slow to respond to 2- and 3-step directions at home, even in the primary language
___Responds inappropriately when others tell her things (e.g., says something that is off topic and unrelated to what was just said; ignores others)
___Has difficulty staying on topic and "wanders" during conversations
___Has difficulty with basic routines, appearing disorganized and confused
___Needs a lot of repetitions (more than siblings) to remember or learn new information
___Has trouble finding the right word for things
___Sounds like a younger child when she talks; has sentences that seem too short and simple for her age
___Seems to have difficulty understanding what people say to her

Other Comments and Concerns

Chapter 2
Navajo Speech and Language Evaluation:
Difference vs. Disorder

Christine B. Vining
University of New Mexico, USA

Davis E. Henderson
Northern Arizona University, USA

EXECUTIVE SUMMARY

The case study highlights the importance of culturally and linguistically appropriate assessment of young Navajo/American Indian children and the importance of alternative assessment procedures to support appropriate diagnoses and recommendations. The case also illustrates systemic issues that result in lack of coordinated care, appropriate diagnosis, and lack of American Indian speech-language pathologists who understand linguistic and cultural differences. The case is based on a typical experience when clinicians who are not familiar with the Navajo language perform speech-language evaluations in Navajo-speaking communities.

INTRODUCTION

The background for the case study focuses on: (1) geographic context; (2) cultural and linguistic context; and (3) educational context.

Geographic context. This case study highlights a clinical experience on the Navajo Nation in New Mexico. New Mexico is rich in cultural and linguistic diversity, including 22 different federally recognized tribes. The case involves a young Navajo boy who lives on the Navajo reservation with his family. The Navajo reservation is the size of West Virginia and spans into four states, including Arizona, New Mexico, Utah and Colorado. The Navajo Nation is one of the largest tribes in the nation.

DOI: 10.4018/978-1-7998-2261-5.ch002

Cultural and linguistic context. The Navajo Nation has a strong history of retaining its language and culture. Maintaining cultural identity has been associated with the vitality of the native language and cultural practices in Navajo homes and communities. Tribal leaders have advocated for culturally and linguistically responsive teachings in the home and school. Some schools provide instruction in Navajo language and culture. There are Navajo dual language learners who are acquiring various levels of English and Navajo proficiencies on the reservation. The term English Language Learner (ELL) describes children who are not fully proficient in English. English may be the primary language for some children, yet they may not be proficient in it. In this case, understanding dialectal differences or Navajo-influenced English will be helpful in determining whether a Navajo student is exhibiting a speech and/or language disorder.

A brief description of the Navajo language and the influence of Navajo on English provides some background. The Navajo (Diné) language is a branch of Athabaskan language family. Almost 150,000 people still speak the Navajo language (Grimes, 1996). In the Navajo speech community, there are monolingual speakers of both Navajo and the Navajo variety of English as well as the majority of adults who are bilingual, more or less fluent in both languages. The traditional elders are often monolingual speakers of Navajo. Children on the Navajo Nation live in homes where they are hear Navajo, English or a combination of both.

Young and Morgan (1987) have described the Navajo language extensively. Their descriptions of the Navajo verb are complex. For example, one unique feature of Navajo is that many meaningful units are compounded together to form a single word, and often elements, such as the subject and object of the verb, aspect, mode, and direction, etc., are embedded in verbs. Within the verb-word there are both derivational and inflectional morphemes. Attached to the end of the verb-word also may be directional and locational morphemes. The morphological markers used in English (i.e., verb tenses) are not used in the same manner. Nouns can be inflected for possession with a personal pronoun prefix ("**shi**chidí" "my car" and "**ni**má" "your mother"). Nouns are not generally marked for number. The sentence in Navajo incorporates a SOV (subject-object-verb) word order.

Young and Morgan (1987) have also developed a Navajo Consonant Inventory (standard orthography) which include nasals, laterals, affricates, fricatives, stops, bilabials, alveolars and velars. A unique feature is that some consonant are glottalized including glottalized t' and k' (velars) and glottalized ts' and ch' (affricates). They also noted that Navajo vowels contrast in length and pitch, and correspond approximately with English /i, e, o, and a/. They describe Navajo phonology, grammar, and syntax extensively, and their work is a valuable resource for speech-language pathologists who wish to understand the Navajo language more in depth.

Linguists such as Leap (1993) have documented linguistic differences and the unique characteristics of the influence of Native American languages on English. The rules that govern phonology, grammar and syntax differs between English and Navajo. Navajo English may include the following examples. Navajo has only a glottal final voiceless stop, so speakers of Navajo English may not distinguish differences in final voiceless stops. They may delete them entirely or substitute one for the other, so "truck" is pronounced "truʔ"; "test" is pronounced "tess"; and "mit" is pronounced "miʔ". Leap claims that reduction in consonant clusters is a general feature of American Indian English (Leap, 1982). For example, "cold" is pronounced col". Navajo has no velar nasal so /n/ replaces /ŋ/ (ng). Speakers of Navajo English say "thin" for "thing" and "walkin" for "walking". There are many more examples that Leap (1982) provides to illustrate the uniqueness of Navajo influenced English.

Educational Context: Historically, Navajo children have often been over referred to special education and related services due to academic difficulties related to limited skills in English. The public education departments have put forth policies and practices to ensure appropriate referrals, assessments and accommodations, and intervention when students struggle in school. Navajo students who do not speak English well are at risk for inappropriate referral to and identification for special education and related services, such as speech-language therapy. This case touches on issues related to determining educational eligibility for speech-language pathology (SLP) services. It is incumbent upon speech-language pathologists to collaborate with educators to gather information, determine educational need, and recommend appropriate educational supports and services. It is also important for SLPs to distinguish language differences from disorders and to make appropriate recommendations whether or not students meet the eligibility of speech and/or language impairments. The Response to Intervention (RTI) process has helped to ensure appropriate referrals and access to supports within special education and related services. However, one of the challenges SLPs continue to face with Navajo children is the lack of research on the tools they administer to assess speech and language skills.

CASE STUDY

The case study focuses on a young five-year old Navajo boy, named Carl, who lives on the reservation in New Mexico with his Navajo-speaking family members. Carl speaks English primarily with exposure to Navajo and English in his home and small, rural community. Carl's pediatrician referred him to a speech-language pathologist at the local Indian Health Service for further testing after failing an initial developmental screening at his well-child check visit. Carl and his family moved to Arizona before the SLP could complete an evaluation. His family moved back to New Mexico when he was four years of age. He did not attend preschool or Head Start. When Carl started kindergarten, his regular education teacher noted concerns with speech, language and literacy skills and consulted with the school support team. After limited progress with regular education recommendations, the student's assistance team determined that the speech-language pathologist could help ascertain Carl's current speech and language skills. Although both of Carl's parents are bilingual in Navajo and English, they reported that the home language was English. Assuming Carl primarily spoke English, the SLP proceeded with the evaluation in English.

Background Information: History

Factors to consider

- English Language Learner (ELL)
- Speech-Language Impairment (SLI)
- Dialectal differences

History and Referral

Carl is a male, age 5 years, 7 months, who was referred for an evaluation by his, kindergarten teacher, Mrs. Catie Smith for speech and language concerns. He is attending Eagle Ranch Elementary School. The evaluator obtained a case history at intake and by review of medical records.

Birth History

According to his medical records, Carl was born at a local Indian Health Hospital in Round Rock, NM. He was born full term to his 25-year old mother. His gestational age was 38 weeks. He weighed 8 pounds and 5 ounces. His vitals and physical exam were within normal limits. He had mild jaundice but otherwise was healthy. At one month, he received medical treatment at the community clinic for fever and coughing, a rash on his face at 3 months, and stomach flu at 10 months. At 2 years of age, his parents were concerned about ear infections and received medication four times for otitis media between 2 and 3 years of age. At 4 years of age, he received a fluoride varnish treatment and was referred to the dentist. Carl had multiple dental work for his cavities under general anesthesia. Growth charts revealed normal growth. He has not had any hospitalizations or serious injuries. He does not have any known allergies. There is no concern for seizures. He currently eats and sleeps well.

Developmental History

According to medical records, Carl's 6-month developmental screen was normal for his age, sitting independently, crawling, transferring objects hand to hand and babbling. He passed the developmental screen for 18 month-olds. He walked backwards, climbed stairs, threw a ball, knew his body parts and fed himself with a spoon. He spoke in words and phrases. Carl's father spoke to his pediatrician about his concerns that Carl had periodic ear infections that began around 2 years of age. At 3 years of age, Carl failed the developmental screening. He did not pass the language items but had adequate fine motor, gross motor skills, and adaptive skills (e.g., dressing, brushing his teeth, and feeding). On the speech and language items, he was able to point to pictures but had trouble understanding spatial concepts (in, on), follow 2-part commands, using verb tenses, naming concepts (e.g., colors), and mispronouncing some sounds. The family moved to Arizona when he was 3 years of age. The family moved back to New Mexico when he was four years old.

Family History

Carl currently lives with his parents and both parents speak English and Navajo. Both parents completed high school. Records indicated Carl's father has a diagnosis of Attention-Deficit/Hyperactivity Disorder (ADHD) - Combined type. The evaluator was not able to obtain any more information about paternal and maternal history.

Educational History

Carl did not attend preschool or Head Start. He is in a regular education classroom at Eagle Ranch as a kindergartener. Carl reportedly did not say much and his teacher described him as a quiet boy. His teacher, Mrs. Smith indicated that Carl does not produce some sounds correctly. He sometimes has trouble following classroom routines and attending to classroom activities. Parents reported that Carl learns best through observation, or modeling, from family members; therefore, parents requested peer modeling within the academic classrooms. Peer modeling appears to be helping him adapt to the structure and expectations of the classroom. With regard to his social development, Carl reportedly gets along with other students. He does not have any major behavior problems such as tantrums in the school setting. Carl enjoys active play and likes to draw on his dry erase board.

SPEECH-LANGUAGE EVALUATION

General Observations

The evaluation took place in a small, quiet room at Eagle Ranch Elementary School. Assessment information included a combination of methods: records review, teacher interview, classroom observation, standardized testing, spontaneous language sample, and clinical observation. Carl came willingly to the testing room and completed all tasks requested of him. He was very active and interactive throughout testing. He squirmed in his seat and got out of his seat to look under the table several times. Breaks included play with a ball and bubbles.

Classroom Observation

Carl's observation took place in his classroom and at recess. To get his teacher's attention, he tapped on her arm and said, "teacho, look" and pointed to another child. He took another student's balloon, and said, "Mine." When the student started to cry and asked for his balloon, Carl gave it back. During lunch, he requested milk, "I want milk." He opened his own milk carton, said, "I did it", and smiled at his teacher. Another student hit him and he hit back as he walked back to his table. After lunch, he dumped his tray and immediately got a book. As he sat turning pages, he said, "Oh no!" "Uh-oh look at pubby/puppy." At times, he looked at the picture closely. Several students crowded around him as he sat with his book. He pushed one student away. He tried to imitate his teacher when she said "caterpillar." He said, "Cadepilla". When the students lined up to go to recess, he rubbed another student's head. As the class walked out, Carl walked his fingers along the wall. Once outside, he ran to the swing and his teacher lifted him into the swing. He then looked for ants on the ground by getting very close to the ground. When other students crowded around him, he pushed them away. When recess ended, he held the door open while the students lined up. Next, the students sat in half-circle for a language lesson on corn. Carl started to take his boot off and his teacher told him to put it back on. He said, "My boot is tight" and showed his boot. He exhibited off-task behaviors during the lesson: looking around, burping, pulling up his shirt, closing his eyes, talking to a peer, and making playful sounds. He moved a lot in his seat when the group moved from the floor to the table. The teacher asked questions ("What color?" "What shape?"); however, Carl did not respond.

Teacher Interview

Carl's teacher reported that he uses gestures and simple sentences to communicate his needs. He plays with others as well as alone. He enjoys building with Legos and he likes to draw. She is concerned that he does not always attend, follow directions, and communicate clearly. He looks at objects closely and, at times, he touches other students a lot and hits the other children when they are too close.

Clinical Procedures

- Hearing Screening
- Clinical Evaluation of Language Fundamental – Fifth Edition (CELF – 5) (Wiig, Semel, & Secord, 2013)
- Goldman-Fristoe Test of Articulation – Third Edition (GFTA – 3) (Goldman & Fristoe, 2015)
- Spontaneous speech-language sample
- Voice
- Fluency
- Oral mechanism exam

CLINICAL FINDINGS

Hearing

Carl passed a bilateral pure tone hearing screening that was administered at 20 dB HL for 500, 1000, 2000, and 4000 Hz. Results indicate that Carl's hearing is within normal limits in both ears. An otoscopic examination revealed no obstructions in the ear canal.

General Test Results

Standardized tests provide one or more derived scores. Derived scores show how a child's performance compares with others in the same age range on the same test.

- **Standard Score (SS):** Standard scores have a mean of 100, and a standard deviation of 15 points. Most people earn scores between 85 and 115. Standard scores may also be Index or Composite scores.
- **Scaled Score (ss):** Scaled scores have a mean of 10 and a standard deviation of 3; scores between 7 and 13 are in the average range.
- **Percentile (% ile):** A percentile rank is the percent of cases that are at or below a score.

Table 1. Language test results

Clinical Evaluation of Language Fundamentals, Fifth Edition (CELF-5) Ages 5-8				
Areas Assessed	**Scores**	**Confidence Interval**	**Percentile Rank**	**Description**
Sentence Comprehension	10	8 to 12	50	Average
Linguistic Concepts	6	2 to 6	9	Below average
Word Structure	6	4 to 8)	9	Below average
Word Classes	9	6 to 10	37	Average
Following Directions	6	5 to 7	9	Below average
Formulated Sentences	5	3 to 7	5	Below average
Recalling Sentences	6	6 to 7	9	Below average
Pragmatics Profile	8	7-9	25	Average
Core Language Score (SS)	81	75 to 87	10	Marginal/Mild
Receptive Language Score (SS)	89	82 to 96	23	Average
Expressive Language Score (SS)	76	70 to 82	5	Low/Moderate
Language Content Index (SS)	82	77 to 87	12	Marginal/Mild
Language Structure Index (SS)	81	75 to 87	10	Marginal/Mild

Language Test Results

Carl's standard scores on the *Clinical Evaluation of Language Fundamentals – Fifth Edition (CELF-5)* can be found in Table 1. The Core Language is a measure of general ability when compared to the norm. A Core Language Score of 81 placed Carl's overall performance in the marginal range. His Receptive Language Index score of 89 is in the average and his Expressive Language Index score of 76 is in the low range. The 13-point difference between the Receptive Language Index and Expressive Language Index scores occurs rarely and is clinically significant ($P<0.05$), indicating greater difficulties with expressive language. The Language Content Index score of 82 and the Language Structure Index score of 81 are in the marginal range, indicating that Carl had mild difficulties with vocabulary, word knowledge and sentence structure. The 1-point difference between Language Content Index score and Language Structure Index score is not significant (<0.05). Based on the profile of Index scores, Carl has a mild-moderate language disorder involving his expressive modalities.

The test scaled scores range from a low of 5 to a high of 10. Scaled scores for Sentence Comprehension (10), Word Classes (9) and Pragmatics Profile (8) are in the average range and indicate areas of strength for Carl. In comparison, scores for Linguistic Concepts (6), Word Structure (6), Following Directions (6), Formulated Sentences (5), and Recalling Sentences (6) are in the below average range and indicate areas of weaknesses.

Analysis of the response pattern for receptive tasks indicated strong ability in sentence comprehension and understanding word associations. On the Sentence Comprehension subtest, Carl did well in choosing one of four pictures that matched the meaning of sentences and understanding grammar. On the Word Classes subtest, Carl was able to understand relationships between words such as *"cat"/"kitten"*, *"marker"/"pencil"*, and *"socks"/"shoes"*. However, Carl struggled executing directions as the directions became longer and more complex on the Following Directions subtest. He was able to complete one-step directions such as, *"Point to white triangle."* He had difficulty following multiple-step directions, such as *"Point to a square, a circle, and a triangle."* He also performed poorly on the Linguistic Concepts, which assessed following oral directions including basic linguistic concepts, such as coordinating conjunctions, references to inclusion or exclusion, time, condition, or quantity. He had trouble with directions containing inclusion/exclusion words (*either…or*) and conditional words (*if* … and *unless*).

Analysis of expressive language items indicated weaknesses related to grammar and sentence structure. The Word Structure subtest required Carl to complete sentences with correct grammatical markers (i.e., past-tense, plural, possessive, etc.) that matched the presented picture. He had difficulty with irregular plurals, third person, pronouns, comparatives and superlatives. Carl was able to understand the rules of regular plurals; however, he had difficulty understanding irregular plurals. For example, he used *"mouses"* rather than *"mice"* and stated, *"childs"* rather than *"children"*. He also had difficulty with the rules of the third person. For example, he said, *"Everyday he is reading"* rather than "*Everyday he reads*". Sometimes he used pronouns incorrectly (e.g., him/her). Instead of *"She does,"* he said, *"The girl has a hamburger."* Carl struggled with comparatives and superlatives. For example, he stated "really fast" instead of "*faster*" and "really big one" instead of "*the biggest*"). Carl's use of verb tenses was also inconsistent. For example, he was capable of using irregular verb tenses, however, he said, "She runned to the bus" on one item on the Formulated Sentences subtest. Carl's difficulty with grammar contributed to weak performance on the Recalling Sentences and Formulated Sentences subtests.

Language Sample

The clinician obtained a corpus of 200 utterances for analysis during free play. Carl's Mean Length of Utterance (MLU) was 5.24 in words and 5.33 in morphemes. According to Brown's Stages of Syntactic and Morphological Development (Brown, 1973), Carl demonstrates skills consistent with stage V+.

Syntax: Carl spoke in five- to six-word utterances; however, his difficulty with grammatical markers sometimes interfered with his ability to formulate complex sentences. He produced various wh-questions. For example, he asked, "Where did the doggie go?" His use of *yes/no* questions were sometimes not grammatical such as "See hims running?" and "You going now?"

Morphology: Carl used several tense markers (irregular past tense, future tense, copula (is, are), and present progressive (-ing). He sometimes omitted the copula (e.g., "Where you going?"). He was inconsistent in using past tense (-ed) and present tense (3rd person –s). For example, he stated, "He ranned really fast," and "Him sister drewed the picture." His errors with pronouns (his, her him, them, they) were evident in spontaneous speech (e.g., "My kitty cat found the house but him got lost first" and "The boy is running to her mom"). He sometimes used the noun instead of a pronoun (e.g., "The boy is sad"). He used plurals and sometimes had trouble with irregular plurals ("sheeps", "childrens"). He used negatives and articles.

Semantics: Carl used nouns, verbs, adjectives, and adverbs. He used words to denote time (later), place (in, on, by, inside), and quantity (lots, ten).

Social Language: Carl used language for a variety of purposes including commenting, describing, greeting, asking questions and answering to others. Carl was able to answer *wh-* and *yes/no* questions appropriately during conversation. For example, "What animal jumps on two legs? [Kangaroo] and "Do you need to feed your cat now?" [Yes]. He told about recent experiences and stayed on topic as he talked about his pets. He was able to engage in conversation.

Table 2. Articulation test results

Goldman-Fristoe Test of Articulation-3 (GFTA-3)		Areas Assessed		Scores
IF "x_-3" "Confidence Interval (90%)	Percentile Rank	Description	Sounds-in-Words	91
86-98	27	Average	Sounds-in-Sentences	95

90-101
37
Average

Table 3. Sounds-in-words phonetic error analysis

Single Consonants		
Initial	Medial	Final
b/v, d/ɵ, d/ð, l/j	ʔ /k, -/t, -/g, n/ŋ, b/v, d/ ð	ʔ /k, n/ŋ, f/ɵ, o/l, o/ɚ

Speech

The evaluator used the *Goldman-Fristoe Test of Articulation – Third Edition* (GFTA – 3) to assess Carl's articulation of the consonant and consonant cluster sounds of Standard American English in Sounds-in-Words and Sounds-in-Sentences subtests (see Table 2 for *GFTA-3* test results and Table 3 for Phonetic Error Analysis). Carl's Sounds-in-Words standard score of 91 (confidence interval = 86 to 98 at 90% level) is in the average range. His Sounds-in-Sentences standard score of 95 (confidence interval 90-101at 90% level) is also in the average range. The Sounds-in-Sentences results indicate that Carol demonstrates the same error patterns in connected speech as he does in single-word productions. The overall intelligibility rating was 85% indicating good speech intelligibility.

The Phonetic Error Analysis (Table 3) based on Carl's responses on the Sounds-in-Words test indicates that he has mastery over stops (p, b, d) in all word positions; however, he produces velars (/k/ and /g/ inconsistently in medial and final word positions. Carl substitutes the glottal stop /ʔ/ for /k/ and /g/ (e.g., dʌʔ/dʌk, kuʔi/kuki, trʌʔ/ trʌk). He produces nasals (/m/, /n/) correctly; however, occasionally he replaces /ŋ/ with /n/ (e.g., swɪn/swɪŋ, finer/fɪŋger). He produces glides (/w/ and /j/) correctly but in one instance he produced (/j/) as /l/ (e.g. lelo/jelo). He inconsistently produces vowels for liquids in the final word position (e.g., titʃo/titʃɚ, pʌzo/pʌzəl). He produces affricates (/dʒ/ and /tʃ/) and most fricatives (/f/, /s/, /z/, and /ʃ/) correctly. He has difficulty producing the /v/ in the initial and medial positions (e.g., bækjum/vækjum, bɛʒdəbəl/vɛdʒtəbəl, and ʃʌbəl/ʃʌvəl). He also has trouble producing fricatives (/ɵ/ and /ð/). For example, d/ɵ (dʌm/ɵʌm) and d/ð (daet/ðaet, brʌdɚ/brʌðɚ).

Carl was administered the stimulability task to determine if he could imitate the sounds children his age have mastered. Carl is able to imitate the sounds /k/, /t/, /j/, /v/, /ŋ/, /ɚ/, /l/ in all positions of syllables and words. He is not stimulable for /ɵ/ and /ð/. Errors with /ɵ/ and /ð/ sounds appear to be developmental in that 95% of children master /ɵ/ at age 7:0-7:11 and master /ð/ at age 6:0-6:11 according *GFTA-3*.

Voice: An informal assessment of spontaneous connected speech indicated that Carl's loudness and pitch were within normal limits for his age and gender.

Fluency: Informal assessment during spontaneous connected speech indicated that Carl's rate, rhythm, and prosody to be within normal limits for his age and gender.

Oral Mechanism Examination: The clinician used a clinic-specific checklist to exam Carl's oral mechanism. Carl has capped upper incisors. His oral motor structures and function were within normal limits.

IMPRESSIONS

The non-Native SLP concluded that Carl's overall language performance is in the marginal range. His receptive language skills are in the average range while his expressive language skills are in the low range. There is a significant difference between his receptive and expressive language abilities indicating moderate difficulties in the area of expressive language. Carl struggles with word knowledge, grammar and syntax, which sometimes limits his communication including his ability to follow directions. He shows adequate pragmatic skills although peers bother him when they get too close. His articulation skills are in the average and his oral motor skills are adequate for speech production. Given this profile, the SLP made the following recommendations to support expressive language deficits.

Recommendations

- Provide language intervention to support Carl's expressive language abilities. The results of testing indicate that Carl would benefit from language therapy focusing on expressive language. Therapy may target Carl's ability to understand and use grammar and syntax including verb tenses and pronouns. He may also benefit from working on language concepts to help him understand and formulate sentences.
- Refer for psycho-educational testing to determine whether there is an underlying learning disorder and to make recommendations for appropriate academic supports.
- Refer for occupational therapy evaluation to assess sensory integration.

Questions for the Reader about Speech

1. How can an SLP who is unfamiliar with the Navajo language develop speech assessment practices that recognizes patterns of speech that reflect the influence of Navajo on speech production?
2. Do the errors produced suggest a pattern reflective of an articulation disorder?
3. Were there examples of errors related to dialectal differences (i.e., sounds that are influenced by his Navajo speech sounds)?
4. Was the GFTA – 3 the best assessment tool to evaluate Carl's speech production?

Discussion of the Questions for the Reader About Speech

1. When a Navajo child comes from a Navajo-speaking home, information on language use in English and Navajo is helpful. A language survey of language use is helpful in determining whether a dialectal differences impacts articulation. In Carl's case, the parents did not complete the form correctly and the SLP erroneously assumed Carl was proficient in English. A Navajo teacher or aide could have been helpful in informing the SLP on whether Carl's speech was similar to those in his speech community. An SLP who is not familiar with the Navajo speech sounds may also consult with a Navajo-speaking SLP or other bilingual staff. The SLP may also need to become familiar with Navajo phonology and its influence on English. An interview with the parents could have been beneficial; however, in this case the parents were not available.
2. Articulation testing assessed the student's speech production in Standard American English. An evaluator who is not familiar with Navajo-influenced speech may interpret Carl's speech errors as indicated of an articulation disorder if his score fell below the mean. The SLP should interpret Carl's articulation errors related to dialectal difference with caution.
3. The speech errors reflected dialectal differences. Following are examples of the dialectal differences:
    a. Use of glottal stops replacing final consonants (/k/, /t/, /d/, /g/, etc.,),
    b. While fricatives exist in the Navajo language, there are no /v/, /ɵ/, /ð/ sounds in the Navajo language and stops sometimes replace /v/ and /ð/ (e.g., b/v, d/ð).
    c. There is also no /r/ is the Navajo language so vocalic /r/ may be problematic.

    Carl's exposure to his native speech sounds may have influenced his English speech production.
4. The *Goldman-Fristoe Test of Articulation-Third Edition (GFTA-3)* is a standardized instrument used to assess speech sound development in children as well as adults (Goldman & Fristoe, 2015). It is a commonly used instrument for articulation assessment. The error patterns at the word and sentence levels are helpful in determining whether speech errors are developmental in nature or related to dialectal differences. In addition, stimulability testing is helpful to determine intervention targets when articulation therapy is necessary. Carl was stimulable for correct production on several sounds in words, which suggests he is capable of correct productions.

While Carl's score is in the average range, his performance should not negate the possibility of linguistic and content bias that may exist in *GFTA-3*. Documentation of the use of *GFTA-3* with Navajo children and descriptions of possible phonemic productions for Navajo-Influenced English are lacking in the extant literature as well as the *GFTA-3*.

Questions for the Reader About Language

1. Carl's parents are bilingual and it is possible that they speak with Navajo-Influenced English. Were Carl's spontaneous communication and responses on the *CELF-5* reflective of dialectal differences? If so, what are some examples?
2. Would it be appropriate for Carl to receive speech and language therapy?

Discussion of the Questions for the Reader about Language

1. Carl demonstrated grammatical and syntactical errors on the language sample and the *CELF-5* subtests that were indicative of Navajo-influenced English. The Navajo language does not have specific gender pronouns but a more generalized pronoun *bi-* (he, she, him, her, it). There are no plural markers as in English and generally, the verb contains information about whether there is one object or several objects. The Navajo verbs are not consistent with the English tense markers, including past tense (–ed), present tense (-s), irregular past tense, and copula (is, are). These English constructions pose a challenge for children who are exposed to Navajo or Navajo-influenced English.

Below are examples from the *CELF-5* subtests that illustrate linguistic differences in morphological markers and syntax:

a. The Formulated Sentences task required Carl to form a grammatically correct sentence given a target word or words while using an illustration as a reference. Carl struggled with verb tenses. For example, he stated, "She runned to the bus."

b. The Word Structure task involved completing sentences with correct grammatical markers (i.e., past-tense, plurals, possessives, etc.) that matched the picture presented by the clinician. Carl was able to understand the rules of regular plurals; however, he had difficulty understanding irregular plurals. For example, he stated, "mouses" rather than "mice" and "childs" rather than "children". He had difficulty with present tense markers (third person –s). For example, he said, "Every day he is reading" instead of "Every day he reads". He also had trouble using pronouns correctly. For example, he substituted "him" for "her" in completing this sentence ("The girl has a guitar. The guitar belongs to him"). Carl also struggled with comparatives and superlatives. For example, his response for "faster, fastest" was "really fast" and his response for "bigger, biggest" was "really big one."

c. In addition, Navajo is verb-based language in that the verbs carry the message of quantity, quality, and composition. Adults may give oral directions in a sequential order or break down the directions. It is not surprising that Carl had trouble on the Following Directions task. He was able to complete one-step directions such as "Point to white triangle;" however, he had difficulty following complex directions, such as "Point to a square, a circle, and a triangle."

2. Standardized testing with Navajo children has been problematic historically. The use of standardized, norm-referenced assessments could overidentify Navajo children with typically developing language as having language impairment (Henderson & Restrepo, 2016). American Indian children who are dual language learners, in particular, are at risk for inappropriate language assessment and identification as children with language impairment due to dialectal variations influenced by their native languages (Vining, Edgarita, Inglebret, & Brendal, 2017). The *Clinical Evaluation of Language Fundamentals, Fifth Edition* (Wiig, Semel, & Secord, 2013) does not describe inclusion of Navajo children in its normative sampling nor does it provide grammatical contrasts between Navajo-influenced English and Mainstream American English. This may pose a challenge for an SLP who lacks knowledge of cultural and linguistic differences when assessing Navajo children. Henderson and Restrepo (2016) conducted a study using the *Clinical Evaluation of Language Fundamental – Fourth Edition (CELF-4)* (Semel, Wiig, & Secord, 2003) with 5- to 8-year old

reservation-residing Navajo children. They found that the mean of typically developing Navajo children fell 1 SD below the test mean. They reported that difficulty with grammatical skills such as plurals, pronouns, comparatives, and vocabulary differences contributed to language errors (Henderson & Restrepo, 2016). Therefore, Carl's speech and language development should take into consideration communication patterns typically used by his speech community. Based on the error patterns, Carl would not qualify for speech-language pathology services. There were many examples of dialectal differences. He also needs time to gain experience and learn skills expected in a new learning environment. The SLP's interpretation of findings and recommendations should reflect that.

Questions for the Reader about Treatment Options

1. Should the SLP explore Dynamic Assessment?
2. What would you recommend as next steps?

Discussion of Questions for the Reader about Treatment Options

1. Dynamic assessment is a test-retest method that rules out lack of experience with test stimuli and tasks. Carl may benefit from the application of dynamic assessment as he has had little academic experience. Results from dynamic assessment could help the SLP validly differentiate whether Carl has a language learning disorder or whether he has learning differences. There has been very little research in the application of dynamic assessment with Navajo children. However, recently Henderson, Restrepo, and Aiken (2018) conducted a study on dynamic assessment using narrative skills with Navajo preschool children (4-5 years of age). Henderson et al. (2018) found that the Predictive Early Assessment of Reading and Language (PEARL) (Petersen & Spencer, 2014), a dynamic assessment of narratives that measures language comprehension and production, could differentiate Navajo children with language impairment from those with typically developing language. The study showed that modifiability was the best discriminator between Navajo children with and without language impairment. It is possible that if Carl completed the PEARL pretest and posttest, his score could reflect learnability to mediation. Dynamic assessment using the PEARL could confirm that Carl demonstrates typically developing language ability in comparison to his speech community.
2. Recommendations for next steps:
    a. Monitor Carl's articulation and language skills to ensure he is developing appropriately for his age and gender. Carl may benefit from in-class monitoring and consultation with his teacher.
    b. Consult with the bilingual education teacher and/or the English as a Second Language teacher who may provide additional resources that Carl could benefit from to help him develop both languages.
    c. Provide medical follow-up to obtain glasses to improve his vision, and refer to a clinical psychologist to determine if Carl exhibits ADHD.

CONCLUSION

This case highlights the importance of considering dialectal differences when assessing Native American children. As authors for this case study, we incorporated problem-based learning strategies so that the reader can think of ways to access information about differences between the Navajo and English language and ways the Navajo language influences English.

In this scenario, Carl is exposed to both English and Navajo in the home; therefore, his English is likely influenced by the Navajo phonology, lexicon, syntax and grammar. Carl's speech and language patterns are typical of Navajo children who speak with Navajo-Influence English (or nonstandard American English) in both structure and phonology (Henderson et al., 2018). For example, the Navajo language is structured as subject-object-verb (SOV) as opposed to subject-verb-object (SVO). Due to this difference, Carl appears to use verb tenses incorrectly. Relative to phonology, Carl uses several Navajo-Influence English speech sounds. For example, he produces the following as a common speech error pattern among Navajo children: /dæn/ for /ðæn/, /dæt/ for / ðæt/. Carl exhibits Navajo-Influence English sounds and language structure that are common among Navajo children his age and gender (Henderson & Restrepo, 2016; Henderson et al., 2018).

This case study heightens the need for the profession of speech-language pathology to expand research to document linguistic variations in Native American communities so that clinical applications can improve with all tribal speech communities. In addition, this case study calls for explicit ways to share dialectal differences with SLPs who are not familiar with Native languages or the characteristics of American Indian English. Most importantly, this case study should challenge SLPs to ask more questions, search for answers, and develop alternative strategies to ensure that all SLPs are distinguishing linguistic differences from language disorders in Native speech communities.

KEY POINTS

When providing services to Navajo children, speech-language pathologists need to:

- Differentiate language differences from disorders
- Take into account cultural differences
- Consider opportunities for educational experiences on these topics prior to assessment
- Implement alternative assessments
- Understand the characteristics of Navajo phonology and language and their influence on English speech and language skills

REFERENCES

Brown, R. (1973). *A first language: The early stages*. London: George Allen & Unwin. doi:10.4159/harvard.9780674732469

Goldman, R., & Fristoe, M. (2015). *Goldman-Fristoe Test of Articulation* (3rd ed.). Bloomington, MN: NCS Pearson, Inc.

Grimes, B. F. (1996). *Ethnologue: Languages of the world*. Dallas, TX: Summer Institute of Linguistics, Inc.

Henderson, D. E., & Restrepo, M. A. (2016, November). *Navajo student's performance on the CELF – 4*. Paper presented at the American Speech-Language-Hearing Association Convention, Philadelphia, PA.

Henderson, D. E., Restrepo, M. A., & Aiken, L. S. (2018). Dynamic assessment of narratives among Navajo preschoolers. *Journal of Speech, Language, and Hearing Research: JSLHR*, *61*(10), 2547–2560. doi:10.1044/2018_JSLHR-L-17-0313 PMID:30304364

Leap, W. L. (1993). *American Indian English*. Salt Lake City, UT: University of Utah Press.

Petersen, D. B., & Spencer, T. D. (2014). *The Predictive Early Assessment of Reading and Language (PEARL): Screener.* Available from www.LanguageDynamicsGroup.com

Semel, E., Wiig, E. H., & Secord, W. A. (2003). *Clinical Evaluation of Language Fundamentals* (4th ed.). Bloomington, MN: NCS Pearson, Inc.

Vining, C., Edgarita, L., Inglebret, E., & Brendal, M. (2017). Speech-language assessment considerations for American Indian and Alaskan Native Children who are dual language learners. *Perspectives of the Special Interest Groups, 2*(Sig 14), 29–40.

Wiig, E. H., Semel, E., & Secord, W. A. (2013). *Clinical Evaluation of Language Fundamentals* (5th ed.). Bloomington, MN: NCS Pearson, Inc.

Young, R. W., & Morgan, W. (1987). *The Navajo language: A grammar and colloquial dictionary*. Albuquerque, NM: University of New Mexico Press.

ADDITIONAL READING

Banks, S. R., & Neisworth, J. T. (1995). Dynamic assessment in early intervention applications for serving American Indian/Alaska Native families. *Journal of American Indian Education*, *34*(2), 27–43.

Begay-Vining, C. (1997). Clinical issues providing speech and language services to Native American children with disabilities. *Communication Disorders and Sciences in Culturally and Linguistically Diverse Populations*, *3*(3), 4–6. doi:10.1044/cds3.3.4

Bialystok, E. (2001). *Bilingualism in development: Language, literacy, and cognition*. New York: Cambridge University Press. doi:10.1017/CBO9780511605963

Cummins, J. (1984). *Bilingualism and special education: Issues in assessment and pedagogy*. San Diego, CA: College-Hill Press.

House, D. (2002). *Language shift among the Navajos: Identity politics and cultural continuity*. Tucson: University of Arizona Press.

Royer, J. M., & Carlo, M. S. (1993). Assessing language comprehension skills in cross-cultural settings. In J. Altarriba (Ed.), *Cognition and culture: A cross-cultural approach to cognitive psychology* (pp. 157–175). Amsterdam: Elsevier Science Publishers. doi:10.1016/S0166-4115(08)61662-3

Spivey, M., & Marian, V. (1999). Cross talk between native and second languages: Partial activation of an irrelevant lexicon. *Psychological Science*, *10*(3), 281–284. doi:10.1111/1467-9280.00151

Ukrainetz, T. A., Harpell, S., Walsh, C., & Coyle, C. (2000). A preliminary investigation of dynamic assessment with Native American kindergartners. *Language, Speech, and Hearing Services in Schools*, *31*(2), 142–154. doi:10.1044/0161-1461.3102.142 PMID:27764386

KEY TERMS AND DEFINITIONS

Attention-Deficit/Hyperactivity Disorder (ADHD) – Combined Type: ADHD-Combined presentation is a neurobehavioral disorder that is characterized by both hyperactivity (moving constantly including in situations where this is not appropriate, fidgeting, excessive talking, restlessness) and impulsivity (making hasty, unplanned actions such as interrupting others or making decisions without considering consequences) as well as inattention (difficulty concentrating or sustaining attention, and forgetfulness).

Dialectal Differences: For individuals learning English as a second language, it is common for the phonemic system of their first language to influence the production of sounds in English.

Dynamic Assessment: Dynamic assessment (DA) is a method of conducting a language assessment which seeks to identify the skills that an individual child possesses as well as their learning potential. The dynamic assessment procedure emphasizes the learning process and accounts for the amount and nature of examiner investment. It is highly interactive and process-oriented.

English Language Learner (ELL): ELL describes children who are not fully proficient in English.

Navajo Nation: The Navajo Nation is one of the largest tribes in the U.S. The Navajo reservation spans four states, including Arizona, New Mexico, Utah and Colorado. The Navajo Nation has a strong history of retaining its language and culture.

Navajo-Influenced English: Navajo-influenced English is a variety of English whose features have been influenced by the phonology and grammar of the Navajo language.

Native Speech Communities: The definition of a speech community is a group of people who speak the same language and share the same words and grammar rules. Native speech communities include members of an indigenous people of North or South America.

Speech-Language Impairment (SLI): Speech-language impairments embrace a wide range of conditions. As the term implies, they include speech disorders which refer to impairments in the articulation of speech sounds, fluency, and voice as well as language disorders which refer to impairments in receptive skills (i.e., the ability to understand what is said or to integrate and organize what is heard) and expressive skills (i.e., the ability to articulate sounds, and use sounds, words, and sentences in meaningful contexts).

Chapter 3
Intervention Services for a Child With Multiple Disabilities

Yolanda D. Keller-Bell
North Carolina Central University, USA

EXECUTIVE SUMMARY

This chapter will focus on providing intervention services for an eight-year-old African-American female, Dawn, with multiple disabilities. Dawn has been diagnosed with Down syndrome, a comorbid diagnosis of an intellectual disability, and exhibits behavior problems at home and school. In this scenario, she has been evaluated within the school system to determine eligibility for services, and the speech-language pathologist needs to develop intervention goals and select therapy strategies to provide appropriate services. While both parents are involved in the child's care, the family does not have permanent housing and moves frequently. Information from actual cases has been incorporated into this chapter.

INTRODUCTION

Down syndrome

Down syndrome (DS) is a chromosomal genetic disorder that occurs in an estimated 1 in 700-750 live births in the United States (Parker et al., 2010). Trisomy 21 is the most common form of Down syndrome, accounting for 95% of cases. It occurs when there is a complete reduplication of Chromosome 21, resulting in three copies of the chromosome instead of two. DS is a commonly identified cause of intellectual disability (Sherman, Allen, Bean, & Freeman, 2007), and individuals with Down syndrome can demonstrate difficulty with phonological memory, attention, and weaknesses in communication.

Speech and Language Characteristics of Children with DS

A specific behavioral phenotype characterizes the communication ability of individuals with DS, in particular, deficits in expressive language ability (Abbeduto, Brady, & Kover, 2007; Chapman, 2006; Roberts et al., 2007; Roberts, Price, & Malkin, 2007). Studies of individuals with Down syndrome have

DOI: 10.4018/978-1-7998-2261-5.ch003

found greater deficits in receptive syntax than in receptive vocabulary (Abbeduto et al., 2003; Loveall, Channell, Phillips, Abbeduto, & Conners, 2016). Cuskelly, Povey, and Jobling (2016) examined the receptive vocabulary ability of individuals with Down syndrome, ranging in age from age 2;7 to 29;7, on the Peabody Picture Vocabulary Test- Revised (PPVT-R; Dunn & Dunn, 1981) or the Peabody Picture Vocabulary Test- Third Edition (PPVT-III; Dunn & Dunn, 1997). Nonverbal cognitive ability, measured by the Pattern Analysis subtest of the Stanford–Binet Intelligence Scale: Fourth Edition (Thorndike, Hagan, & Sattler, 1986), was related to receptive vocabulary; however, surprisingly, maternal education was not associated with performance. Receptive vocabulary continues to increase for individuals with Down syndrome until approximately 20 years of age, although the rate of increase is slower for individuals with Down syndrome than their typically developing peers (Cuskelly et al., 2016).

Findings regarding expressive language ability have been consistent. Berglund, Eriksson, and Johansson (2001) found that more than half of the children with DS did not have a spoken vocabulary of two words until two-years of age, and a majority did not have a spoken vocabulary of 50 words until four-years of age. Studies report difficulties in expressive morphology and syntax relative to expectations for chronological age and cognitive ability (Chapman, Hesketh, & Kistler, 2002; Chapman, 2006; Fowler, Gelman, & Gleitman, 1994; Miller, 1999). Individuals with Down syndrome are delayed in expressive syntax when compared to other populations with intellectual disabilities such as Fragile X syndrome (Abbeduto et al., 2001; Bellugi, Lichtenberger, Jones, Lai, & St. George, 2000; Ring & Clahsen, 2005; Vicari, Caselli, Gagliardi, Tonucci, & Volterra, 2002), and unknown etiologies (Chapman, 2006). In conversational samples, participants with Down syndrome achieved lower scores on the total score and each of the subscales of the Index of Productive Syntax (IPSYN; Scarborough, 1990) than typically developing (TD) children and males with Fragile X syndrome (FXS) matched for nonverbal cognitive ability.

Similar to receptive vocabulary, studies indicate that children with DS continue to develop expressive language skills throughout adolescence, albeit at a slow pace. In a longitudinal study, 84% of participants with DS showed a positive growth trajectory over six years as measured by mean length of utterance in morphemes (MLUm) in narrative samples (Chapman et al., 2002). Adolescents with DS and TD children matched for MLUm produced narrative samples that were similar in the number of different types of complex sentences as well as the percentage of complex utterances (Thordardottir, Chapman, & Wagner, 2002).

Individuals with DS demonstrate significant delays in speech sound development and production (Dodd & Thompson, 2001; Kent & Vorperian, 2013; Kumin, 2001; Wild, Vorperian, Kent, Bolt, & Austin, 2018). Individuals with DS exhibit delays in the acquisition of speech sounds, particularly consonants, and demonstrate disordered speech production (Kent & Vorperian, 2013). Poor speech intelligibility is a consistent finding in the literature (Kent & Vorperian, 2013; Kumin, 2001; Wild et al., 2018); however, there is some evidence that speech intelligibly may continue to improve over the individual's life span (Wild et al., 2018). The age at which infants use canonical babbling may be delayed but the delay is relatively smaller when compared to the degree of delay in the acquisition of other developmental milestones for gross motor skills (e.g., walking, standing) (Cobo-Lewis, Oller, Lynch, & Levine, 1996; Kent & Vorperian, 2013; Palisano et al., 2001).

Biological/Physical Characteristics of DS

In addition to an increased risk for communication disorders, individuals with DS are at risk for cardiovascular defects. Approximately 50% of infants with DS are diagnosed with a cardiovascular defect (Bergstrom et al., 2016; Kucik et al., 2013; Vis et al., 2000). Individuals with DS who also have a heart defect have an increased risk of death in the postneonatal period nearly five times that of those children with DS who do not have a heart defect (Kucik et al., 2013). The presence of a heart defect continues to be a significant predictor of mortality through 20 years of age. While the mortality rates have improved across racial and ethnic groups, non-Hispanic White children with Down syndrome continue to have a higher survival rate beyond infancy than non-Hispanic Black children with DS (Kucik et al., 2013).

Studies have also reported that children with DS are at higher risk of hearing loss (Nightengale, Yoon, Wolter-Warmerdam, Daniels, & Hickey, 2017; Phelan, Pal, Henderson, Green, & Bruce, 2016). A retrospective database study of children with DS indicated that 9% of the children had a unilateral hearing loss while 91% had a bilateral hearing loss (Kreicher, Weir, Nguyen, & Meyer, 2018). The most common types of hearing loss were pure conductive and "undefined." Approximately 19% of the children with DS had a moderate or more severe hearing loss, and 75% of the children had chronic otitis media or multiple episodes of acute otitis media (Kreicher et al., 2018).

Service Provision

Federal and state mandates require collaboration between professionals and parents to develop plans such as an Individualized Family Service Plan or Individual Education Plan (IEP) for individuals with disabilities. The purpose of these plans is to facilitate growth in academic, communication, social, and vocational skills (Olivos, Gallagher, & Aguilar, 2010; Turnbull, Turnbull, Erwin, & Shogren, 2015). One factor that professionals should consider when developing and implementing these plans is the parental level of stress. Naniwadekar (2018) reported that parents of children with communication disorders reported high levels of stress. Parents of children with autism spectrum disorders, followed by intellectual disabilities, multiple disabilities, and hearing loss reported the highest levels of stress. Individuals with DS are at risk for a comorbid diagnosis of each of these disabilities (Naniwadekar, 2018), which may compound the levels of stress these families may experience and increase the need for support services for parents.

Factors such as race, ethnicity, culture, and geographic location can influence the number and types of sources of support for caregivers of children with disabilities (Darling & Gallagher, 2004; Lynch & Hanson, 2011). For example, African-American caregivers in urban locations have reported higher levels of needs in terms of personal and family growth than African-American caregivers in rural locations or European-American caregivers in rural or urban locations (Darling & Gallagher, 2004). Darling and Gallagher (2004) reported that African-American families who reported the higher levels of need also reported lower levels of support and that families that reported lower levels of need indicated higher levels of support. In qualitative interviews, African American mothers of sons with autism spectrum disorders (ASD) reported a lack of awareness of ASD by immediate family members (Lovelace, Tamayo, & Robertson, 2018). The lack of awareness negatively impacted the mothers' levels of stress and their willingness to access support services (Lovelace, Tamayo, & Robertson, 2018). This contrast indicates that access to resources for family support may have a significant role in the experiences of family caregivers.

High Mobile Students and the Presence of a Disability

The home environment, such as stability of the home, can impact a child's academic, cognitive, and social development. Between 2014 to 2017, the number of students enrolled in public schools and reported as being homeless increased by 7% in the United States, with a total of 1,355,821 homeless students in the 2016-2017 school year (National Center for Homeless Education, 2019). According to the McKinney-Vento Homeless Education Assistance Improvements Act of 2001 ("Subtitle VII-B of the McKinney-Vento Homeless Assistance act (42 u.S.C. 11431 et seq.),"), children of a homeless parent or youth who are homeless must have access to a free, public education including preschool services. "Homeless" is defined as people who lack a fixed, regular, and adequate nighttime residence ("Subtitle VII-B of the McKinney-Vento Homeless Assistance act (42 u.S.C. 11431 et seq.),"). In addition, students at risk for enrolling in multiple schools or have enrolled in multiple schools in grades kindergarten through high school are known as Highly Mobile students (Costley, 2012). Unfortunately, children who are homeless or highly mobile (HHM) are at greater risk for poor academic and social development due to the instability of their family circumstances (Masten, 2012; Masten et al., 2014; Masten, Fiat, Labella, & Strack, 2015).

Although 13% of total children enrolled in public schools in the U.S. have a disability, 62% of states report that 20% of children who are homeless have a disability (NCHE, 2019). States and local education systems must fulfill the requirements of the McKinney-Vento Act and the Individuals with Disabilities Education Act (IDEA) ("Individuals with Disabilities Education Act, 20 u.S.C. § 1400 ", 2004) when working with children who are homeless and have a disability, but those who have a disability and transient residencies encounter several barriers to service access. These barriers include a) lack of a caregiver to accompany the child or youth to appointments; b) lack of timely enrollment in school; c) an untimely diagnosis or not being diagnosed; d) not being identified as needing special services when they have a disability and; e) lack of timely or continuity of service provision (National Center for Homeless Education at SERVE, 2015).

CASE STUDY

Clinical Evaluations

Dawn is an 8;2 year old African American female enrolled in the third grade at a public elementary school. She lives in an urban area with her mother, father, an older brother, and a younger sister. English is the primary language spoken in the home. Both of her parents completed high school and a year of community college. This is Dawn's third elementary school in two years as she has lived in various apartment complexes or hotels. A comprehensive speech and language evaluation was completed at her previous school at the beginning of the school year; however, Dawn transferred to her current school before services were implemented. She is in a self-contained classroom for children with intellectual disabilities.

Dawn's mother, Mrs. Williamson, is the primary caregiver and provided background information and history. Mrs. Williamson stated that her physician recommended that she have prenatal testing due to her age (maternal age of 30 years) and she was informed that Dawn was at risk for having Down syndrome. The diagnosis was confirmed at birth. Dawn had a congenital heart defect, an Atrioventricular Septal Defect (also referred to as an Endocardial Cushion Defect). She was hospitalized for the first six months of her life, has had two cardiovascular surgeries, and sees a cardiologist twice a year. Dawn goes to the local community health center for annual check-ups. According to Mrs. Williamson, Dawn takes medication for her heart condition, but she does not know the names of each of them.

Mrs. Williamson noted that Dawn's developmental, motor, and feeding milestones were not met as expected. Dawn did not say her first words until she was approximately two years old. Dawn started therapy at her home when she was 18 months, but it was hard to maintain the therapy schedule. Dawn received physical therapy until she was five, and her mother stated that she is supposed to receive occupational therapy at school. Mrs. Williamson does not know if this has started yet. Upon recommendation from a psychologist in her former school district, Dawn currently takes Ritalin to maintain attentiveness at school.

Mrs. Williamson reported that her daughter has had a lot of "ear problems" and suggested that recurrent ear infections and a tympanostomy tube influenced her ability to acquire age-appropriate language. She said she wants Dawn to "talk more" but noted that Dawn produces mostly short sentences (two to four words). She stated that Dawn is friendly, plays with her siblings, and likes to look at books, but that reading is challenging. Dawn can have difficulty "doing what she is supposed to do sometimes," and Mrs. Williamson wants her to be more independent.

Her mother reports that she goes to "lots of meetings at school" but does not always understand what is being discussed. Mr. Williamson, Dawn's father, cannot attend most meetings because of his work schedule. The mother stated that the family frequently moves because "it is hard to keep up with the rent," but they try to find apartments in "good" school districts because education is important to the family.

School Psychologist

The school psychologist completed an evaluation two months ago, and results indicated that Dawn met the criteria for an intellectual disability (American Psychiatric Association, 2013). The Wechsler Intelligence Scale for Children – Fifth Edition (Wechsler, 2014) was administered to assess cognitive ability and Dawn earned a standard score of 68 (-2.13 standard deviations (SD) below the mean). On a measure of adaptive ability, the Vineland Adaptive Behavior Scales (Sparrow, Cicchetti, & Saulnier, 2016), Dawn earned a standard score of 66 (-2.27 SD below the mean) on the Adaptive Behavior Composite and a standard score of 65 (-2.33 SD below the mean) on the Communication Domain. These scores indicate that Dawn's cognitive and adaptive functioning skills are poorer than typically developing peers. The school psychologist reports that Dawn has been referred to administration by teachers for behavior problems three times in two months. Dawn demonstrated disruptive behaviors when transitioning between classroom activities and settings.

Classroom Report

Dawn's teacher, Ms. Hopson, indicated that Dawn has difficulty following directions, reading comprehension (e.g., understanding what is read, finding the main idea), and writing. She expressed significant concern regarding Dawn's ability to produce complete sentences and her limited expressive vocabulary skills. Dawn has difficulty communicating her wants and needs and becomes frustrated easily. When frustrated, Dawn may cry or throw objects. Ms. Hobson stated that the school has behavioral expectations, but they are not posted in her room. She indicated that she has tried to meet with Mrs. Williamson, but it is difficult to coordinate schedules. Dawn does have friends in the class and likes to play with her peers. She believes that Dawn is supposed to receive occupational therapy but is unaware of the therapy goals.

Assessment Procedures

A hearing screening was administered to test for any hearing difficulties. An oral-motor exam was also administered to examine Dawn's oral-facial structure and musculature. Speech sound development was assessed using the Arizona Articulation and Phonology Scale Fourth Revision (Arizona-4) (Fudala & Stegall, 2017). The Peabody Picture Vocabulary Test Fourth Edition (PPVT-4, Dunn & Dunn, 2007) was administered to assess receptive vocabulary. The Oral and Written Language Scale, Second Edition (OWLS-II) (Carrow-Woolfolk, 2011) was administered to test receptive and expressive language. An informal language sample was conducted to assess sounds in sentences as well as receptive and expressive language.

Hearing Screening

A pure tone hearing screening was conducted at 20 dB HL and Dawn did not respond at the following frequencies in either ear: 1000 Hz, 2000 Hz, and 4000 Hz. She was referred for a full audiological evaluation and the audiologist confirmed a mild conductive hearing loss, primarily due to a malformation of the external ear canal and otitis media, an infection of the middle ear. The audiologist referred Dawn to a physician at a community clinic to address the otitis media. The physician recommended the placement of bilateral tympanostomy tubes, and upon placement, the audiologist approved the continuation of the rest of the evaluation.

Oral-Facial Mechanism Examination

An informal oral-facial mechanism examination revealed mouth breathing and a relatively small oral cavity with an enlarged tongue. Tongue movement was limited in range and speed of movement. Epicanthus folds, a skin fold of the upper eyelid that covers the inner corner of the eye, were noted on both eyes. Epicanthus folds can be found in typically developing individuals but are characteristic of DS. Mild hypotonia (a.k.a. "floppy muscles") facial muscles were observed. Evaluation of Dawn's mandible revealed normal symmetry with limited range of motion. The maxilla, the upper jaw, is relatively smaller than the mandible, the lower jawbone. Evaluation of the detention revealed missing teeth and uneven spacing, but missing teeth at age 8;7 is normal, as children's adult teeth emerge. Her pharynx has the typical pink or red color, and the tonsils are still present and not occluding the pharynx. Dawn's hard and soft palate revealed normal color, symmetry, arch height, but a narrow width. In sum, the results of the oral-facial mechanism exam revealed concerns about the structural and functional integrity of Dawn's oral musculature that could hinder her speech production and intelligibility.

Voice and Resonance

Voice production for pitch and loudness were judged appropriate for age and sex. Breathiness was noted in conversational speech.

Table 1. Summary of Dawn's results from the Arizona-4

Arizona-4			
	Standard Score (Mean = 100, SD = 15)	**Percentile Rank**	**Severity Range**
Word Articulation	≤50	<0.1	Severe
Phonology	≤50	<0.1	Severe

Source: Fudala & Stegall, 2017

Fluency

There were no significant pauses, hesitations, or repetitions observed during the evaluation session. Rate of speech was judged to be appropriate.

Articulation and Phonology

Articulation and phonology were formally assessed via administration of the Arizona-4 (Fudala & Stegall, 2017), a measure of speech production of consonant and vowel sounds in single words. See results in Table 1.

Dawn produced the consonants /p, h, b, d, t, s, w, k, f, n/ correctly in the initial and final position of words. She substituted [f] for /θ/ and [d] for /ð/ in words and conversation. Dawn's speech was considered unintelligible by an unfamiliar listener who comprehended approximately 70% of words in conversational speech. Results of this analysis indicated a significant delay in her speech sound production which impacts her communication with others (see Table 2).

COMPREHENSIVE LANGUAGE

The Listening Comprehension and Oral Expression Scales from the OWLS-II (Carrow-Woolfolk, 2011) were administered to test receptive and expressive language abilities. Dawn earned the following scores (see Table 3):

Language Sample Analysis

Non-standardized methods were also used to assess Dawn's language skills during a twenty-minute play session. A conversational sample of utterances was obtained during free play, and a narrative sample was obtained while reviewing a wordless picture book. Dawn exhibited the communicative functions of requesting and commenting, and also initiated a topic during the activities. She did not, however, ask for clarification or attempt to repair breakdowns in communication. Instead, she cried or threw the object (e.g., book or toy) on the floor.

Table 2. Phonological process analysis from the Arizona-4

Phonological Processes	Percent of Occurrence
Syllable Reduction	50%
Cluster Simplification	91%
Initial Consonant Deletion	0%
Final Consonant Deletion	44%
Fronting	25%
Deaffrication	0%
Stopping	36%
Gliding	75%
Vowelization	89%
Prevocalic Voicing	0%
Postvocalic Devoicing	36%

Source: Fudala & Stegall, 2017

Table 3. Dawn's results from the OWLS-II

OWLS-II		
COMPOSITE SCORES	**Standard Score Mean= 100; SD=15; (Severity; 90% Confidence)**	**Percentile Rank**
Oral Language Composite Score	65 (Deficient; Confidence Interval = 61-69)	1%
Oral Expression Scale (Assesses ability to answer questions, finish sentences, and generate sentences)	71 (Below Average; Confidence Interval = 68-74)	5%
Listening Comprehension Scale (Measures receptive language presented verbally)	75 (Below Average; Confidence Interval = 71-79)	3%

Source: Carrow-Woolfolk, 2011

Mean Length of Utterance (MLUm) refers to the average number of morphemes that a client produces in an utterance, while Mean Length of Utterance (MLUw) refers to the average number of words produced in an utterance. A total of 60 utterances were obtained; however, only 30 utterances were complete and intelligible.

For Dawn's age, MLUm scores between 4.7 and 6.64 are within one standard deviation of the mean of 5.67 and therefore considered to be within normal limits (Rice et al., 2010). A mean MLUw of 5.08, with a one standard deviation range of 4.24 to 5.92 is also within normal limits (Rice et al., 2010). Dawn produced a MLUm of 3.11 and a MLUw of 2.84, indicating MLUs outside normal limits. The Number of Total Words (NTW) and the Number of Different Words (NDW) reflect the quantity and diversity of words produced in a language sample. Typically developing eight-year olds have a mean NTW of 137 and NDW of 67 (Justice, Bowles, Kaderavek, Ukrainetz, Eisenberg, & Gillam, 2006). Dawn's NTW was 86 and her NDW was 40. The clinician noted that Dawn used "sposta", "fixin", and omitted plurals when describing the quantity of an item, e.g., "two book".

Questions for the Reader

1. Are the results of Dawn's evaluation consistent with the phenotype of DS? What are her strengths and weaknesses?
2. In addition to speech-language pathology, should there be a referral(s) to other professionals or resources? Who and why?
3. How might Dawn's home life impact her academic and communication development?

Discussion of the Questions for the Reader

1. The results of the evaluation are consistent with the communication pattern for DS reported in the literature. The literature indicates that individuals with DS are at greater risk for delays in speech and language, particularly expressive language, cognitive delays, and hearing loss. There are physical characteristics that are associated with DS as well such as malformations of the ear and epanthical folds.

In this case example, Dawn did not respond at any frequency at 20 dB HL in either ear. Her background indicates delays in cognitive, speech, and language development. The results from the language sample analysis, the OWLS-II, and the teacher report present converging evidence that Dawn's language ability falls below the normal limits for her age and indicate greater delays in expressive language in comparison to receptive language. The sound substitutions of [f] for /θ/ and [d] for /ð/ for are consistent with dialectal variations of African American English and are not considered speech errors (Bland-Stewart, 2003; Pearson, Velleman, Bryant, & Charko, 2008; Stockman & Kamhi, 1996). Pragmatic skills are an area of strength for Dawn.

2. Dawn's hearing should be monitored on a routine basis by the audiologist and family physician. A referral to the school's social worker for family resources and information regarding the behavioral expectations for the school and classroom would be beneficial. A dental consultation to evaluate dental spacing and confirmation of occupational therapy services is needed.
3. Children who are homeless or highly mobile are at increased risk for emotional and behavioral problems, and poor academic development, as inconsistency in school enrollment disrupts continuity of educational and therapeutic services.

TREATMENT OPTIONS

A comprehensive approach to service provision should be used to address the needs of the family and Dawn as an individual. Lo and Hiatt-Michael (2014) recommend strategies to increase the involvement of families from culturally and linguistically diverse backgrounds in the education of their children, such as providing parent education, facilitating mentorship relationships between families, and providing formal support at Individualized Education Program (IEP) meetings. For example, another parent or community stakeholder could attend the meeting to describe the IEP process, access to community resources, and rights and services afforded by the McKinney-Vento Act ("Subtitle VII-B of the McKinney-Vento Homeless Assistance act (42 u.S.C. 11431 et seq.),") . A referral to the school's social worker and counselor should be made to address concerns regarding the family's transient housing.

Behavior

IDEA requires public school systems to consider the use of Positive Behavior Interventions and Supports (PBIS) for any student whose behavior impedes their learning or the learning of others (IDEA, 2004). PBIS is a prevention-oriented approach for organizing evidence-based behavioral strategies within a tiered continuum to facilitate the academic and behavioral performance of all students- with or without a disability (Lewis & Sugai, 1999; Sugai & Horner, 2002 (Technical Assistance Center on Positive Behavioral Intervention and Supports, 2010)).

PBIS is typically conceived as having three tiers and is based on continual collection and evaluation of data regarding a child's behavior. Primary interventions are provided in Tier 1. These supports and strategies successfully address the behavioral management needs of approximately 80% of all students with or without a disability. (Spaulding, Horner, May, & Vincent, 2008). Tier 2, secondary interventions, addresses those students considered to be at risk for developing significant behavioral or academic problems or have been identified as having significant needs. Serving approximately 15% of all students, Tier 2 interventions are often delivered as small group strategies and procedures (Simonsen et al., 2015). When primary- and secondary-level interventions are not successful in reducing or eliminating the undesirable behavior, Tier 3 interventions are implemented. Students in Tier 3, approximately 1-5% of all students, may have significant histories of academic and behavioral difficulties (Simonsen et al., 2015). Tier 3 interventions are individualized for the specific needs of the child. It is important to note that all children, including those who may have a disability that puts them at higher risk for behavioral disturbances, such as autism spectrum disorders (ASD) or emotional disturbance, should still be considered for PBIS.

The speech-language pathologist should collaborate with the family, teacher (Ms. Hopson), and the school psychologist to develop a behavioral intervention plan to reduce the number of disruptive behaviors. A positive behavior intervention and support (PBIS) framework should be used to a) identify antecedents or triggers to disruptive behaviors; b) explicitly teach behavioral expectations and; c) provide culturally appropriate responses to decrease inappropriate referrals to school administrators (Keller-Bell & Short, 2019). In order to establish a foundation for Tier 1 supports, the physical environment should be arranged to minimize distractions and facilitate learning (Simonsen, Fairbanks, Briesch, Myers, & Sugai, 2008; Simonsen et al., 2015). The school has three behavioral expectations (e.g., *I will be respectful, I will be ready to learn, I will be responsible*) that should be prominently displayed in Dawn's classroom, the cafeteria, and therapy rooms. Using role play (Simonsen et al., 2015), explicit examples of appropriate and inappropriate behavior for each behavioral expectation should be discussed with Dawn's class. The teacher and the SLP should identify and create school routines for Dawn and provide visual schedules to increase the predictability of routines (Bopp, Brown, & Mirenda, 2004).

The next step in PBIS implementation is to use responsive and positive preventative strategies to reduce the number of behavioral disruptions. Verbal, behavior-specific acknowledgments will be used each time Dawn or any child demonstrates the behavioral expectations (Bambara, Janney, & Snell, 2015; Bambara & Kern, 2005). Ms. Hopson reported that Dawn likes to win prizes, so a token economy system was developed. Each time Ms. Hopson, the SLP, or other school personnel observe a child exhibiting one of the behavioral expectations, the child should receive a ticket which can be redeemed for a prize at the end of the year. As the final step of implementation, collected data can be analyzed to determine if the number of behavioral disruptions is reduced (Simonsen et al., 2015). These strategies should be shared with Dawn's mother to facilitate continuity between home and school.

Speech and Language

In terms of communication, the SLP should prioritize the following targets for intervention: 1) improving speech intelligibility and sound production; 2) increasing and diversifying her semantic abilities and; 3) increasing Dawn's mean of length of utterance. The *Naturalistic Intervention for Speech Intelligibility and Speech Accuracy* (Camarata, 2010) protocol should be used in conjunction with the *Cycles Phonological Approach* (Hudson, 2010; Prezas & Hodson, 2010).

Naturalistic Intervention for Speech Intelligibility and Speech Accuracy (Camarata, 2010), designed to improve speech intelligibility, incorporates two stages of intervention by a) increasing overall intelligibility and b) increasing accuracy of individual speech phonemes. Rather than focusing on single-sound production, the emphasis is on whole-word production and does not require detailed phonetic transcription. Thus, while the SLP coordinates the service delivery, the naturalistic approach can be implemented by Dawn's teachers, parents, and other stakeholders (Camarata, 2010). The approach should be implemented in an interactive activity, e.g., playing with toys, conversation, or reading books. No specific materials or toys are required; however, having a defined set of activities may facilitate understanding of highly unintelligible children (Bauman-Waengler, 2015). The activities should elicit spontaneous productions which the adult should recast using the appropriate speech production (Camarata, 2010). For example, if the child points to a baby doll and says "bobo', the adult responds by saying "baby".

Children with significant speech sound errors who are highly unintelligible are candidates for the *Cycles Phonological Approach* (Hudson, 2010; Prezas & Hodson, 2010). The approach targets speech sound patterns the child cannot produce spontaneously in connected speech, but are stimulable; meaning they can say the sounds when prompted. Specific phonological patterns are targeted during each cycle, and each target phoneme per cycle should be targeted for 60 minutes per week (Prezas & Hodson, 2010). The cycles range in length for five to sixteen weeks but may last longer for children with intellectual disabilities. Following the completion of a cycle for one or more targeted phonological patterns, another cycle for different phonological patterns is introduced. This rotation continues until the phonological patterns emerge in conversational speech (Prezas & Hodson, 2010).

Throneburg, Calvert, Sturm, Paramboukas, and Paul (2001) compared the effects of collaborative, classroom-based, and traditional pull-out service delivery models for semantic development/curriculum based vocabulary. All three were effective but the greatest effect sizes were seen with collaborative and classroom-based services. Thus, the SLP should work with Ms. Hopson to identify books and vocabulary aligned with the curriculum and incorporate curriculum-based materials into the speech-language therapy sessions. The SLP should also work with Dawn once a week in the classroom during English Language Arts.

Indirect language stimulation should be used to augment language skills. Similar to the *Naturalistic Intervention for Speech Intelligibility and Speech Accuracy* (Camarata, 2010), these strategies are used in the context of naturalistic, child-directed activities (Paul & Norbury, 2012). While these strategies have been used with children chronologically younger than Dawn, the SLP considered them to be appropriate, given Dawn's current language level and cognitive ability. Expansions occur when the adult adds semantic details and grammatical markers to a child's utterance to create a grammatically acceptable utterance. A recast sentence is similar to an expansion, except the child's utterance is changed into a different type of utterance, e.g., a child's declarative statement is recast as a question, or made into an elaborated sentence (Paul & Norbury, 2012). If only semantic information is added to a child's utterance, it is known as an extension (Paul & Norbury, 2012).

Aspects of the robust vocabulary approach will be used to improve semantic abilities by categorizing words into tiers for instruction. Robust vocabulary instruction provides an explicit, child- friendly definition of an unfamiliar word by providing additional information, such as visual or semantic information, to increase the child's engagement with the word (Beck, McKeown, & Kucan, 2013). This approach has been used with children from diverse backgrounds who were at-risk for or not meeting academic benchmarks (Apthorp, 2006; Lovelace & Stewart, 2009) The SLP should collaborate with Ms. Hopson to select Tier 1 and Tier 2 vocabulary words focusing on Dawn's comprehension of the words. Tier 1 vocabulary words are high-frequency words that usually occur in conversation, e.g., *happy*, while Tier 2 words are less likely to be used in conversation or learned on their own. These words need specific instruction and exposure to convey that the meaning of the word "delighted" is similar to "happy" (Beck et al., 2013; Beck, McKeown, Kucan, Hiebert, & Kamil, 2005). Robust vocabulary activities should take place in the context of shared storybook reading (Lovelace & Stewart, 2009).

Outcomes

An IEP meeting was scheduled at the end of the school year, and another mother of a child with a developmental disability attended the IEP meeting with Mrs. Williamson, Dawn's mother. Mrs. Williamson initially expressed reluctance to contact the social worker but has made an appointment to meet with the social worker. The family may need to move again but Mrs. Williamson says the family will try to stay in the same area to remain at the school. The number and frequency of Dawn's inappropriate behaviors have steadily decreased, and she has responded well to the token economy system being used in the classroom. Ms. Hopson and Mrs. Williamson both reported an improvement in Dawn's behavior.

Dawn's speech intelligibility has improved to 80% intelligibility in words; however, she still demonstrates significant delays in her production of sounds. Thus, the Cycles Phonological Approach should continue to be used. Dawn has exhibited improvement in her receptive and expressive language skills, increasing her MLUw and MLUm. While her language skills remain delayed, she has shown improvement in all aspects of communication.

Children with multiple disabilities such as the Dawn require a holistic approach to assessment and intervention. While the child may have a primary diagnosis such as DS, there may be comorbid diagnoses such as intellectual disabilities, hearing loss, and behavior problems that need to be considered when providing services. The compounding effect of multiple disabilities can exacerbate levels of parent stress. Further, factors such as a transient home environment and cultural-linguistic differences may impact the ability of the family to identify and access appropriate support services. A holistic approach to services takes into consideration each of these factors when interacting with the families and when providing direct services to the child.

Additional Questions for the Reader

1. What is the prognosis for Dawn's receptive and expressive language ability?
2. What impact does Dawn's limited speech sound production ability have on her expressive language skills?
3. Children with disabilities are expected to meet educational goals and standards. What other needs may Dawn have in the future?

Discussion of the Additional Questions for the Reader

1. Based on the research, Dawn's receptive and expressive language abilities should continue to develop into adulthood albeit at a slower pace than her typically developing peers. Her receptive language skills may become commiserate with her nonverbal cognitive ability.
2. Dawn exhibits several phonological processes such as cluster reduction and final consonant deletion that impact the ability to assess her expressive language skills accurately. For example, omission of plurals could be attributed to a speech sound error, an expressive language error, or both. As Dawn's intelligibility increases, she should produce more complete and intelligible utterances, which will improve her conversational skills and facilitate the use of language sample analysis to monitor her progress.
3. IDEA (2004) indicates that children with disabilities are expected to meet educational benchmarks. As literacy expectations increase, Dawn may need specific instruction in reading.

KEY POINTS

- Down syndrome is a genetic, chromosomal disorder that is a common cause of intellectual disability. Individuals with DS exhibit a common pattern of associated disorders, including hearing loss, cardiovascular impairments, delays in speech sound production, and language impairments.
- The number of homeless or highly mobile children enrolled in public schools in the United States has increased from 2014 to 2017. These children are at higher risk for poor academic and emotional outcomes. Services should take a holistic approach by considering the support systems needed by the child and the family.
- Children with multiple disabilities from culturally and linguistically diverse families and transient home environments may face additional barriers to access services, and these barriers need to be explicitly addressed by the intervention team.

REFERENCES

Abbeduto, L., Brady, N., & Kover, S. T. (2007). Language development and Fragile X Syndrome: Profiles, syndrome-specificity, and within-syndrome differences. *Mental Retardation and Developmental Disabilities Research Reviews*, *13*(1), 36–46. doi:10.1002/mrdd.20142 PMID:17326110

Abbeduto, L., Murphy, M. M., Cawthon, S. W., Richmond, E. K., Weissman, M. D., Karadottir, S., & O'Brien, A. (2003). Receptive language skills of adolescents and young adults with Down syndrome or Fragile X Syndrome. *American Journal of Mental Retardation*, *108*(3), 149–160. doi:10.1352/0895-8017(2003)108<0149:RLSOAA>2.0.CO;2 PMID:12691594

Abbeduto, L., Pavetto, M., Kesin, E., Weissman, M. D., Karadottir, S., O'Brien, A., & Cawthon, S. (2001). The linguistic and cognitive profile of Down syndrome: Evidence from a comparison with fragile x syndrome. *Down's Syndrome: Research and Practice*, *7*(1), 9–15. doi:10.3104/reports.109 PMID:11706811

American Psychiatric Association. (2013). *Diagnostic and statistical manual of mental disorders* (5th ed.). Arlington, VA: American Psychiatric Publishing.

American Speech-Language-Hearing Association (ASHA). (2019). *Practice portal: Speech sound disorders-articulation and phonology*. Retrieved from https://www.asha.org/PRPSpecificTopic.aspx?folderid=8589935321&section=Treatment

Apthorp, H. S. (2006). Effects of a supplemental vocabulary program in third-grade reading/language arts. *The Journal of Educational Research, 100*(2), 67–79. doi:10.3200/JOER.100.2.67-79

Bambara, L. M., Janney, R., & Snell, M. (2015). *Behavior support: Teachers' guides to inclusive practices* (3rd ed.). Baltimore, MD: Brookes.

Bambara, L. M., & Kern, L. (2005). *Individualized supports for students with problem behaviors: Designing positive behavior plans*. New York, NY: Guilford.

Bauman-Waengler, J. (2015). *Articulatory and phonological impairments: A clinical focus* (5th ed.). Boston, MA: Pearson, Allyn, & Bacon.

Beck, I. L., McKeown, M. G., & Kucan, L. (2013). *Bringing words to life: Robust vocabulary instruction*. New York, NY: Guilford.

Beck, I. L., McKeown, M. G., Kucan, L., Hiebert, E. H., & Kamil, M. L. (2005). Choosing words to teach. In *Teaching and learning vocabulary: Bringing research to practice* (pp. 209–222). Mahwah, NJ: Lawrence Erlbaum Associates.

Bergstrom, S., Carr, H., Petersson, G., Stephansson, O., Bonamy, A. K., Dahlstrom, A., ... Johansson, S. (2016). Trends in congenital heart defects in infants with Down syndrome. *Pediatrics, 138*(1), e20160123. doi:10.1542/peds.2016-0123 PMID:27252035

Bland-Stewart, L. M. (2003). Phonetic inventories and phonological patterns of African American two-year-olds: A preliminary investigation. *Communication Disorders Quarterly, 24*(3), 109–120. doi:10.1177/15257401030240030201

Bopp, K. D., Brown, K. E., & Mirenda, P. (2004). Speech-language pathologists' roles in the delivery of positive behavior support for individuals with developmental disabilities. *American Journal of Speech-Language Pathology, 13*(1), 5–19. doi:10.1044/1058-0360(2004/003) PMID:15101810

Camarata, S. (2010). Naturalistic intervention for speech intelligibility and speech accuracy. In A. L. Williams, S. McLeod, & R. McCauley (Eds.), *Interventions for speech sound disorders in children* (pp. 381–406). Baltimore, MD: Brookes.

Carrow-Woolfolk, E. (2011). *Oral and Written Language Scales* (2nd ed.). Torrance, CA: Western Publishing Services.

Chapman, R. S. (2006). Language learning in Down Syndrome: The speech and language profile compared to adolescents with cognitive impairment of unknown origin. *Down's Syndrome: Research and Practice, 10*(2), 61–66. doi:10.3104/reports.306 PMID:16869363

Cobo-Lewis, A. B., Oller, D. K., Lynch, M. P., & Levine, S. L. (1996). Relations of motor and vocal milestones in typically developing infants and infants with Down syndrome. *American Journal of Mental Retardation: AJMR*, *100*(5), 456–467. PMID:8852298

Costley, K. C. (2012). *Learners on the move: Responsive teachers fill in the gap for highly mobile students*. Retrieved from http://eric.ed.gov/?id=ED533514

Cuskelly, M., Povey, J., & Jobling, A. (2016). Trajectories of development of receptive vocabulary in individuals with Down syndrome. *Journal of Policy and Practice in Intellectual Disabilities*, *13*(2), 111–119. doi:10.1111/jppi.12151

Darling, S. M., & Gallagher, P. A. (2004). Needs of and supports for African American and European American caregivers of young children with special needs in urban and rural settings. *Topics in Early Childhood Special Education*, *24*(2), 98–109. doi:10.1177/02711214040240020501

Dodd, B., & Thompson, L. (2001). Speech disorder in children with Down syndrome. *Journal of Intellectual Disability Research*, *45*(4), 308–316. doi:10.1046/j.1365-2788.2001.00327.x PMID:11489052

Dunn, L. M., & Dunn, D. M. (2007). *Peabody Picture Vocabulary Test-4*. Minneapolis, MN: Pearson.

Dunn, L. M., & Dunn, L. M. (1981). *Peabody Picture Vocabulary Test- Revised*. Circle Pines, MN: American Guidance Service.

Dunn, L. M., & Dunn, L. M. (1997). *Peabody Picture Vocabulary Test-III* (3rd ed.). Circle Pines, MN: American Guidance Service.

Fudala, J. B., & Stegall, S. (2017). *Arizona Articulation and Phonology Scale* (4th ed.). Torrance, CA: Western Psychological Services.

Hudson, B. (2010). *Evaluating and enhancing children's phonological systems: Research and theory to practice*. Wichita, KS: PhonoComp.

Individuals with Disabilities Education Act, 20 u.S.C. § 1400 (2004).

Individuals with Disabilities Education Improvement Act of 2004 (IDEA). (2004). *Public Law 108-446, 108th Congress*. Retrieved from https://sites.ed.gov/idea/

Keller-Bell, Y., & Short, M. (2019). Positive behavioral interventions and supports in schools: A tutorial. *Language, Speech, and Hearing Services in Schools*, *50*(1), 1–15. doi:10.1044/2018_LSHSS-17-0037 PMID:30950772

Kent, R. D., & Vorperian, H. K. (2013). Speech impairment in Down syndrome: A review. *Journal of Speech, Language, and Hearing Research: JSLHR*, *56*(1), 178–210. doi:10.1044/1092-4388(2012/12-0148) PMID:23275397

Kreicher, K. L., Weir, F. W., Nguyen, S. A., & Meyer, T. A. (2018). Characteristics and progression of hearing loss in children with Down syndrome. *The Journal of Pediatrics*, *193*, 27–33. doi:10.1016/j.jpeds.2017.09.053 PMID:29174076

Kucik, J. E., Shin, M., Siffel, C., Marengo, L., & Correa, A. (2013). Trends in survival among children with Down syndrome in 10 regions of the United States. *Pediatrics*, *131*(1), e27–e36. doi:10.1542/peds.2012-1616 PMID:23248222

Kumin, L. (2001). Speech intelligibility in individuals with Down syndrome: A framework for targeting specific factors for assessment and treatment. *Down Syndrome Quarterly, 6*(3), 1-8.

Lo, L., & Hiatt-Michael, D. (2014). *Promising practices to empower culturally and linguistically diverse families of children with disabilities*. Charlotte, NC: Information Age Publishing.

Loveall, S. J., Channell, M. M., Phillips, B. A., Abbeduto, L., & Conners, F. A. (2016). Receptive vocabulary analysis in Down syndrome. *Research in Developmental Disabilities*, *55*, 161–172. doi:10.1016/j.ridd.2016.03.018 PMID:27084992

Lovelace, S., & Stewart, S. R. (2009). Effects of robust vocabulary instruction and multicultural text on the development of word knowledge among African American children. *American Journal of Speech-Language Pathology*, *18*(2), 168–179. doi:10.1044/1058-0360(2008/08-0023) PMID:19106209

Lovelace, T. S., Tamayo, S., & Robertson, R. E. (2018). Experiences of African American mothers of sons with autism spectrum disorder: Lessons for improving service delivery. *Education and Training in Autism and Developmental Disabilities*, *53*(1), 3–16.

Lynch, E. W., & Hanson, M. J. (2011). *Developing cross-cultural competence: A guide for working with young children and their families* (4th ed.). Baltimore, MD: Paul H. Brookes.

Masten, A. S. (2012). Risk and resilience in the educational success of homeless and highly mobile children: Introduction to the special section. *Educational Researcher*, *41*(9), 363–365. doi:10.3102/0013189X12467366

Masten, A. S., Cutuli, J. J., Herbers, J. E., Hinz, E., Obradovic, J., & Wenzel, A. J. (2014). Academic risk and resilience in the context of homelessness. *Child Development Perspectives*, *8*(4), 201–206. doi:10.1111/cdep.12088 PMID:29623104

Masten, A. S., Fiat, A. E., Labella, M. H., & Strack, R. A. (2015). Educating homeless and highly mobile students: Implications of research on risk and resilience. *School Psychology Review*, *44*(3), 315–330. doi:10.17105pr-15-0068.1

Naniwadekar, K. (2018). Stress and anxiety among parents of children with communication disorders. In *Handbook of research on psychosocial perspectives of human communication disorders* (pp. 141–156). Hershey, PA: Information Science Publishing/IGI Global. doi:10.4018/978-1-5225-4955-0.ch008

National Center for Homeless Education at SERVE. (2015). *Navigating the intersections of the Mckinney-Vento Act and Individuals with Disabilities Education Act: Coordination to help homeless children and youth with disabilities. Best practices in homeless education brief series.* Retrieved from http://www.nclive.org/cgi-bin/nclsm?url=http://search.ebscohost.com/login.aspx?direct=true&db=eric&AN=ED574610&site=ehost-live

National Center for Homelessness. (2019). *Federal data summary: School years 2014-15 to 2016-17*. Retrieved from https://nche.ed.gov/wp-content/uploads/2019/02/Federal-Data-Summary-SY-14.15-to-16.17-Final-Published-2.12.19.pdf

Nightengale, E., Yoon, P., Wolter-Warmerdam, K., Daniels, D., & Hickey, F. (2017). Understanding hearing and hearing loss in children with Down syndrome. *American Journal of Audiology*, *26*(3), 301–308. doi:10.1044/2017_AJA-17-0010 PMID:28854301

Olivos, E. M., Gallagher, R. J., & Aguilar, J. (2010). Fostering collaboration with culturally and linguistically diverse families of children with moderate to severe disabilities. *Journal of Educational & Psychological Consultation*, *20*(1), 28–40. doi:10.1080/10474410903535372

Palisano, R. J., Walter, S. D., Russell, D. J., Rosenbaum, P. L., Gemus, M., Galuppi, B. E., & Cunningham, L. (2001). Gross motor function of children with Down syndrome: Creation of motor growth curves. *Archives of Physical Medicine and Rehabilitation*, *82*(4), 494–500. doi:10.1053/apmr.2001.21956 PMID:11295010

Parker, S. E., Fau, M. C., Canfield, M. A., Fau, C. M., Rickard, R., Fau, R. R., . . . Correa, A. (2010). *Updated national birth prevalence estimates for selected birth defects in the United States, 2004-2006*. (1542-0760 (Electronic)).

Paul, R., & Norbury, C. (2012). *Language disorders from infancy through adolescence: Listening, speaking, reading, writing, and communicating* (4th ed.). St. Louis, MO: Elsevier.

Pearson, B., Velleman, S., Bryant, T., & Charko, T. (2008). Phonological milestones for African American English-speaking children learning Mainstream American English as a second dialect. *Language, Speech, and Hearing Services in Schools*, *40*(3), 229–244. doi:10.1044/0161-1461(2008/08-0064) PMID:18952815

Phelan, E., Pal, R., Henderson, L., Green, K. M. J., & Bruce, I. A. (2016). The management of children with Down syndrome and profound hearing loss. *Cochlear Implants International*, *17*(1), 52–57. doi:10.1179/1754762815Y.0000000019 PMID:26252564

Prezas, R. F., & Hodson, B. W. (2010). The Cycles Phonological Remediation approach. In A. L. Williams, S. McLeod, & R. McCauley (Eds.), *Interventions for speech sound disorders in children* (pp. 137–158). Baltimore, MD: Brookes.

Rice, M. L., Smolik, F., Perpich, D., Thompson, T., Rytting, N., & Blossom, M. (2010). Mean length of utterance levels in 6-month intervals for children 3 to 9 years with and without language impairments. *Journal of Speech, Language, and Hearing Research: JSLHR*, *53*(2), 333–349. doi:10.1044/1092-4388(2009/08-0183) PMID:20360460

Roberts, J., Price, J., Barnes, E., Nelson, L., Burchinal, M., Hennon, E. A., ... Hooper, S. R. (2007). Receptive vocabulary, expressive vocabulary, and speech production of boys with Fragile X Syndrome in comparison to boys with Down Syndrome. *American Journal of Mental Retardation*, *112*(3), 177–193. doi:10.1352/0895-8017(2007)112[177:RVEVAS]2.0.CO;2 PMID:17542655

Roberts, J. E., Price, J., & Malkin, C. (2007). Language and communication development in Down Syndrome. *Mental Retardation and Developmental Disabilities Research Reviews*, *13*(1), 26–35. doi:10.1002/mrdd.20136 PMID:17326116

Simonsen, B., Fairbanks, S., Briesch, A., Myers, D., & Sugai, G. (2008). Evidence-based practices in classroom management: Considerations for research to practice. *Education & Treatment of Children*, *31*(3), 351–380. doi:10.1353/etc.0.0007

Simonsen, B., Freeman, J., Goodman, S., Mitchell, B., Swain-Bradway, J., Flannery, B., . . . Putman, B. (2015). *PBIS technical brief on classroom PBIS strategies.* Retrieved from https://www.pbis.org/common/ cms/files/pbisresources/Supporting%20and%20Responding% 20to%20Behavior.pdf.

Sparrow, S. S., Cicchetti, D., & Saulnier, C. (2016). *Vineland Adaptive Behavior Scales* (3rd ed.). Bloomington, MN: Pearson.

Spaulding, S. A., Horner, R. H., May, S. L., & Vincent, C. G. (2008). *Evaluation brief: Implementation of school-wide PBS across the United States*. Retrieved from http://pbis.org/evaluation/evaluation_briefs/default.aspx

Stockman, I. (1996). Phonological development and disorders in African American children. In A. G. Kamhi, K. E. Pollock, & J. L. Harris (Eds.), *Communication development and disorders in African American children: Research, assessment, and intervention* (pp. 117–153). Baltimore, MD: Paul H. Brookes.

Subtitle VII-B of the McKinney-Vento Homeless Assistance Act (42 u.S.C. 11431 et seq.).

Technical Assistance Center on Positive Behavioral Intervention and Supports. (2010). *SWPBIS implementation blueprint and self-assessment. Positive behavioral intervention and supports.* Retrieved from http://www.pbis.org/Common/Cms/files/pbisresources/SWPBS_ImplementationBlueprint_vSep_23_2010.pdf

Technical Assistance Center on Positive Behavioral Interventions and Supports. (2017). *Student-sample behavior expectations.* Retrieved from https://www.pbis.org/training/staff/student

Thorndike, R. L., Hagan, E. P., & Sattler, J. M. (1986). *The Stanford-Binet Intelligence Scale* (4th ed.). Chicago, IL: Riverside Publishing.

Throneburg, R., Calvert, L., Sturm, J., Paramboukas, A., & Paul, P. (2001). A comparison of service delivery models: Effects on curricular vocabulary skills in the school setting. *American Journal of Speech-Language Pathology*, *9*(1), 10–20. doi:10.1044/1058-0360.0901.10

Turnbull, A., Turnbull, H. R., Erwin, E. J., & Shogren, K. A. (2015). *Families, professionals, and exceptionality: Positive outcomes through partnerships and trust* (7th ed.). Bloomington, MN: Pearson.

Vis, J. C., Duffels, M. G., Winter, M. M., Weijerman, M. E., Cobben, J. M., Huisman, S. A., & Mulder, B. J. (2009). Down syndrome: A cardiovascular perspective. *Journal of Intellectual Disability Research*, *53*(5), 419–425. doi:10.1111/j.1365-2788.2009.01158.x PMID:19228275

Wechsler, D. (2014). *Wechsler Intelligence Scale for Children-V* (5th ed.). San Antonio, TX, US: Psychological Corporation.

Wild, A., Vorperian, H. K., Kent, R. D., Bolt, D. M., & Austin, D. (2018). Single-word speech intelligibility in children and adults with Down syndrome. *American Journal of Speech-Language Pathology, 27*(1), 222–236. doi:10.1044/2017_AJSLP-17-0002 PMID:29214307

KEY TERMS AND DEFINITIONS

Acute Otitis Media (AOM): Rapid onset of one or more symptoms of middle ear inflammation and the presence of fluid in the middle ear fluid.

Adaptive Behavior: An individual's ability to independently demonstrate social and cognitive skills and perform activities of daily living.

Down Syndrome: A genetic chromosomal disorder where an individual has three copies of chromosome 21 and is known as Trisomy 21.

Homeless: Individuals who do not have an adequate, fixed, and consistent nighttime residence.

Individual Education Plan (IEP): A written document that is designed by school personnel and parents to improve the educational outcomes of a student in the general curriculum and meets the requirements of the Individuals with Disabilities Education Act.

Individualized Family Service Plan (IFSP): A written treatment plan for young children who have a developmental disability that outlines early intervention services from birth to three years of age.

Intellectual Disability: A significant limitation in an individual's adaptive behavior and intellectual functioning that originates before 18 years of age.

Otitis Media With Effusion: The presence of fluid in the middle ear without evidence of an ear infection.

Positive Behavioral Interventions and Supports: A prevention-oriented approach for organizing evidence-based behavior strategies within a tiered continuum to facilitate the academic and behavioral performance of all students.

Chapter 4
Language, Social Pragmatic Communication, and Childhood Trauma

Yvette D. Hyter
https://orcid.org/0000-0002-6910-8576
Western Michigan University, USA

EXECUTIVE SUMMARY

This case focuses on the effects of trauma on the language and social pragmatic communication of a 10-year-old girl who was one of the many children separated from familial caregivers between 2016 and 2019 when she and her parents came to the U.S. from Central America seeking asylum due to gang violence and economic reasons. The child spent 8 months in the detention center without her parents and then was transferred to a foster home where she suffered neglect as well as physical and psychological abuse. This case study focuses on the long-term effects of structural violence and maltreatment on child development, and specifically on language and social pragmatic communication.

INTRODUCTION

Disclaimers: The case discussed in this chapter contains facts from a real case; however, some of the events were changed and others were added. The events that were added are actual events from a compilation of real cases occurring in the current U.S. news or seen at a midwestern transdisciplinary clinic that provides comprehensive assessments to children and adolescents with histories of maltreatment and prenatal alcohol exposure. All names have been changed to protect the privacy of those involved with the case. Some parts of this case were presented in the article and presentations cited below, and have been used in Dr. Hyter's course on Disordered Language Development:

DOI: 10.4018/978-1-7998-2261-5.ch004

- Hyter, Y.D. (2012). Complex trauma and prenatal alcohol exposure: Clinical implications. *ASHA Perspectives on School-Based Issues, 13*(2), 32 – 42. doi/10.1044/sbi13.2.32
- Hyter, Y.D. & Ciolino, C. (2017, November). Providing SLP services through a trauma informed lens. Seminar presented at the annual convention of the American Speech-Language-Hearing Association, Los Angeles, CA.
- Hyter, Y.D., Henry, J., Sloane, M., Suarez, M., & Ciolino, C. (2018). The effects of complex trauma and alcohol exposure: The brain, language and skills for daily living. Short course presented at the Annual Convention of the Michigan Speech-Language-Hearing Association, Kalamazoo.

Global Connections

How Isidra came to live in the U. S. from Guatemala is a story of how all humans on earth are all linked through global connections. Isidra was one of the many children separated from familial caregivers between 2016 and 2019. Isidra and her parents came to the U.S. from Central America seeking asylum due to gang violence and economic reasons. The CAFTA (Central American Free Trade Agreement – implemented in 2006) has had outcomes in Guatemala and other Central American countries that are not equivalent to the results CAFTA has had in the U.S.

CAFTA was designed to eliminate "barriers to U.S. exports, improving U.S. competitiveness against Central American and third country [*sic*] suppliers" (Office of the U.S. Trade Representative, 2004; Perla, 2016; U.S. Customs and Border Protection, 2019). In the U.S. CAFTA has helped to create new jobs and has benefited small companies (Murphy & Busch, 2015). CAFTA, however, has resulted in limited governmental basic services for populations in Central America, displaced farmers who cannot compete with low prices of goods imported from the U.S., high levels of unemployment, poor working conditions for laborers, and low wages (Beneria, Berik, & Floro, 2016; Burgos, 2007; Perez-Rocha & Paley, 2014). CAFTA is the context in which powerful gangs have risen, and has motivated migration to the U.S.

Migration by the Numbers

While in Guatemala, Isidra's home country, her family began receiving threats from gangs to pay a protection price. Her father and mother worried about Isidra's safety and made the decision to leave their home country for the U.S., which they perceived as a safer place to raise a family and one that would provide a future for Isidra. Upon arrival at the U.S. border, Isidra was separated from her parents.

Although there is no U.S. law or court ruling that requires systematic removal of children from their families, and detention of children (Binford, 2019; Rizzo, 2018), according to the ACLU (2019), as of October 2018, there were 2654[1] children determined to be separated from their parents. Of these 2654 children, 525 (20%) were girls like Isidra, 10-years-old or older (ACLU, 2019). Some of these children were detained without their parents for up to a year (ACLU, 2019). An executive order ending the current federal administration's policy of separating migrant children from their parents was signed on 19 June 2018 (Gonzales, 2018); nevertheless, family separations continued well into 2019 with at least 700[2] more children being separated from parents or grandparents (Human Rights Watch, 2019).

Maltreatment and Adverse Childhood Experiences

Isidra spent eight months in the detention center without her parents, in "facilities without enough food or toothbrushes – going days without showering, overcrowded and undercared for" (Binford, 2019; Lind, 2019). When she left the detention center, Isidra lived with two foster families, both who lost their rights to care for her following substantiated physical and emotional abuse, and neglect. Sexual abuse is suspected but not yet substantiated. Isidra is currently residing in a residential center; the U. S. government has not yet been able to reunite Isidra with her biological parents.

According to the U.S. Department of Health and Human Services, Administration for Children and Families (ACF, 2019), 3.5 million children were investigated for abuse in 2017.[3] Of these 3.5 million children, about 674,000 cases were substantiated, which is a rate of 9.1 victims per 1000 children. Of these substantiated cases, 505,000 (74.9%) were cases of neglect, 123,342 (18.3%) were of physical abuse, and 57,964 (8.6%) were of sexual abuse. In 2017, approximately 1700 children died as a result of their experience of maltreatment.

Maltreatment is pervasive across socioeconomic and racial lines; that is, wealthy people engage in child maltreatment as well as those who are impoverished. The same can be said for people who identify as White, and those who identify as People of Color. Yet, there is agreement in the literature that African American and Latinx[4] children are overrepresented in the U.S. Child Welfare System and that Asian and White families are underrepresented (Anyon, 2010; Child Welfare Information Gateway, 2016). Although there are likely many reasons for this disproportional representation in Child Welfare, some causes may be due to racism and elitism[5], which both lead to ill-informed assumptions about the "fitness" of families of color and/or those families that are impoverished (Simon, 2018).

Adverse Childhood Experiences (ACEs), first introduced in the 1990s, refer to the types of adversities people face throughout childhood (Felitti, Nordenberg, Williamson, Spitz, Edwards, Kross . . ., 1998). ACEs included events such as emotional, physical, or sexual abuse, physical or emotional neglect, substance abuse in the household, mental illness in the household, physical abuse of a parent, divorce, and criminal behavior in the household (Burke-Harris, 2018). Burke-Harris (2018) reports that her patients with "4 or more ACEs were 32.6 times as likely to have been diagnosed with learning and behavioral problems" (p. 66).

The Impact of Trauma on Child Development

Traumatic stressors could be due to complex trauma (maltreatment occurring within a caregiving context), or to structural violence – the indirect kind of violence that is not caused by individuals but by structures and institutions within a society (Farmer, 2005; Galtung, 1969). It is the "violence exerted systematically" (Farmer, 2004, p. 307), that can serve to deny some of their basic human rights (Ho, 2007, p. 1; Ortega, Graybill, & Lasch, 2015). Structural violence occurs when families are forced into the uncertainty and chaotic situation of being displaced from their natural environment as a result of armed conflict, natural disasters (Perez Foster, 2001), global development-based causes (Farmer, 2005) and/or immigration policies (Escobar, 2018; Ortega et al., 2015). Structural violence imposes material conditions on the way some groups of people are forced to live such as:

- Food deserts (i.e., the absence of places to purchase fresh food but the overabundance of places to purchase fast food, liquor or processed foods) (American Nutrition Association, 2019);
- Lack of clean and safe water to consume (e.g., water crises in Flint, Michigan);
- Limited safe and clean places to play;
- Unequal access to affordable health care;
- Chronic stress of low paying jobs, unreliable transportation;
- Living in areas where high levels of toxic fumes are expelled (e.g., near a bus depot or landfill).

Trauma Effects on the Brain

Some of the effects of maltreatment include a reduction in electrical brain activity, changes or disruptions in the development of neurons, and the production and pruning of synapses, and myelination (Burke-Harris, 2018; Cook, Blaustein, Spinazzola, & van der Kolk, 2003; DeBellis, 2001). Traumatic experiences processed in the brain bypass the thalamus to cortex to amygdala neural pathway; but rather, the thalamus to amygdala pathway is sensitized (Henry, Sloane, & Black-Pond, 2007) causing elevated cortisol responses that provoke involuntary physiological behaviors (DeBellis, 2001; DeBellis, Woolley & Hooper, 2013). These physiological behaviors include increased heart rate and blood pressure, hypervigilance (i.e., elevated alertness), impaired sleeping and attention abilities, and problems with sensory modulation (Henry et al., 2007; Hyter, Henry, Sloane, Suarez & Ciolino, 2018; Steele & Malchiodi, 2016). As a result of these physiological changes, children develop psychological issues that may serve as protective behaviors, but these protective behaviors (e.g., dissociation, distrust, self-harm, behaviors perceived as aggressive, engaging in high-risk behaviors) are not often effective for functioning in daily life (Atchison, 2007; Hyter et al., 2018; SAMHSA, 2014). Developmental deficits occur in the areas of social cognition, executive functions, affect regulation, working memory and social pragmatic communication (Hyter, 2012; Hyter et al., 2018).

Child traumatic experiences exist both within the caregiving (i.e., family) system (Henry et al., 2007), as well as in institutional settings, such as in state and government systems (Spratt, Freidenberg, Swenson, LaRosa, De Bellis, Macias et al., 2012). Nevertheless, little empirical research has focused on the effects of trauma on child communication and language development.

Trauma Effects on Cognition, Communication, Language and Social Pragmatic Abilities

Trauma experiences negatively affect language development. In a study of 74 preschool aged children with histories of trauma, Culp, Watkins, Lawrence, Letts, Kelly, and Rice (1991) compared the results of language (using the *Preschool Language Scale* [*PLS*, Zimmerman Steiner, & Pond, 1979]), speech (using the *Goldman-Fristoe Test of Articulation* [*GFTA*, Goldman & Fristoe, 1972]), and cognitive (using the *Early Intervention Development Profile* [*Profile*, Schafter & Moesch, 1981]) outcomes for children with different types of trauma histories, namely those with histories of physical abuse, those with histories of neglect but not physical abuse, and those with histories of both physical abuse and neglect. They found that the language skills of children with histories of neglect were the most delayed of the three groups, and this group also showed difficulty demonstrating age-appropriate language skills. All three groups showed delays in speech and cognitive development (Culp et al., 1991).

Research conducted by Spratt et al. (2012) confirm that children with histories of neglect present with more impaired cognitive and language skills than those who do not experience neglect. These authors state that neglect caused by "low stimulation environments and inconsistent parenting," (p. 176) can result in lower cognitive and language outcomes. Parent-child interpersonal interactions support language acquisition, and if these interactions are absent or inconsistent, child language development will be at risk (Spratt et al., 2012).

In a meta-analytic review, Sylvestre, Bussiéres, and Bouchard (2016) compared the language skills of children with histories of trauma (abuse and/or neglect) with those who had not experienced trauma and found that the language skills of children with histories of trauma are delayed. The language skills primarily examined in this study were syntax and semantics. Similarly, Richardson, Black-Pond, Sloane, Atchison, Hyter and Henry (2015) showed that children with histories of trauma presented with both receptive and expressive syntactic and semantic deficits.

Several published studies have identified social pragmatic communication as an area of difficulty for children with histories of trauma (De Sante, Sylvestre, Bouchard, & Leblond, 2019; Hyter, 2010; Hyter, 2012; Hyter & Ciolino, 2017; Moreno, Garcia-Baamonde, Guerrero, & Blazquez, 2010; Moreno Manso, García-Baamonde Sánchez, Blázquez Alonzo, and Pozueco Romero, 2012; Moreno-Manso, García-Baamonde, Blázquez-Alonzo, Pozueco-Romero, & Godoy-Merino, 2016; Yehuda, 2016).

In the transdisciplinary trauma clinic where the author works, they have found that children with histories of maltreatment appear to have more difficulties in the area of social pragmatic language than in the areas of language structure and meaning (Ciolino, 2018; Hyter, 2010; Hyter & Ciolino, 2017), such as difficulty with discourse skills (Ayoub et al., 2006; Ciolino, 2018; Hyter, 2012; Sylvestre et al. 2016), perspective taking, with particular difficulty in second order belief attribution (Ciolino, 2018; Hyter, 2012; Luke & Banerjee, 2013); and difficulty identifying communitive intentions of others (Ciolino, 2018).

Why Should Maltreatment and Trauma be of Interest to SLPs?

Speech-language pathologists frequently encounter children with histories of traumatic stress and maltreatment on their caseloads even when the children do not have an official diagnosis of complex trauma. Due to the numerous difficulties experienced by this population in the areas of pragmatics and social communication, they are frequently referred for speech-language services (Westby, 2007; Yehuda, 2016). Children with histories of maltreatment may have language delays in the areas of syntax and semantics, but frequently in social communication and pragmatics (Ciolino, 2018; Hyter et al., 2018; Hyter, Henry, Atchison, Sloane, Black-Pond, & Shangraw, 2003).

CASE STUDY

Isidra is a 10;3-year-old third grader with a history of trauma caused by structural violence, as well as complex trauma. Trauma is an event or series of events that take place and leave a person feeling helpless, vulnerable (Black-Pond & Henry, 2008; Cook, Blaustein, Spinazzola, & van der Kolk, 2003; NCTSN, 2016, Steele & Malchiodi, 2012), and overwhelmed (van der Kolk, 2015; Yehuda, 2016). Complex trauma is the chronic maltreatment (abuse or neglect) that takes place within the caregiving system, and the long-lived effects that these experiences have on the child's development (Black-Pond & Henry, 2008; Henry, Sloane, & Black-Pond, 2007; NCTSN, 2016).

In addition to complex trauma, Isidra has experienced at least five Adverse Childhood Experiences (ACEs, Burke-Harris, 2018; Felitti et al., 1998) – the abuse, neglect, household dysfunction and "potentially traumatic experiences that occur to people under the age of 18" (CDC, 2019). Some of those other potentially traumatic experiences may include exposure to such events as *community violence*[6], domestic violence, substance abuse of family members, mental illness of family members, *separation from family members* and/or a parent, divorce of parents, incarcerated household member, *outside-of-home placement, loss of significant people in one's life*, and substance abuse of a family member (Burke-Harris, 2018; CDC, 2019; Ciolino, 2018; Felitti et al., 1998).

Isidra understands some words in Garifuna (the first language [L1] of her parents) but is proficient[7] in Spanish and English having used both languages at home and school for the first seven years of her life. Currently, Isidra is dominant in English because for the last three years while in the U.S., she has exclusively heard and spoken English at the detention center, in her foster homes, and while at school (Bedore et al., 2011; Grosjean, 2010).

Family History

Isidra's biological parents are from Guatemala. Isidra and her family identify as Latinx and Garifuna[8], and racially identify as of African descent or Black. Isidra's parents are proficient speakers of Garifuna[9], Spanish, and English. While in Guatemala, Garifuna was used primarily when Isidra's parents spoke to each other. Her parents used Spanish primarily for interacting with community members in Guatemala, and both Spanish and English were used when they were speaking with Isidra.

Isidra's parents were repeatedly threatened by the maras (i.e., gangs in Central America specifically in Guatemala, Honduras, and El Salvador); therefore, the family fled to the U. S. but were caught up in the immigrant detentions. When they arrived at the U.S. border the family was separated, and Isidra eventually ended up in her first foster home – the Maddens. The Madden family consisted of the foster mother, foster father who was a physician, and a teen-aged son. This foster family's rights were terminated having been found guilty of neglect, physical and psychological abuse. It is suspected that Isidra also was sexually abused by her foster brother, based on Isidra's sexualized behaviors[10]; however, sexual abuse was never substantiated. While living with the Maddens, Isidra had multiple visits to the hospital emergency room for fractured and/or broken bones in her limbs and face; 24 emergency room visits were recorded in the span of one year.

After being removed from the Madden's home, Isidra spent 18 months in her second foster home placement with the "Redding family." This foster home included two other children (biological son and daughter), the foster mother, and foster father. This family of five had an income of $28,000 per year, which is less than 100% of the current national poverty level of $30,170[11] for a family of five (ASPE, 2019). The Redding family had a history with Child Protective Services (CPS) after fostering Isidra, and they eventually lost rights to parent her over a year ago, when Isidra was 9 years old. During a CPS visit, she was found locked in a cage 3.5 feet high [12] and 4 feet wide in the dark basement of the Redding's home. She was described as being emaciated with a "gaunt face," "thin arms," appearing to have "limited energy and minimal coordination" and being "extremely small for her age." She was rated at the 10th percentile for weight (i.e., 60 lb [average for a 10.3-year-old is 75 lb]) (CDC, 2000a). Her height was rated at the 5th percentile for height (i.e., 50.5 inches [average for a 10.3-year-old is 55 inches]) (CDC, 2000b). Isidra was not permitted to eat regularly, was dirty from not being allowed take a bath or shower daily, her hair was matted having not been combed or washed in several months, and her skin was extremely dry and cracked. The Reddings stated that they had difficulty managing Isidra's behaviors, that she was "always running away," and that is why they "needed" to lock her in a cage.

Currently, Isidra is living in a residential center and seems to be thriving there. She exhibits social confidence, although she frequently misinterprets facial expressions and the intentions of her peers. Isidra is currently going to school within the residential center and is receiving psychological counseling. She was brought to the transdisciplinary clinic for further assessment.

Clinical Evaluations

The following evaluations were completed with Isidra and her foster family members. Each of these assessments and the results are discussed below.

1. *Ethnographic interviews* with Isidra, her foster parents (Mr. and Mrs. Redding), and the case worker focused on Isidra's strengths and challenges from their respective perspectives. Ethnographic interviewing is a valuable tool for understanding how Isidra and her foster family members and teachers conceptualize her "communication needs, strengths, and challenges" (Hyter & Salas-Provance, 2019, p. 145).
2. *Hearing Screening* to rule out concerns with hearing acuity.
3. *Universal Nonverbal Intelligence Test* (Bracken & McCallum, 1998) was used to measure general cognition without placing undue demands on receptive and expressive language (DeThorne & Schaefer, 2004).
4. *Sensory Profile - 2* (Dunn, 2014) was completed by Isidra's foster mother to determine if there were sensory modulation concerns.
5. *Narrative Scoring Scheme* (NSS, Heilmann, Miller & Dunaway, 2010).[13] A narrative retelling was collected from Isidra in both Spanish and English.
6. *Second Order Belief Attribution and Intention Reading* tasks from the Hyter Pragmatic Protocol-Revised: 9-15-years-old (Hyter & Jackson, 2010) (collected in both Spanish and English).
7. *Self-Report subtest of the Assessment of Pragmatic Language and Social Communication* (APLSC, Hyter & Applegate, 2012) (collected in both Spanish and English).
8. *Behavior Rating Inventory of Executive Function* (BRIEF; Gioia, Isquith, Guy, & Kenworthy, 2010).

Note that some of the assessments were administered in both Spanish and English. Although Isidra is reported to be proficient in both languages, she may not have the same linguistic skills in each language. Narrative was assessed because it is reported to present less test bias than standardized norm-referenced testing (Cleve, Girolametto, Chen, & Johnson, 2010; Peña, Gillam, & Bedore, 2014).

ETHNOGRAPHIC INTERVIEW DATA

Ethnographic Interview of the Foster Mother (Ms. Redding)

Isidra's foster mother participated in an interview about Isidra although she no longer has "parental" rights. About participating in the interview, Ms. Redding said *"I still love Isidra, and we didn't mean to harm her, but we just couldn't take good care of her with all of those behaviors she had."* When asked about Isidra's strengths, Ms. Redding said that *"she is funny. She sees the world in such a special way – as if everyone and everything is here to serve her. I got to hand it to the girl, she knows how to get what she wants."* When asked about challenges, Ms. Redding stated, *"she put our lives in danger by all that running away and the boy-crazy-act she put on. She ran away every week, you know."* When asked what the "boy-crazy-act" looked like Mrs. Redding said that *"she's not the sweet little girl she used to be. She jumps in the lap of any man or boy that comes to the house – it's embarrassing. She thinks she's the center of attention all of the time. I still want to help her be a better person."* Ms. Redding expressed concerns about Isidra's behavior and memory skills. She indicated that Isidra often ran away and was picked up by strangers who brought her back to the house late at night, and that she saw that as *"very dangerous behavior,"* and that *"nothing has happened yet, but it's just a matter of time."* Ms. Redding also shared that she thought Isidra *"was having difficulty adjusting to life as a third grader, cause she thinks she's the boss. She talks to me and my husband like we're supposed to be kids,"* and thought that Isidra was not experiencing academic or social success because "*she did not have any friends – other kids don't like her and don't want to be around her."*

Ethnographic Interview of Isidra's Case Worker (Sindy Case)

Isidra's case worker said that her strengths were her "*upbeat personality. Everything just rolls off her back*." When asked to describe that statement in another way, Ms. Case said, *"nothing gets her down – absolutely nothing bothers her. Isidra, can have not one friend, hasn't talked to her parents – her biological parents, but believes she is loved by everyone."* Ms. Case expressed worry for Isidra stating that Isidra *"has no friends,"* and that Isidra *"gets into fights at the drop of a hat."* The case worker also views Isidra as a *"very literal thinker,"* and that Isidra *"doesn't seem to understand what's real vs. what's pretend. Someone can be joking, and she'll take it too seriously, or something can be really serious, and she takes it to lightly."* Ms. Case also stated that *"she* [Isidra] *has some very violent behaviors, does not seem to have respect for authority, and even threatened to kill me, her foster and her teacher."* Ms. Case raised concerns about Isidra's progress in school stating that she *"is disruptive in class by constantly talking and arguing, and steals from everyone."*

Ethnographic Interview with Isidra

During her ethnographic interview, Isidra made the following statement when asked about her strengths, *"I am very smart. I can figure almost everything out. I know a lot."* When asked about her experiences with other kids in her class, she said, *"They don't think I'm cool because I am very smart. I'm smarter than they are, and I tell them so."* She was also asked if there might be reasons that the other kids did not like her, she responded with, *"Nope. They can only be jealous because I'm just too smart for them."* She stated, *"people play tricks on me."* When asked to give an example of how people play tricks on her

Table 1. List of concerns (red flags) and areas you would like to assess

Domain (Semantics, Pragmatics, Syntax, etc.)	Concerns or Red Flags & Why	What measures you would use to assess

she stated that, *"they say I take things from their bags, but I don't. The stuff just falls out and I find it."* When asked about how she manages when others play tricks on her, she responded with, *"I get angry, and when I get angry, I run away. I run away because that's the only thing I can do to help myself. If they want to keep playing tricks on me, that's ok because I know how to take care of myself. My parents taught me how."*

Assignment 1: Based on the information presented in the ethnographic interviews, use Table 1 to identify concerns or red flags that were revealed in the history and interview data, why those are concerns, and what assessment measures you would likely employ.

Assignment 2: Review Isidra's assessment data, comprised of a hearing screening, a nonverbal intelligence test, an informal narrative analysis, and social pragmatic communication assessments.

Assessment Results

Hearing Screening: Isidra passed a binaural hearing screening that tested 1000, 2000, and 4000 Hz signals at 20 dB HL.

Universal Nonverbal Intelligence Test-Second Edition (UNIT-2, Bracken & McCallum, 2016) is used to assess general cognitive skills, and is comprised of six subtests that comprise seven composite scores, each with a mean of 100 and a standard deviation of 15. Isidra received the following standard scores:

Memory – 88

Isidra's memory score indicates that she performed below average on tasks that required her to "recall multiple salient features simultaneously, including content, color, number, location and sequence" (Bracken & McCallum, 2016, p. 3). This lower memory score may be due to the effects of complex trauma on the areas of the brain involved with emotional regulation (limbic system) and memory (amygdala, hippocampus, cerebellum and prefrontal cortex). There are some data that suggest that childhood trauma interrupts one's ability to understand, recognize, and express emotions, to show empathy, engage in prosocial behavior (Young & Widom, 2014), and negatively affects memory (The National Scientific Council of the Developing Child, 2012).

Reasoning – 97

Isidra's reasoning score corresponds with the average descriptive classification. Her reasoning score shows that she demonstrated strengths in "pattern processing, awareness of visual-spatial juxtapositions, and understanding geometric relationships" (Bracken & McCallum, 2016, p. 4). Her reasoning score is significantly different from her memory score.

Quantitative – 100

Her quantitative score of 100 corresponds to average performance on tasks requiring numerical reasoning and relationships and numerical sense (Bracken & McCallam, 2016, p. 4). Her quantitative score is significantly different from her memory score. Isidra's memory score does vary from the reasoning and quantitative score. These results suggest that her short-term and working memory skills may be less developed than her reasoning or quantitative skills.

Sensory Profile – 2 (Dunn, 2014), is a group of assessments, completed by a parent or guardian, that evaluate sensory processing patterns as exhibited in various contexts, e.g., home, school, community. The results of the Sensory Profile-2 determine whether the child of interest is much less likely, less likely, as likely, more likely, or much more likely to be overwhelmed by sensory input than others. Children with trauma histories typically have attachment systems that have been interrupted, which negatively affect familial relationships, and efforts to establish relationships with peers (Warner, Loomar, Lary, & Cook, 2013). Biological systems are affected (Atchison, 2007; DeBellis & Zisk, 2014; Warner et al., 2013, p. 730), but what is often most affected is behavior regulation (Warner et al., 2013; van der Kolk, 2015), which often presents as adaptive or maladaptive responses (Atchison, 2007). Specifically, the body's primary biological stress system - limbic-hypothalamic pituitary adrenal axis (LHPA) – is overstimulated, resulting in hyper- or hypo-arousal and behavioral dysregulation (Burke-Harris, 2018; DeBellis & Zisk, 2014; Henry et al., 2007; Warner et al., 2013; van der Kolk, 1994; 2015). Adolescents with behavioral regulation concerns subsequent to trauma often present with high levels of emotional lability, impulsiveness or withdrawn behaviors, as well as depression or disassociation (Warner et al., 2013).

- Isidra's profile showed a number of concerns with sensory processing suggesting that sensory inputs may be overwhelming her brain. If a person has difficulty processing sensory input, their ability to engage in daily life experiences can be interrupted (Henry, 2016).
- Isidra's results showed that she
    - Was much more likely to be overwhelmed by sensory experiences than her peers;
    - Detects more sensory cues than her peers; and
    - Misses many more sensory cues than her peers (Dunn, 2014).
- Sensory processing difficulties may contribute to Isidra's perceived aggressive behavior, which is more likely adaptive (i.e., protective) rather than maladaptive in response to incoming sensory stimuli.

Narrative Scoring Scheme (NSS, Heilmann, Miller & Dunaway, 2010) is used to assess narrative skills. Narrative discourse is produced by many cultural groups; therefore, narrative assessment may be one of the least biased forms of assessment (Peña et al., 2014). Therefore, this narrative assessment measure was used rather than a standardized norm-reference language assessment measure.

There are some data to support that children with histories of trauma may exhibit difficulties with narrative discourse. Some children with histories of trauma exhibited difficulty organizing their ideas into a narrative, which was attributed to producing non-causal utterances (Toth, Stronach, Rogosch, Caplan, & Cicchetti, 2011), and producing less-complex narratives than peers without trauma histories (Ayoub, 2006). Hyter (2012) found similar characteristics – that children with histories of trauma demonstrated limited narrative cohesion and organization. Ciolino (2018) found that almost 52% of the children in her sample of 79 children did not adequately include landscape of consciousness (i.e., mental, emotional states) of characters, 33.9% exhibited difficulty with narrative cohesion, and 29.8% presented with narratives that did not exhibit coherence or informativeness. Being able to present an organized narrative is important in the lives of children so they can make sense of past experiences, but additionally, children may need to recount what happened to them in a way that is organized and detailed.

The NSS includes micro- and macro-structure analyses; yet, goes beyond story grammar to include other areas of advanced narrative skills for example the use of literate language, such as "metacognitive (e.g., think or know) or metalinguistic (e.g., say or talk) verbs" (p. 156), as well as cohesive devices that help "carry concepts across individual utterances" (p. 156) such as referential, conjunctive, and lexical cohesion. Isidra produced two narratives both in Spanish and English. One narrative was a retelling of her favorite movie (Narrative Retell), and the other was a generated narrative about a personal event (Personal Narrative).

- Isidra received proficient scores across all of the narrative characteristics for the Narrative Retell.
- During the personal narrative activity in both Spanish and English, Isidra received proficient scores for all narrative characteristics except for Mental States (she used a minimal number of mental states words and these words were used inconsistently), Conflict Resolution (the resolution Isidra offered was anti-social), and Cohesion. It is important to keep in mind, however, that some research has shown that for bilingual children, narrative macrostructure (i.e., overall narrative organization) told in both languages may be the same, but microstructure (e.g., lexical content) may be different (Iluz-Cohen & Walters, 2012; Simón-Cereijido & Gutiérrez-Clellen, 2009; Silliman, Bhar, Hnath-Chisolm & Mahecha, 2002).

The outcome of Isidra's narrative assessment is consistent with the difficulties that she presented with other assessment measures. Complex trauma creates a series of events in the brain that affect functioning. Major changes to the structure of the brain includes reduced size of the corpus callosum resulting in limited transfer of information between hemispheres, and diminished development of the "neocortex, hippocampus, and amygdala" (Teicher, Andersen, Polcari, Anderson, Navalta, & Kim, 2003, p. 33) resulting in social cognitive difficulties and impaired executive functioning. Hyter (2012) found that children with histories of complex trauma exhibited impaired narrative cohesion and organization and presented with limited abilities to provide prosocial outcomes to personal narratives. Additionally, Hyter (2012) reports that children who have experienced maltreatment exhibited deficits in understanding others' communicative intentions. Ciolino (2018) found that this population exhibited high rates of difficulties in understanding mental states of others and using narrative cohesion and second order belief attributions.

Hyter Pragmatic Protocol-Revised (Hyter & Jackson, 2010). The Pragmatic Protocol collects data on social pragmatic communication skills, which are the ability to understand a social situation and then to respond appropriately for that social situation. These skills allow a child to successfully engage in conversations, initiate, as well as to develop, and maintain positive social relationships. Additionally, social pragmatic communication skills support the ability to understand the perspectives and intentions of others, which is instrumental in predicting others' motivations and can be useful in modifying one's own behavior. Social pragmatic communication skills were examined through three of the six subtests that are part of this protocol – (a) participating in Conversations, (b) the Theory of Mind tasks focused on Second Order Belief Attribution, and (c) Intention Reading.

Cicchetti, Rogosch, Maughan, Toth and Bruce (2003) found that children with histories of maltreatment performed less well on false belief tasks than their non maltreated peers. A preliminary study conducted by Hyter (2012) found that children with histories of complex trauma and prenatal alcohol exposure exhibited difficulty with the aforementioned social pragmatic communication skills. Children with both complex trauma and prenatal alcohol exposure performed poorer in conversational discourse, second order belief attribution, and intention reading than those children with only exposure to maltreatment (trauma) (Hyter, 2012). Ciolino (2018) found that school age children exhibited relatively intact conversational skills, although 26% of study participants had difficulty providing sufficient information and on-topic comments during conversations. Additionally, school-age children presented greater difficulty with second order belief attribution tasks than first order belief attribution tasks.

Isidra's ability to participate in *conversations* were observed throughout the assessment day when engaged in conversation with examiners. A simple rubric was used to determine the presence or absence of conversational moves including starting a conversation, maintaining a topic, asking relevant questions, the use of nonspecific words (e.g., this, that, thing), making minimal revisions, and being a reciprocal conversational partner (Hyter & Jackson, 2010).

- Isidra demonstrated age appropriate conversation skills by following the conversational topic, effective use of shading to change topics, providing sufficient information for the conversational partner to follow, and engaging as a reciprocal conversational partner with the clinician.

Second Order Belief Attribution is the ability to separate one's own knowledge from what others might believe. This skill is important for understanding social interactions (Perner, 1988), and occurs when individuals consider "what people think about other people's thoughts" (Perner & Wimmer, 1985, p. 438). Specifically, it is the ability to understand embedded mental states such as, "he thinks that she thinks" (Sullivan & Tager-Flusberg, 1999, p. 524) or "Tom believes that John thinks it is raining . . " (Hollebrandse, van Hout, & Hendriks, 2014, p. 322). The "John and Mary" task (Perner & Wimmer, 1985) was used to assess this skill, and was administered in both Spanish and English.

- Isidra did not demonstrate an ability to correctly respond to a second order belief question. This skill is typically emerging by 5 or 6 years of age and present by 7 or 8 years of age (Hollebrandse, et al., 2014; Perner & Wimmer, 1985). This outcome suggests that Isidra may have difficulty seeing the perspective of others, particularly if it differs from her own. This result is consistent with her own reports and those of others in her life, that she has difficulty understanding others' intentions (why others do what they do), how her own behavior may affect others, and how to have reciprocal social relationships.

Intention Reading was assessed using a task developed by Happé (1994) designed to determine if the responder was able to attribute mental states, e.g., intentions and desires, to others. Happé developed 24 vignettes called "Strange Stories," which were read to Isidra who was asked to explain why a character in the vignette said something that was not true, such as why a character in a vignette may have said a banana was a telephone while holding the banana to his ear (e.g., pretending). Children with trauma histories have more difficulty with belief attribution tasks, and have more difficulty understanding the meanings of emotions and facial expression in others.

- Isidra did not demonstrate the ability to attribute intentions to the characters in the vignette particularly if the intention was a "joke," "lie," or the use of "sarcasm."

Assessment of Pragmatic Language and Social Communication (APLSC, Hyter & Applegate, 2012). The APLSC is a battery of assessments that include parent, teacher, and self-report checklists, and an SLP observation report that includes a narrative re-tell task and a sense making task. The only measure from the APLSC that was used with Isidra was the self-report.

- On the APLSC-Self-Report, Isidra endorsed that she does not have many friends and gets along better with adults than her peers. She reported struggling to engage with peers, to differentiate jokes from serious statements, and with understanding how others might feel or think particularly if those feelings or thoughts are different than her own.

Some children with history of complex trauma exhibit limited social perspective taking skills, and more self-centered thinking (Luke & Banerjee, 2013). Additionally, maltreatment experiences limit the number of positive social relationships experienced.

Behavior Rating Inventory of Executive Function (BRIEF®, Gioia, Isquith, Guy & Kenworthy, 2003). The *Behavior Rating Inventory of Executive Function (BRIEF)* is a group of instruments designed to examine executive function of children and adolescents from the perspectives of the caregiver [*BRIEF-P*], an educator [*BRIEF-T*], and the individual's self-report [*BRIEF-SR*]. Executive functions are cognitive processes that are essential for a person's ability to manage him or herself, to use organized, self-regulated and goal directed processing of behaviors needed to engage in skills such as language and reasoning (McCloskey, Perkins, & Van Diviner, 2009). Caregiver and teacher forms are completed for children and adolescents ages 5-18 years. Self-reports are completed by adolescents between the ages of 11-18 years. The *BRIEF* addresses eight clinical scales that measure different aspects of executive functioning, and also includes two sub scales (Behavioral Shift and Cognitive Shift) and two validity scales. Raw scores are converted into a *T* score, percentile and confidence interval (CI). A *T* score of 65 or higher is 1.5 standard deviations above the mean, which is the recommended threshold for interpretation of a score as abnormally elevated and indicates potential for clinical significance (indicated with an "X" in the charts below). A *T* score of 60 to 64 indicate mildly elevated scores that may reflect areas of concern (indicated with a * in the charts below). The literature suggests that children with histories of trauma may experience executive function deficits (Cook et al., 2003; DePrince, Weinzierl, & Combs, 2009; Henry et al., 2007) in the areas of cognitive flexibility and processing speed (Spann, Mayes, Kalmar, Guiney, Womer, Pittman . .. Blumberg, 2012; Mothes, Kristiensen, Grassi-Oliveira, Fonseca, de Lima Argimon, & Irigaray, 2015).

Figure 1. Brief-P scores, completed by Foster Mother, Ms. Redding

Index/Scale	T Score	*Interpretation*
Inhibit	65	X
Shift	50	
Emotional control	70	X
Behavioral Regulation Index (BRI)		
Initiate	50	
Working Memory	70	X
Plan/Organize	60	*
Organization of Materials	50	
Monitor	64	*

Table 2. Summarize assessment results by indicating strengths and challenges

Assessment Domains	Strengths	Challenges
Hearing		
Nonverbal Intelligence		
Conversational Sample		
Narrative		
• Narrative - Retell		
• Narrative – Generated Personal		
Social Pragmatic Communication		
• Second Belief Attribution		
• Intention Reading		
Executive Functions		

Assignment 3

Use Table 2 to summarize the assessment data, identifying Isidra's strengths and challenges exhibited in the areas of (a) cognition (i.e., social cognition, executive functions, working memory), and (b) social pragmatic communication.

Table 3. Intervention plan for Isidra

Areas of difficulty as determined by assessment results	Potential intervention strategies to address these difficulties. Provide a rationale.
1.	
2.	
3.	

Assignment 4

Use Table 3 to develop an intervention plan for Isidra.

It is imperative that SLPs begin to use a trauma-informed lens when assessing and treating children – all children, not just those with diagnosed complex trauma. Yehuda (2016) is very poignant when she wrote the following:

Children end up at clinics and offices for all manner of reasons. Those who fall behind, forget directions or do not express themselves well often get sent to the speech-language pathologist. Those with misbehaviors, school refusal or anxieties are taken to the psychologist. Children who seem unable to tolerate stimuli may see an occupational therapist. . . Awareness to trauma and communication is important in all cases. (p. 171)

Trauma-Informed Practice

Trauma-informed practice is comprised of the following elements: (1) the recognition of the widespread impact of trauma, while also being aware of the potential for recovery; (2) the ability to identify the signs and symptoms of trauma in those with whom we collaborate in their care; (3) the integration of knowledge about trauma into policies, procedures, and daily practices; and (4) consistently and actively *resisting* re-traumatization (SAMHSA, 2014, p. 11).

A Framework for Trauma-Informed SLP Practice

The author developed a Framework for Trauma-informed SLP Practice (Hyter, 2016; Hyter & Ciolino, 2017; Hyter et al., 2018) to help identify and explain the interconnecting systems that can be affected by trauma and that trauma affects. This framework has not yet been empirically examined but may serve as a guide for highlighting the knowledge and skills needed by SLPs when providing effective trauma-informed practice.

In Figure 2, there are three primary levels: (1) culturally and globally responsive practice, (2) understanding and integrating knowledge about the impact of trauma, and (3) intrapersonal and interpersonal effects of trauma and assessment and intervention practices. Each of the components will be reviewed briefly.

Figure 2. A model of trauma informed SLP practice

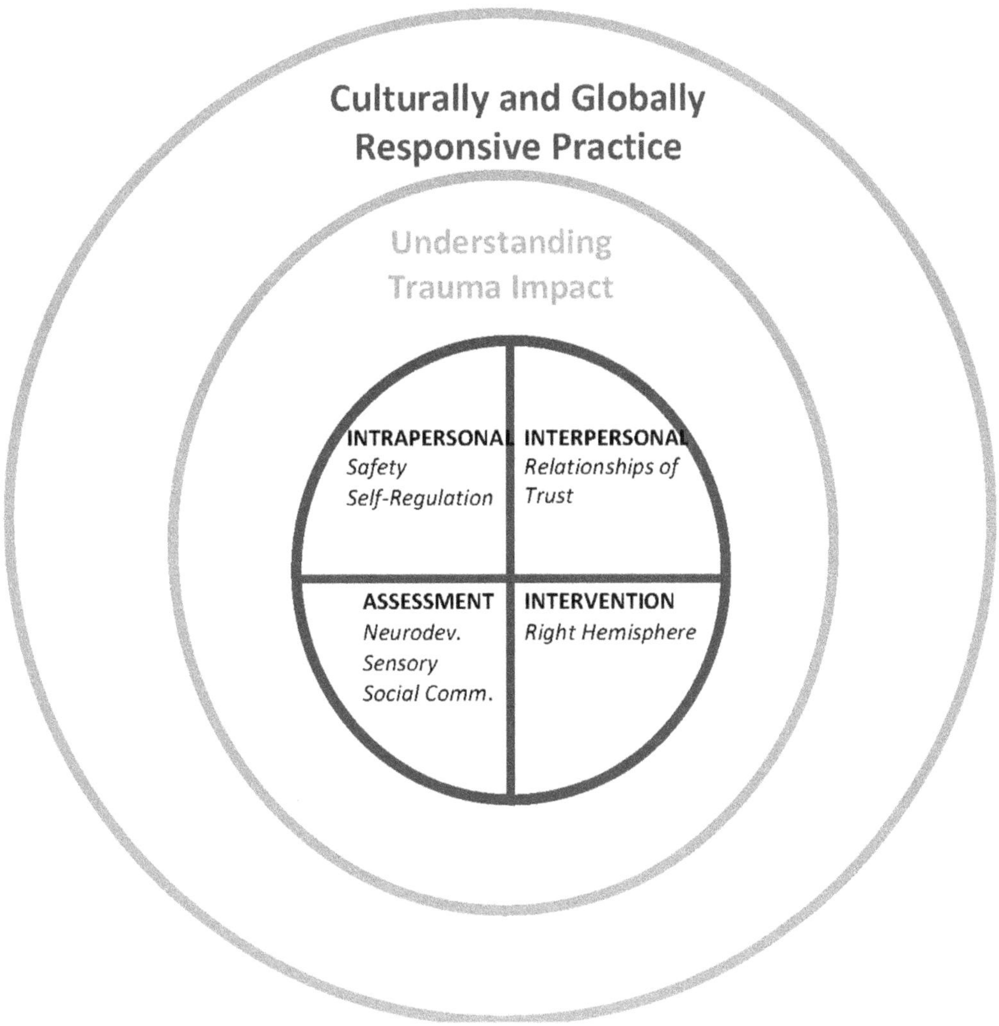

The outer circle of this model represents culturally and globally responsive services, which includes engaging in transdisciplinary praxis (reflective collaboration across disciplines), conceptualizing practice from a global perspective (understanding world events that can be traumatizing such as forced migration), acquiring world literacy (understanding world events and how those events can affect local behaviors), and engaging in macro-practice (focusing on individuals and families but also on communities and policies). Culturally and globally responsive services could include the following steps highlighted in Figure 3 (also see Hyter, 2008, 2014, 2016; Hyter, Roman, Staley, & McPherson, 2017; Hyter & Salas-Provance, 2019):

Figure 3. Level one of the model of trauma informed SLP practice
Soure: Hyter, 2016, 2017

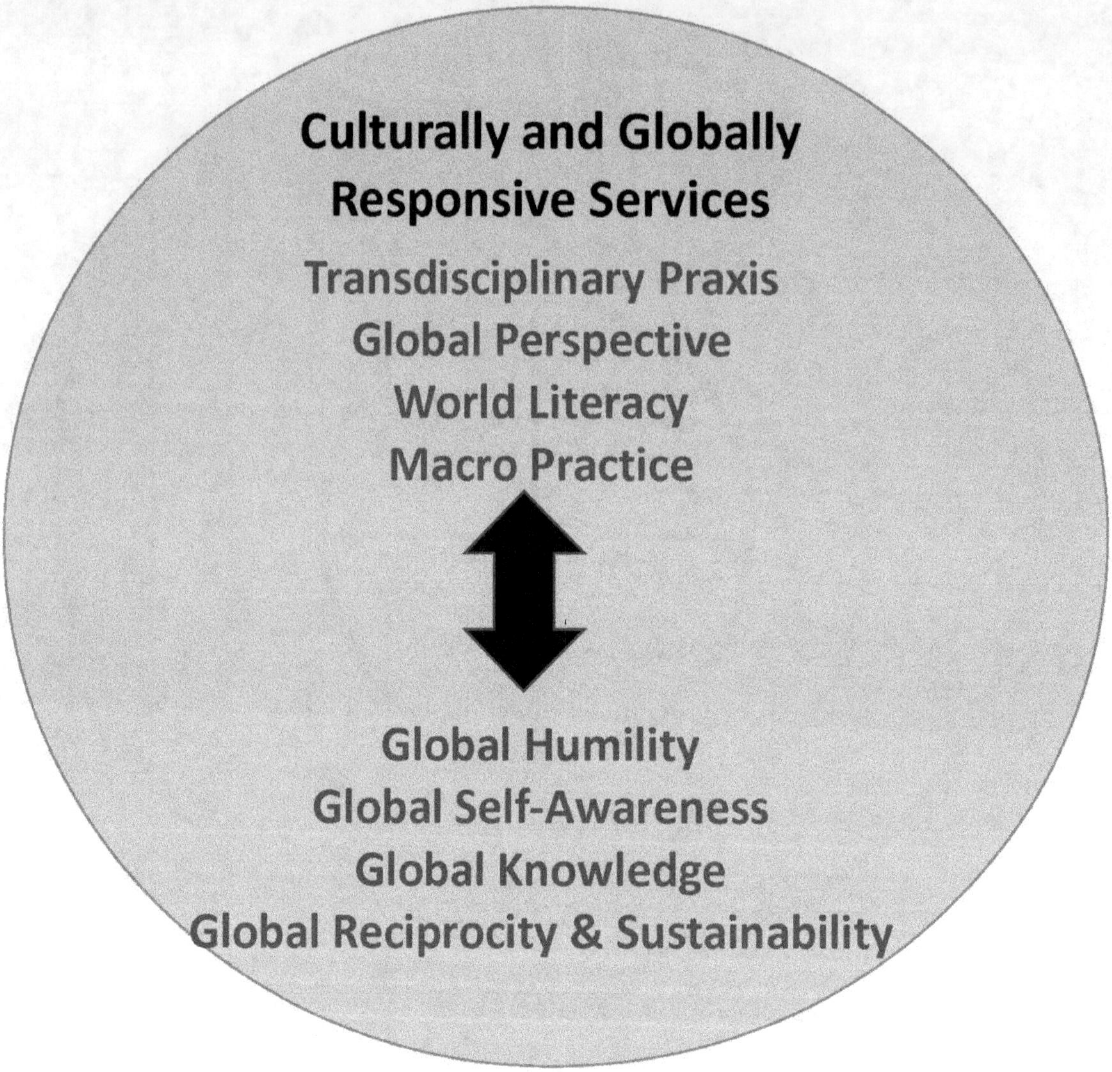
Culturally and Globally
Responsive Services
Transdisciplinary Praxis
Global Perspective
World Literacy
Macro Practice
Global Humility
Global Self-Awareness
Global Knowledge
Global Reciprocity & Sustainability

1. **Global and Cultural Humility:** Knowledge that there are multiple valid and effective ways of arriving at the same end;
2. **Self-Awareness:** Knowledge of your own beliefs, values, assumptions and how they affect your practice;
3. **Global Reciprocity:** Awareness of your own and your professions beliefs, values, assumptions and those of the groups with whom you work, and being able to translate those beliefs, values, assumptions into service that is recognizable by you as a clinician and the families with whom you are collaborating in their care;

Figure 4. The second level of the model of trauma informed SLP practice

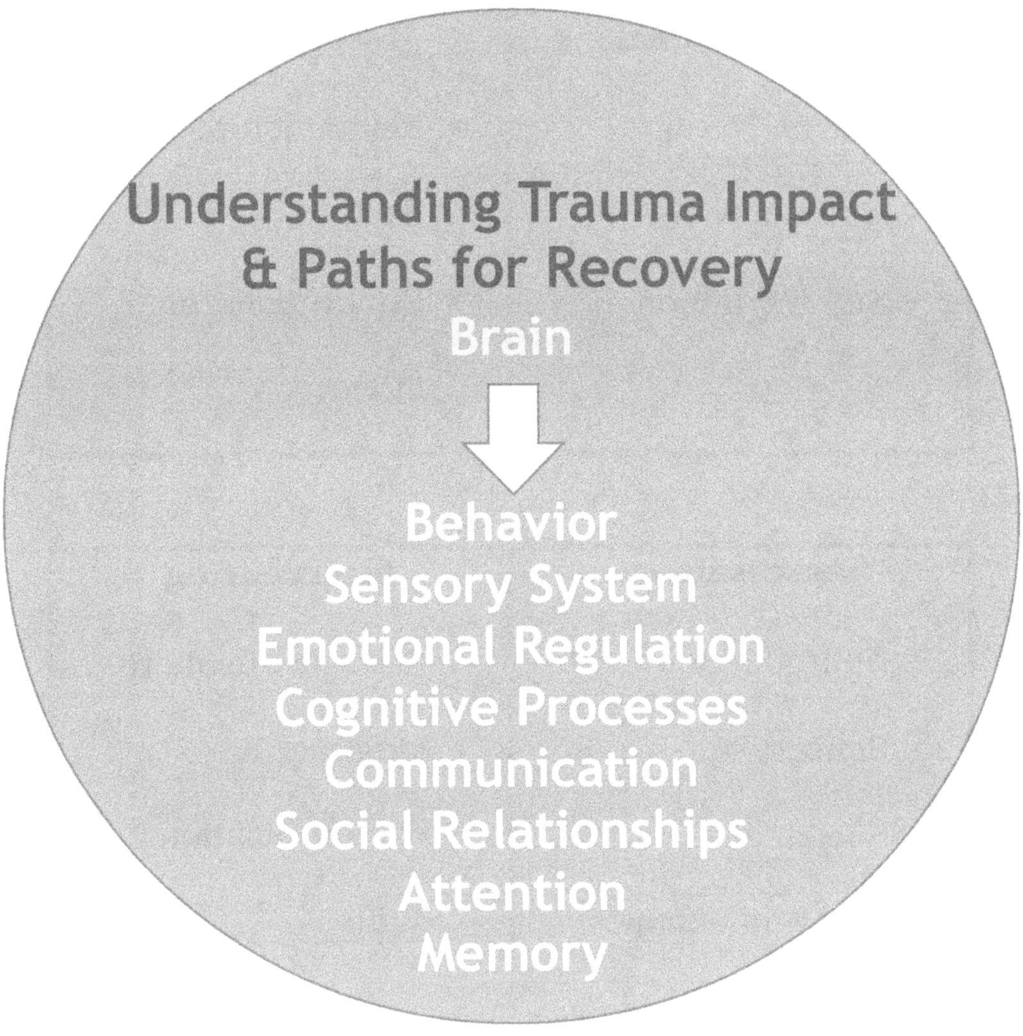

4. **Engaging in Sustainable Practice:** Communities or groups receive long-term benefit through collaboration, which will last beyond your personal involvement (Hyter & Salas-Provance, 2019; Stringer, 2017).

Isidra experienced complex trauma in the care giving system (i.e., foster families), but also as a result of structural violence (i.e., the reasons her family left Guatemala and their treatment upon arriving in the U.S.). Isidra's traumatic experiences began as a result of global processes (the cascade of problems that may have been exacerbated by CAFTA). Then her family had to leave everything and everyone they knew to avoid being killed by gangs. They fled to the U.S. to seek asylum but were retraumatized by being separated. Isidra has not seen her parents in three years, she has been in two foster homes, which were not well vetted, and caused complex trauma.

Figure 5. Third level of the model of trauma informed SLP practice

Intrapersonal	Interpersonal
• Safety • Autonomy • Self-regulation	• Relationships of trust • Environmental integrity

Assessment	Intervention
• Neurodevelopmental • Sensory • Social communication & Pragmatic language	• Right hemisphere language & communication skills • Executive functions • Attunement

The next circle (Figure 4) in the Model of Trauma-informed SLP Practice is understanding the impact of trauma (Henry et al., 2007; Hyter, 2013; Hyter, 2016; Hyter & Ciolino, 2017; Hyter et al., 2018; Steele & Malchiodi, 2016; Yehuda, 2016) in all of its forms within the culturally and globally responsive context. There are life-long consequences that affect child development including brain development and functioning, emotional well-being, communication particularly in the area of social pragmatic communication, and cognitive functioning such as theory of mind, social cognition, executive functioning and working memory.

The third and inner most part of the model is comprised of four components (Figure 5) that should constitute speech-language pathology intervention for those with whom we collaborate. These components are intrapersonal and interpersonal knowledge, assessment, and intervention (Hyter, 2016; Steele & Malchiodi, 2016; Yehuda, 2016).

Intrapersonal Level

Trauma and chronic stress impede one's ability to modulate sensory inputs, which results in limited abilities to self-regulate emotions and behavior and minimizes general coping skills. It also reduces one's autonomy because it is an assault on feelings of safety and self-control. Physical and psychological safety is essential for affect regulation and cognition (Perry, 2006, 2009). Examples of creating safety include:

- Recognizing that what is determined to be safe is based on the child. In other words, you may believe the child is safe, but the child may not perceive safety (Yehuda, 2016);
- Providing the child some control over the context. For example, make sure the child understands (a) why he or she is coming to the clinic, (b) what the plan for the day entails, and (c) let the child choose the order of activities in which he or she will participate; and
- Respecting the child's boundaries by being consistent (e.g., if you say you are going to do something, then do it; if you say the child can choose to not participate in some activity, do not try to convince him or her to participate in that activity later).

Interpersonal Level

Trauma and chronic stress negatively affect our relationships with others. It minimizes the ability to trust; trust is built through reciprocal relationships. Trust is not just dependent on the environments, but also is dependent on actions, interactions and reactions of the people in the environments. Environmental changes may be necessary so that people can thrive (Yehuda, 2016; van der Kolk, 2014). Garcia-Winner's (2019) Social Thinking-Social Competency Model may be helpful at this level. The Social Competency Model includes competencies (social attention, social interpretation, and problem solving), and social behaviors.

Trauma-informed Assessment

The effects of trauma on the development of children are much more complicated than any one profession can manage on its own; consequently, this author strongly urges the involvement of collaborative interprofessional teams using a transdisciplinary model of service for providing comprehensive assessments and interventions. Neurodevelopmental assessments should consist of memory, motor, sensory, language, literacy, visual processing, attention, behavior, cognition, and executive functions. In their arsenal of tools, SLPs need standardized norm-referenced assessments, together with valid and reliable non-standardized descriptive measures (e.g., rating scales, checklists, observations, simulated tasks, narrative and expository analyses, theory of mind) to examine language, literacy, social pragmatic communication, social cognition, executive functions, and working memory (Hyter et al., 2003; Olswang, Coggins & Timler, 2001). Occupational therapists typically assess sensory processing and modulation, motor skills, and visual processing. Social workers or counselors may conduct forensic interviews and/or psychosocial interviews.

Trauma-Informed Intervention

Trauma-informed intervention requires SLPs to focus on the potential for recovery and to address the effects of trauma on language and social pragmatic communication. It is also important to integrate knowledge about the effects of trauma into policies, procedures and practices within clinics and service centers. Listed below are several practices that can be incorporated into SLP trauma-informed intervention. Limited space prevents a detailed description of each practice, but resources are provided where relevant.

1. It is important to be attuned with the child. Attunement is the ability to be in sync or connected with the emotional needs of another (van der Kolk, 2014), so people shape behaviors, tone of voice, etc. in a way that is in sync with another.
2. Change your mind (and everyone else's) about the child's behaviors and needs (Henry et al., 2007; Yehuda, 2016). At the trauma clinic where I work, my colleagues and I often say, rather than asking "what's wrong with the child," ask "what happened to her or to him?" Rather than thinking that the child's behaviors are willful or deliberate, think about how you can provide physical and psychological safety to the child (Henry et al., 2007). Henry et al. (2007) developed a framework for intervention for children with complex trauma and those affected by fetal alcohol spectrum disorders (who have similar behavioral and linguistic profiles). This framework focuses on brain-behavior-based paradigm that recognizes the etiology of the child's behaviors.
3. Establish safety (Henry et al., 2007; van der Kolk, 2014; Yehuda, 2016). Safety is essential for engagement, for making connections, and for learning and is less likely to be established unless the clinician is also attuned with the child. With children who have histories of trauma, safety is not easy to recognize for them or for the service provider. Some examples of ways to establish safety are (1) providing options (e.g., would you like to do A or B?); (2) providing explanations (e.g., first we are going to look at pictures, then we'll read a story); and (3) letting the child have some control (e.g., letting the child remain under the table rather than sitting at the table if the child feels more comfortable under the table).
4. Incorporate art, music and movement into intervention (van der Kolk, 2014). Expressive therapies (Malchiodi, 2005), typically part of psychotherapy or counseling include integrating art, dance, music, play, poetry, storytelling and theater into traditional "talk" therapy, have had some success in facilitating healing among individuals with trauma histories. These therapies are particularly useful for children with histories of trauma who may not be able to put the experiences they have had into words or into a verbal story (van der Kolk, 2014).
5. Model ways to communicate and provide opportunities to practice. Communicate through role-play, scripting, and modeling using puppets, for example (Hyter, 2003; Hyter, Rogers-Adkinson, Self, Friederich Simmons, & Jantz, 2001). Modeling reciprocity in communication (e.g., question/answer skills, exploring opinions, offering suggestions) can help children with trauma histories fill the gaps of some communication opportunities missed (Yehuda, 2016, p. 189).

ISIDRA'S INTERVENTION AND OUTCOMES

Isidra presents with several strengths. She is comical, has a good sense of humor and has a generally positive outlook on life in spite of her trauma history, and in spite of not having seen her parents for three years. She exhibits confidence in herself and in her opinions, and is an engaging, reciprocal conversational partner. She also enjoys being in the company of her peers, although she does not always understand how to connect with them.

Isidra received intervention from a team of professionals including a psychologist, occupational therapist, and speech-language pathologist. The psychologist implemented Trauma-Focused Cognitive Behavior Therapy (TF-CBT), a therapy that is focused on the effects of traumatic stress. This therapy approach has been shown to alter the patient's thinking, which helps to change behaviors associated with the effects of trauma (Cohen, Deblinger, Mannario, & Steer, 2004; Mannario, Cohen, Deblinger, Runyon, & Steer, 2012). Isidra received occupational therapy focused on sensory modulation, specifically sensory avoidance. Some of the environmental changes that were made in her classroom included reducing overhead lighting by changing to soft lighting rather than neon lights, scheduling quiet breaks from the classroom, and choosing a location in the classroom that she felt she could work in best rather than in her typical assigned seat, away from distractions (Jordan, n.d).

The speech-language pathologist focused on social cognitive skills, narrative cohesion, and working memory. Social cognitive impairments resulted in Isidra exhibiting difficulty with making and keeping friends; understanding, recognizing and expressing emotions, and showing empathy; and understanding and recognizing cognitive mental states and emotional affective states in herself and in others. These difficulties in social cognition also affected her ability to engage in prosocial behaviors, which may have also been influenced by her sensory processing impairments. Additionally, Isidra had difficulty understanding why people did or said what they did, which manifested as an inability to identify and differentiate jokes, lies, and sarcasm, and limited abilities to see events from other people's perspectives. Speech-language intervention included the use of social stories (Gray, 2010), role play (Hyter et al., 2001; Hyter, 2003), and the use of age-appropriate literature (Westby & Robinson, 2017) to help develop theory of mind and increase her ability to accurately interpret behaviors and predict the intentions of her peers.

Westby and Robinson (2017) provided examples of how to use age-appropriate literature to model and make explicit the type of inferences that characters may be making in a story. There is literature to support that explanations of mental states increases understanding of mental states (Peterson & Slaughter, 2003). Westby and Robinson (2017) also identified scaffolded techniques that could be used to develop inter- and intra-personal thinking. One strategy included using "think alouds" when looking at a picture and reflecting on what one does or does not know and making inferences about characters' thoughts or feelings. It is predicted that improvement in this area will facilitate Isidra's better understanding of her peers and her ability to build more positive relationships with them.

To address working memory, the SLP followed the framework (five guiding principles) outlined by Sanger and Bashir (2018), in the absence of sufficient evidenced-based interventions for improving working memory. The five principles outlined by Sanger and Bashir are:

Table 4. Isidra's intervention outcomes

Location of Data	Areas of Concern	Intervention Plan	Intervention Outcomes
UNIT-2	Working memory		
Ethnographic Interviewing UNIT-2 NSS APLSC-Self Report	Social cognitive skills showed difficulty: • making and keeping friends (difficulty understanding, recognizing and expressing emotions, & showing empathy) • understanding and recognizing mental states in self and others • engaging in prosocial thinking and behavior • cannot consistently monitor thoughts and behaviors especially when under emotional stress actions, particularly when under		
NSS	• Referential and conjunctive Cohesion		
HPP-R Ethnographic Interview	Social Cognition - difficulties • separating her own knowledge from what others might believe is true (difficulty to see other perspectives) • understanding why people do what they do (particularly joking, lying, or using sarcasm)		

1. The underlying neurodevelopmental status and absolute capacity of working memory cannot be directly manipulated to improve contextualized language;
2. Increasing efficiency and automaticity with language frees up resources in working memory; in turn, the functionally improves working memory capacity;
3. Storage and effective processing of verbal information in working memory can be supported through the use of visual anchors (e.g., graphic organizers) that serve to make language stand still;
4. The verbal working memory demands of real-time language processing can be supported by heightening linguistic structure and salience; and
5. Professional collaboration should seek to identify factors that influence student performance and, in turn, accommodate students' verbal working memory limitations across different language and learning contexts (pp. 451-456).

Assignment 5

Review the resources mentioned in this chapter, identify at least three additional published articles about intervention in the areas in which Isidra presents difficulties, and develop an intervention plan for her using Table 4.

KEY POINTS

- Trauma experiences affect brain growth and functioning.
- Trauma affects brain structures and functioning including the brainstem, limbic system, right hemisphere, and the prefrontal cortex.
- SLPs are highly likely to already have children on their caseloads with ACEs and/or complex trauma who have not been diagnosed (Jonson-Reid, Drake, Kim, Porterfield, & Han, 2004).
- Children with disabilities are more likely to experience complex trauma.
- It is imperative to approach assessment and intervention from a posture of trauma-informed practice to best meet the needs of children and families experiencing adverse childhood experiences and/or traumatic events within the caregiving system.
- Although this case highlighted a child who was from a country other than the U.S., and who spoke languages other than English, it is vital to approach *all* clinical interactions as if they are cross-cultural ones. All interactions are influenced by the linguistic, cultural, social and ethnic complexities brought to the interaction by each interlocutor (Würth, Langewitz, Reiter-Theil, & Schuster, 2018).
- In the era of evidenced based interventions, current interventions that are considered to be evidenced based may be "narrow in its application when addressing the complexities of trauma. . . " (Steele & Malchiodi, 2016, p. 214). SLPs need more evidenced based interventions, particularly in speech-language pathology that are applicable for children with histories of complex, environmental, or structural trauma.

REFERENCES

ACLU. (2019). *Family separation by the numbers*. Retrieved from https://www.aclu.org/issues/immigrants-rights/immigrants-rights-and-detention/family-separation

American Nutrition Association. (2019). USDA defines food deserts. *Nutrition Digest, 38*(2). Retrieved from http://americannutritionassociation.org/newsletter/usda-defines-food-deserts

American Psychiatric Association (APA). (2013). Diagnostic and statistical manual of mental disorders-5. Washington, DC: Author.

Anyon, Y. (2010). Reducing racial disparities and disproportionalities in the child welfare system: Policy perspectives about how to serve the best interests of African American youth. *Children and Youth Services Review*, *33*(2), 242–253. doi:10.1016/j.childyouth.2010.09.007

Arioli, M., Crespi, C., & Canessa, N. (2018). Social cognition through the lens of cognitive and clinical neuroscience. *BioMed Research International*, *2018*, 4283427. doi:10.1155/2018/4283427 PMID:30302338

Bedore, L. M., & Peña, E. D. (2008). Assessment of bilingual children for identification of language impairment: Current findings and implications for practice. *International Journal of Bilingual Education and Bilingualism*, *11*(1), 1–29. doi:10.2167/beb392.0

Bedore, L. M., Peña, E. D., Joyner, D., & Macken, C. (2011). Parent and teacher rating of bilingual language proficiency and language development concerns. *International Journal of Bilingual Education and Bilingualism, 14*(5), 489–511. doi:10.1080/13670050.2010.529102 PMID:29910668

Benarous, X., Guile, J. M., Consoli, A., & Cohen, D. (2015). A systematic review of the evidence for impaired cognitive theory of mind in maltreated children. *Frontiers in Psychiatry, 6*(108). doi:10.3389/fpsyt.2015.00108 PMID:26283975

Beneria, L., Berik, G., & Floro, M. (2016). *Gender, development and globalization: Economics as if all people mattered* (2nd ed.). New York: Routledge.

Binford, W. (2019, June 21). A firsthand report of 'inhumane conditions' at a migrant children's detention center. *Interview on PBS News Hour*. Retrieved from https://www.pbs.org/newshour/show/a-firsthand-report-of-inhumane-conditions-at-a-migrant-childrens-detention-facility

Black-Pond, C., & Henry, J. (2008). A trauma-informed Child Welfare System practice: The essential elements. *The Michigan Child Welfare Law Journal, 11*(2), 11–23.

Borella, E., Carretti, B., Cornoldi, C., & De Beni, R. (2020). Working memory training from an individual differences perspective: Efficacy in older adults. In J. M. Novick, M. F. Bunting, M. R. Dougherty, & R. W. Engle (Eds.), *Cognitive and working memory training: Perspectives from Psychology, Neuroscience, and Human Development* (pp. 14–39). New York, NY: Oxford University Press.

Bracken, B. A., & McCallum, R. S. (2016). Universal Nonverbal Intelligence Test – Second Edition (UNIT-2). Austin, TX: Pro-Ed.

Burgos, V. (2007, November 14). Mexico-Guatemala: The other border. *Upside Down World.* Retrieved from http://upsidedownworld.org/archives/mexico/mexico-guatemala-the-other-border/

Burke-Harris, N. (2018). *The deepest well: Healing the long-term effects of childhood adversity.* New York: Houghton Mifflin Harcourt.

Centers for Disease Control and Prevention (CDC). (2000a). *Weight-for-age percentiles: Girls, 2 to 20 years.* CDC Growth Charts: United States. Retrieved from https://www.cdc.gov/growthcharts/data/set2/chart-08.pdf

Centers for Disease Control and Prevention (CDC). (2000b). *Stature-for-age percentiles: Girls, 2 to 20 years.* CDC Growth Charts: United States. Retrieved from https://www.cdc.gov/growthcharts/data/set2/chart-08.pdf

Centers for Disease Control and Prevention (CDC). (2019). *Adverse childhood experiences.* Retrieved from https://www.cdc.gov/violenceprevention/childabuseandneglect/acestudy/index.html

Child Welfare Information Gateway. (2016). *Racial disproportionality and disparity in child welfare.* Retrieved from https://www.childwelfare.gov/pubpdfs/racial_disproportionality.pdf

Cicchetti, D., Rogosch, F. A., Maughan, A., Toth, S. L., & Bruce, J. (2003). False belief understanding in maltreated children. *Development and Psychopathology, 15*(4), 1067–1091. doi:10.1017/S0954579403000440 PMID:14984138

Ciolino, C. (2018). *Language profiles of children who have experienced complex trauma and fetal alcohol spectrum disorders* (Unpublished master's thesis). Western Michigan University, Kalamazoo, MI.

Cohen, J. A., Deblinger, E., Mannarino, A. P., & Steer, R. (2004). A multi-site, randomized controlled trial for children with abuse-related PTSD symptoms. *Journal of the American Academy of Child and Adolescent Psychiatry, 43*(4), 393–402. doi:10.1097/00004583-200404000-00005 PMID:15187799

Cook, A., Blaustein, M., Spinazzola, J., & Van Der Kolk, B. (2003). *Complex trauma in children and adolescents*. National Child Traumatic Stress Network. Retrieved from http://www.NCTSNet.org

Culp, R. E., Watkins, R. V., Lawrence, H., Letts, D., Kelly, D. J., & Rice, M. L. (1991). Maltreated children's language and speech development: Abused, neglected, and abused and neglected. *First Language, 11*(33), 377–389. doi:10.1177/014272379101103305

Curenton, S. (2015). African American preschooler' emotion explanations can provide evidence of their pragmatic skills. *Topics in Language Disorders, 35*(1), 46–60. doi:10.1097/TLD.0000000000000045

DeBellis, M. D. (2001). Developmental traumatology: The psychobiological development of maltreated children and its implications for research, treatment and policy. *Development and Psychopathology, 13*, 537–561. PMID:11523847

DeBellis, M. D., Woolley, D. P., & Hooper, S. R. (2013). Neuropsychological findings in pediatric maltreatment: Relationship of PTSD, dissociative symptoms, and abuse/neglect indices to neurocognitive outcomes. *Child Maltreatment, 18*(3), 171–183. doi:10.1177/1077559513497420 PMID:23886642

DeBellis, M. D., & Zisk, A. (2014). The biological effects of trauma. *Child and Adolescent Psychiatric Clinics of North America, 23*(2), 185–222. doi:10.1016/j.chc.2014.01.002 PMID:24656576

DeThorne, L. S., & Schaefer, B. A. (2004). A guide to child nonverbal IQ measures. *American Journal of Speech-Language Pathology, 13*(4), 275–290. doi:10.1044/1058-0360(2004/029) PMID:15719895

Di Sante, M., Sylvestre, A., Bouchard, C., & Leblond, J. (2019). The pragmatic language skills of severely neglected 420month old children: Results of the ELLAN study. *Child Maltreatment, 24*(3), 244–253. doi:10.1177/1077559519828838 PMID:30782015

Dunn, W. (2014). *Sensory Profile-2*. New York: Pearson.

English, L. H., Wisener, M., & Bailey, H. N. (2018). Childhood emotional maltreatment, anxiety, attachment and mindfulness: Associations with facial emotion recognition. *Child Abuse & Neglect, 80*, 146–160. doi:10.1016/j.chiabu.2018.02.006 PMID:29605464

Escobar, N. (2018, August 14). Family separation isn't new: U. S. Immigration policy has traumatized migrant children and parents for nearly a century. *The Atlantic*. Retrieved from https://www.theatlantic.com/family/archive/2018/08/us-immigration-policy-has-traumatized-children-for-nearly-100-years/567479/

Farmer, P. (2004). An anthropology of structural violence. *Current Anthropology, 45*(3), 305–325. doi:10.1086/382250

Farmer, P. (2005). *Pathologies of power. Health, human rights, and the new war on the poor*. Berkeley, CA: University of California Press.

Felitti, V. J., Nordenberg, A. R. F., Williamson, D. F., Spitz, A. M., Edwards, B., Kross, M. P., & Marks, J. S. (1998). Relationship of childhood abuse and household dysfunction to many of the leading causes of death in adults. The Adverse Childhood Experiences (ACE) Study. *American Journal of Preventive Medicine, 14*(4), 245–258. doi:10.1016/S0749-3797(98)00017-8 PMID:9635069

Fraser, K., MacKenzie, D., & Versnel, J. (2017). Complex trauma in children and youth: A scoping review of sensory-based interventions. *Occupational Therapy in Mental Health, 33*(3), 199–216. doi:10.1080/0164212X.2016.1265475

Galtung, J. (1969). Violence, peace, and peace research. *Journal of Peace Research, 6*(3), 167–191. doi:10.1177/002234336900600301

Gillam, R. B., & Pearson, N. (2017). Test of Narrative Language, Second Edition (TNL-2). Austin, TX: Pro-Ed.

Gillam, S., Gillam, R. B., Fargo, J., Olszewski, A., & Segura, H. (2016). Monitoring Indicators of Scholarly Language (MISL): A progress-monitoring instrument for measuring narrative discourse skills. *Communicative Disorders and Deaf Education Faculty Publications. Paper 494*. Retrieved from https://digitalcommons.usu.edu/comd_facpub/494

Gioia, G. A., Isquith, P. K., Guy, S. C., & Kenworthy, L. (2003). *Behavior Rating Inventory of Executive Function (BRIEF)*. Lutz, FL: PAR, Inc.

Gonzales, R. (2018, June 20). Trumps' executive order on family separation: What it does and doesn't do. *NPR News*. Retrieve from https://www.npr.org/2018/06/20/622095441/trump-executive-order-on-family-separation-what-it-does-and-doesnt-do

Gray, C. (2010). *The new social story book*. Arlington, TX: Future Horizons.

Grosjean, F. (2010). *Bilingual life and reality*. Cambridge, MA: Harvard University Press. doi:10.4159/9780674056459

Gross, M., Buac, M., & Kaushanskaya, M. (2014). Conceptual scoring of receptive and expressive vocabulary measures in simultaneous and sequential bilingual children. *American Journal of Speech-Language Pathology, 23*(4), 574–586. doi:10.1044/2014_AJSLP-13-0026 PMID:24811415

Happé, F. (1994). An advanced test of theory of mind: Understanding of story characters' thoughts and feelings by able autistic, mentally handicapped, and normal children and adults. *Journal of Autism and Developmental Disorders, 24*(2), 129–154. doi:10.1007/BF02172093 PMID:8040158

Heilmann, J., Miller, J. F., & Dunaway, C. (2010). Properties of the Narrative Scoring Scheme using narrative retells in young school-age children. *American Journal of Speech-Language Pathology, 19*(2), 154–166. doi:10.1044/1058-0360(2009/08-0024) PMID:20008470

Henry, J. (2016). The CTAC in Action. In W. Steele, & C. Malchiodi (Eds.), Trauma-informed practices with children and adolescents (pp. 36 – 40). New York: Routledge.

Henry, J., Richardson, M., Black-Pond, C., Sloane, M., Atchison, B., & Hyter, Y. D. (2011). A grass-roots prototype for trauma-informed child welfare system change. *Child Welfare, 90*(6), 169–186. PMID:22533048

Henry, J., Sloane, M., & Black-Pond, C. (2007). Neurobiology and neurodevelopment of childhood traumatic stress and alcohol exposure. *Language. Speech and Hearing in Schools*, *38*, 99–108. doi:10.1044/0161-1461(2007/010) PMID:17428956

Ho, K. (2007). Structural violence as a human rights violation. *Essex Human Rights Review*, *4*(2), 1–17.

Hollebrandse, B., van Hout, A., & Hendriks, P. (2014). Children's first and second-order false belief reasoning in a verbal and a low-verbal task. *Synthese*, *191*(3), 321–333. doi:10.100711229-012-0169-9

Human Rights Watch. (2019, July 11). *US: Family separation harming children, families*. Retrieved from https://www.hrw.org/news/2019/07/11/us-family-separation-harming-children-families

Hyter, Y. D. (2003). Language intervention for children with emotional and behavioral disorders. *Behavioral Disorders*, *29*(1), 65–76. doi:10.1177/019874290302900104

Hyter, Y. D. (2008, January 22). Considering conceptual frameworks in communication sciences and disorders. *ASHA Leader*, *13*(1), 30–31. doi:10.1044/leader.FMP.13012008.30

Hyter, Y. D. (2010 April). Prenatal alcohol exposure, complex trauma and language outcomes. Seminar presented at the annual conference of the National Black Association of Speech-Language and Hearing, Tampa, FL.

Hyter, Y.D. (2012). Complex trauma and prenatal alcohol exposure: Clinical implications. *ASHA Perspectives on School-Based Issues, 13*(2), 32 – 42. doi/ doi:10.1044bi13.2.32

Hyter, Y. D. (2014). Conceptual framework for responsive global engagement in communication sciences and disorders. *Topics in Language Disorders*, *34*(2), 103–120. doi:10.1097/TLD.0000000000000015

Hyter, Y. D. (2017). Pragmatic assessment and intervention in children. In L. Cummings (Ed.), *Research in clinical pragmatics* (pp. 493–526). New York: Springer International Publishing. doi:10.1007/978-3-319-47489-2_19

Hyter, Y. D., & Applegate, E. B. (2012). *Assessment of Pragmatic Language and Social Communication (APLSC). Unpublished research version*. Kalamazoo: Western Michigan University.

Hyter, Y. D., & Black-Pond, C. (2005). *Juan and Maria Cell Phone Task: Second order belief attribution script. Unpublished assessment protocol*. Kalamazoo: Western Michigan University.

Hyter, Y. D., & Ciolino, C. (2017, November). *Providing SLP services through a trauma informed lens.* Seminar presented at the annual convention of the American Speech-Language-Hearing Association, Los Angeles, CA.

Hyter, Y. D., Henry, J., Atchison, B., Sloane, M., Black-Pond, C., & Shangraw, K. (2003). Children affected by trauma and alcohol exposure. *ASHA Leader*, *8*(21), 6–14. doi:10.1044/leader.FTR2.08212003.6

Hyter, Y. D., Henry, J., Sloane, M., Suarez, M., & Ciolino, C. (2018). *The effects of complex trauma and alcohol exposure: The brain, language and skills for daily living*. Short course presented at the Annual Convention of the Michigan Speech-Language-Hearing Association, Kalamazoo, MI.

Hyter, Y. D., & Jackson, J. J. (2010). *Hyter Pragmatic Protocol Revised: 9 – 15-years old. Unpublished assessment protocol*. Kalamazoo: Western Michigan University.

Hyter, Y. D., Rogers-Adkinson, D. L., Self, T. L., Friederich Simmons, B., & Jantz, J. (2011). Pragmatic language intervention for children with language and emotional/behavioral disorders. *Communication Disorders Quarterly*, *23*(1), 4–16. doi:10.1177/152574010102300103

Hyter, Y.D., Roman, T.R., Staley, B., & McPherson, B. (2017). Competencies for effective global engagement: A proposal for communication sciences and disorders. *Perspectives of the ASHA Special Interest Groups, SIG 17*, *2*(1), 9 – 20.

Hyter, Y. D., & Salas-Provance, M. B. (2019). *Culturally responsive practices in speech, language and hearing sciences*. San Diego, CA: Plural Publishing.

Iluz-Cohen, P., & Walters, J. (2012). Telling stories in two languages: Narratives of preschool children with typical and impaired language. *Bilingualism: Language and Cognition*, *15*(1), 58–74. doi:10.1017/S1366728911000538

Jones, S. (2019, February 4). Trump administration: Reuniting some separated migrant families might be too hard. *Intelligencer*. Retrieved from http://nymag.com/intelligencer/2019/02/hhs-reuniting-separated-migrant-families-hard.html

Jonson Reid, M., Drake, B., Kim, J., Porterfield, S., & Han, L. (2004). A prospective analysis of the relationship between reported child maltreatment and special education eligibility among poor children. *Child Maltreatment*, *9*(4), 382–394. doi:10.1177/1077559504269192 PMID:15538037

Jordan, K. A. (n.d.). *Sensory strategies for classroom sensory avoiders*. Retrieved from https://www.iidc.indiana.edu/styles/iidc/defiles/IRCA/SensoryAvoiders.pdf

Lind, D. (2019, June 25). *The horrifying conditions facing kids in the border detention, explained*. Retrieved from https://www.vox.com/policy-and-politics/2019/6/25/18715725/children-border-detention-kids-cages-immigration

Luke, N., & Banerjee, R. (2013). Differential associations between childhood maltreatment experiences and social understanding: A meta-analysis and systemic review. *Developmental Review*, *33*(1), 1–28. doi:10.1016/j.dr.2012.10.001

Malchiodi, C. A. (2005). Expressive therapies: History, theory, and practice. In C. A. Malchiodi (Ed.), *Expressive therapies* (pp. 1–15). New York: Guilford Publications.

Manarino, A. P., Cohen, J. A., Deblinger, E., Runyon, M. K., & Steer, R. A. (2012). Trauma focused cognitive-behavioral therapy for children: Sustained impact of treatment 6 and 12 months later. *Child Maltreatment*, *17*(3), 231–241. doi:10.1177/1077559512451787 PMID:22763575

McCloskey, G., Perkins, L. A., & Van Diner, B. (2009). *Assessment and intervention for executive function difficulties*. New York: Routledge.

Moreno, J. M., Garcia-Baamonde, M. E., & Blazquez, M. (2010). Desarrollo linguistico y adaptacion escolar en ninos en acogimiento residencial [Linguistic development and adaptation in children in residential care]. *Anales de Psicología*, *26*, 189–196.

Moreno-Manso, J. M., Garcia-Baamonde, M. E., Blazquez-Alonso, M., Pozueco-Romero, J. M., & Godoy-Merino, M. J. (2016). Social communication disorders and social cognitive attitudes in victims of child abuse. *Journal of Child and Family Studies*, *25*(1), 241–250. doi:10.100710826-015-0192-9

Mothes, L., Kristensen, C. H., Grassi-Oliveira, R., Fonseca, R. P., de Lima Argimon, I. I., & Irigaray, T. Q. (2015). Childhood maltreatment and executive functions in adolescents. *Child and Adolescent Mental Health*, *20*(1), 56–62. doi:10.1111/camh.12068

Murphy, J., & Busch, Z. (2015, August 5). *CAFTA-DR Notches 10-year record of success.* Retrieved from https://www.uschamber.com/issue-brief/cafta-dr-notches-10-year-record-success

National Child Traumatic Stress Network (NCTSN). (2016). *Complex trauma.* Retrieved from http://www.nctsn.org/trauma-types/complex-trauma

National Child Traumatic Stress Network (NTCSN). (n.d.). *Complex trauma.* Retrieved from https://www.nctsn.org/what-is-child-trauma/trauma-types/complex-trauma

National Scientific Council on the Developing Child. (2012). *The science of neglect: The persistent absence of responsive care disrupts the developing brain: Working paper 12.* Retrieved from https://developingchild.harvard.edu/resources/the-science-of-neglect-the-persistent-absence-of-responsive-care-disrupts-the-developing-brain/

Office of the U.S. Trade Representative. (2004, February). *Putting CAFTA into perspective: Fact sheet on agriculture.* Retrieved from https://ustr.gov/about-us/policy-offices/press-office/fact-sheets/archives/2004/february/putting-cafta-perspective-fact-sheet-agricu

Olswang, L. B., Coggins, T. E., & Timler, G. R. (2001). Outcome measures for school-age children with social communication problems. *Topics in Language Disorders*, *21*(4), 50–73. doi:10.1097/00011363-200111000-00006

Ortega, D. M., Graybill, L., & Lasch, C. N. (2015). Enacting and sustaining trauma and violence through policy enforcement: Family immigration detention. *Journal of Women and Social Work*, *30*(3), 281–285. doi:10.1177/0886109915595190

Peña, E. D., Gillam, R. B., & Bedore, L. M. (2014). Dynamic assessment of narrative ability in English accurately identifies language impairment in English language learners. *Journal of Speech, Language, and Hearing Research: JSLHR*, *57*(6), 2208–2220. doi:10.1044/2014_JSLHR-L-13-0151 PMID:25075793

Perez Foster, R. (2001). When immigration is trauma: Guidelines for the individual and family clinician. *The American Journal of Orthopsychiatry*, *71*(2), 153–170. doi:10.1037/0002-9432.71.2.153 PMID:11347358

Perez-Rocha, M., & Paley, J. (2014, November 21). What “Free Trade” has done to Central America. *Foreign Policy in Focus.* Retrieved from https://fpif.org/free-trade-done-central-america/

Perla, H. (2016 March 1). *The impact of CAFTA: Drugs, gangs and immigration.* Retrieved from https://www.telesurenglish.net/opinion/The-Impact-of-CAFTA-Drugs-Gangs-and-Immigration-20160301-0008.html

Perner, J. (1988). Higher-order beliefs and intentions in children's understanding of social interaction. In J. W. Astington, P. L. Harris, & D. R. Olson (Eds.), *Developing theories of mind* (pp. 271–294). Cambridge, UK: Cambridge University Press.

Perner, J., & Wimmer, H. (1985). "John thinks that Mary thinks that. . .": Attribution of second order beliefs by 5- to 10-year-old children. *Journal of Experimental Child Psychology*, *39*(3), 437–471. doi:10.1016/0022-0965(85)90051-7

Perry, B. D. (2006). The neurosequential model of therapeutics: Applying principles of neuroscience to clinical work with traumatized and maltreated children. In N. Boyd Webb (Ed.), *Working with traumatized youth in child welfare* (pp. 27–52). New York: Guilford Press.

Perry, B. D. (2009). Examining child maltreatment through a neurodevelopmental lens: Clinical applications of the neurosequential model of therapeutics. *Journal of Loss and Trauma*, *14*(4), 240–255. doi:10.1080/15325020903004350

Peterson, C., & Slaughter, V. (2003). Opening windows into the mind: Mothers' preferences for explanations and children's theory of mind. *Cognitive Development*, *18*(3), 399–429. doi:10.1016/S0885-2014(03)00041-8

Richardson, M., Black-Pond, C., Sloane, M., Atchison, B., Hyter, Y. D., & Henry, J. (2015). Neurodevelopmental impact of child maltreatment. *Mental Health Issues in Childhood Maltreatment*. Retrieved from https://wmich.edu/sites/default/files/attachments/u354/2016/Neurodevelopmental%20Impact%20of%20Child%20Trauma%20Chaper-1.pdf

Rizzo, S. (2018, June 19). The facts about Trump's policy of separating families at the border. *The Washington Post*. Retrieved from https://www.washingtonpost.com/news/fact-checker/wp/2018/06/19/the-facts-about-trumps-policy-of-separating-families-at-the-border/?noredirect=on

Romero, J. M. (2012). Pragmatic communicative intervention strategies for victims of child abuse. *Children and Youth Services Review*, *34*(9), 1729–1734. doi:10.1016/j.childyouth.2012.05.003

Sanger, B. D., & Bashir, A. S. (2018). Wait. What??? Guiding intervention principles for students with verbal working memory limitations. *Language, Speech, and Hearing Services in Schools*, *49*(3), 449–462. doi:10.1044/2018_LSHSS-17-0101 PMID:29978212

Segura, R. (2010). *Central Americans in Los Angeles*. Chicago, IL: Arcadia Publishing.

Silliman, E. R., Bahr, R. H., Hnath-Chisolm, T., & Mahecha, N. R. (2002). Spanish and English proficiency in the linguistic encoding of mental states in narrative retellings. *Linguistics and Education*, *13*(2), 199–234. doi:10.1016/S0898-5898(01)00062-6

Simon, K. B. (2018). Catalyzing the separation of Black families: A critique of foster care placements without prior judicial review. *Columbia Journal of Law and Social Problems*, *51*(3), 347–385.

Simón-Cereijido, G., & Gutiérrez-Clellen, V. F. (2009). A cross-linguistic and bilingual evaluation of the interdependence between lexical and grammatical domains. *Applied Psycholinguistics*, *30*(2), 315–337. doi:10.1017/S0142716409090134 PMID:19444336

Spagat, E., & Galvan, A. (2019, July 31). Over 900 more children separated at the border since a judge halted the practice: ACLU. *Time*. Retrieved from https://time.com/5639549/900-children-separated-border-aclu/

Spann, M. N., Mayes, L. C., Kalmar, J. H., Guiney, J., Womer, F. Y., Pittman, B., ... Blumberg, H. P. (2012). Childhood abuse and neglect and cognitive flexibility in adolescents. *Child Neuropsychology, 18*(2), 182–189. doi:10.1080/09297049.2011.595400 PMID:21942637

Spratt, E. G., Friedenberg, S. L., Swenson, C. C., LaRosa, A., De Bellis, M. D., Macias, M. M., & ... . (2012). The effects of early neglect on cognitive, language and behavioral functioning n childhood. *Psychology (Irvine, Calif.), 3*(2), 175–182. doi:10.4236/psych.2012.32026 PMID:23678396

Steele, W., & Malchiodi, C. A. (2016). *Trauma-informed practices with children and adolescents*. New York: Routledge.

Substance Abuse and Mental Health Services Administration (SAMHSA). (2014). *Treatment improvement protocol (TIP) Series, No. 57. Trauma Informed Care in Behavioral Health Services*. Rockville, MD: Author.

Sullivan, K., & Tager-Flusberg, H. (1999). Second-order believe attribution in Williams Syndrome: Intact or impaired? *American Journal of Mental Retardation, 104*(6), 523–532. doi:10.1352/0895-8017(1999)104<0523:SBAIWS>2.0.CO;2 PMID:10587733

Sylvestre, A., Bussieres, E. L., & Bouchard, C. (2016). Language problems among abused and neglected children: A meta-analytic review. *Child Maltreatment, 2*(1), 47–58. doi:10.1177/1077559515616703 PMID:26620719

Taylor, C. (2012). *The Black Carib wars: Freedom, survival and the making of the Garifuna*. Jackson, MS: University Press of Mississippi. doi:10.14325/mississippi/9781617033100.001.0001

Teicher, M. H., Andersen, S. L., Polcari, A., Anderson, C. M., Navalta, C. P., & Kim, D. M. (2003). The neurobiological consequences of early stress and childhood maltreatment. *Neuroscience and Biobehavioral Reviews, 27*(1-2), 33–44. doi:10.1016/S0149-7634(03)00007-1 PMID:12732221

Toth, S. L., Stronach, E. P., Rogosch, F. A., Caplan, R., & Cicchitti, D. (2011). Illogical thinking and thought disorder in maltreated children. *Journal of the American Academy of Child and Adolescent Psychiatry, 50*(7), 659–668. doi:10.1016/j.jaac.2011.03.002 PMID:21703493

United Nations Children's Fund (UNICEF). (1993). *The teacher's handbook: Teaching the UN Convention Rights of the Child*. Geneva, Switzerland: Author.

U.S. Customs and Border Protection. (2019, August 13). *Central America-Dominican Republic Free Trade Agreement (CAFTA-DR)*. Retrieved from https://www.cbp.gov/trade/free-trade-agreements/cafta-dr

U.S. Department of Health & Human Services, Administration for Children and Families, Administration on Children Youth and Families, Children's Bureau (ACF). (2019). *Child Maltreatment 2017*. Available from https://www.acf.hhs.gov/cb/research-data-technology/statistics-research/child-maltreatment

U.S. Department of Health and Human Services, Office of the Assistant Secretary for Planning and Evaluation (USDHHS – ASPE). (2019). *Poverty guidelines*. Retrieved from https://aspe.hhs.gov/poverty-guidelines

van der Kolk, B. (1994). The body keeps the score: Memory and the emerging psychobiology of post-traumatic stress. *Harvard Review of Psychiatry*, *1*(5), 253–265. doi:10.3109/10673229409017088 PMID:9384857

van der Kolk, B. (2015). *The body keeps the score: Brain, mind and body in the healing of trauma*. New York: Penguin Books.

Wamser-Nanney, R., Sager, J. C., & Campbell, C. L. (2019). Maternal support as a predictor of children's sexualized behaviors following childhood sexual abuse. *Child Maltreatment*, *24*(1), 36–44. doi:10.1177/1077559518786821 PMID:30004257

Warner, E., Koomar, J., Lary, B., & Cook, A. (2013). Can the body change the score? Application of sensory modulation principles in the treatment of traumatized adolescents in residential settings. *Journal of Family Violence*, *28*(7), 729–738. doi:10.100710896-013-9535-8

Westby, C. E. (2007). Maltreatment: A global issue. *Language, Speech, and Hearing Services in Schools*, *38*(2), 140–148. doi:10.1044/0161-1461(2007/014) PMID:17428960

Westby, C.E., & Robinson, L. (2017, October). *Social communication and pragmatic language: Developmental perspective from infancy through adolescence*. Invited Keynote, Van Riper Lecture Series, Western Michigan University, Kalamazoo, MI.

Wiig, E. H., Semel, E., & Secord, W. A. (2013). Clinical Evaluation of Language Fundamentals, Fifth edition (CELF-5). New York: Pearson.

Würth, K., Langewitz, W., Reiter-Theil, S., & Schuster, S. (2018, July 4). Their view: Difficulties and challenges of patients and physicians in cross-cultural encounters and a medical ethics perspective. *BMC Medical Ethics*, *19*(70). Retrieved from https://bmcmedethics.biomedcentral.com/articles/10.1186/s12910-018-0311-4 PMID:29973220

Yehuda, N. (2016). *Communicating trauma: Clinical presentations and interventions with traumatized children*. New York: Routledge.

Young, J. C., & Widom, C. S. (2014). Long-term effects of child abuse and neglect on emotion processing in adulthood. *Child Abuse & Neglect*, *38*(8), 1369–1381. doi:10.1016/j.chiabu.2014.03.008 PMID:24747007

ADDITIONAL READING

Atchison, B. (2007). Sensory modulation disorders among children with a history of trauma: A frame of reference for speech-language pathologists. *Language, Speech, and Hearing Services in Schools*, *38*(2), 109–116. doi:10.1044/0161-1461(2007/011) PMID:17428957

DeBellis, M. D., Woolley, D. P., & Hooper, S. R. (2013). Neuropsychological findings in pediatric maltreatment: Relationship of PTSD, dissociative symptoms, and abuse/neglect indices to neurocognitive outcomes. *Child Maltreatment*, *18*(3), 171–183. doi:10.1177/1077559513497420 PMID:23886642

Fujiki, M., Brinton, B., McCleave, C. P., Anderson, V. W., & Chamberlain, J. P. (2013). A social communication intervention to increase validating comments by children with language impairment. *Language, Speech, and Hearing Services in Schools*, *44*(1), 3–19. doi:10.1044/0161-1461(2012/11-103) PMID:23305940

Henry, J., Sloane, M., & Black-Pond, C. (2007). Neurobiology and neurodevelopmental impact of childhood traumatic stress and prenatal alcohol exposure. *Language, Speech, and Hearing Services in Schools*, *38*(2), 99–108. doi:10.1044/0161-1461(2007/010) PMID:17428956

Lum, J. A. G., Powell, M., & Snow, P. C. (2018). The influence of maltreatment history and out of home care on children's language and social skills. *Child Abuse & Neglect*, *76*, 65–74. doi:10.1016/j.chiabu.2017.10.008 PMID:29073491

Yehuda, N. (2016). *Communicating trauma: Clinical presentations and interventions with traumatized children*. New York: Routledge.

KEY TERMS AND DEFINITIONS

Adverse Childhood Experiences (ACEs): Adverse (and possibly traumatic) events that occur during the life of a child (CDC, 2019).

Complex Trauma: Maltreatment (abuse and neglect) that occurs in the caregiving system (Henry, Sloane, & Black-Pond, 2007) and the long term effects of that maltreatment (NCTSN, n.d.).

Executive Functions: Cognitive skills that allow a person the ability to organize ideas, regulate one's own behaviors and thoughts, and process emotions, and serves as a support for language and reasoning. Executive functions have been characterized to include shifting (flexibility), inhibition, and working memory (McCloskey, Perkins, & Van Divner, 2009).

Social Cognition: Is a cognitive skill that the ability to make sense of (e.g., interpret, analyze) the social world; these processes is the ability to understand why people do what they do (Arioli, Crespi, & Canessa, 2018).

Social Pragmatic Communication: The ability to use verbal and nonverbal language to communicate effectively, and to use language to establish and maintain social relationship (APA, 2013; Hyter, 2017).

Structural Violence: The way systems and social structures (e.g., economics, politics) are organized that cause harm to groups of people, and can deny these groups their human rights (Ortega, Graybill, & Lasch, 2015).

Trauma-Informed Practice: Recognizing the symptoms of trauma, being able to incorporate knowledge about trauma and its effects on development into policies and professional practices (SAMHSA, 2014).

Working Memory: A cognitive skill that allows one to hold on to one piece of information while processing other information. Working memory is involved in skills such as problem solving and reading comprehension (Borella, Carretti, Cornoldi, & De Beni, 2020).

ENDNOTES

1 This figure is likely to be an underestimate (Jones, 2019).

2 Some sources report up to 900 separations (Spagat & Galvan, 2019).

3 These are the latest figures available.

4 Latin Americans with African ancestry. The 'x' or '@' at the end of Latino or Latina is the gender-neutral version of the words (Hyter & Salas-Provance, 2019).

5 Or classism - the unmerited discrimination against people who are impoverished.

6 The italicized events are those that are consistent with Isidra's history.

7 Defined as how well children speak the language . . . as defined by their parents and teachers (Bedore, Peña, Joyner, &. Macken, 2011, p. 493).

8 The Garifuna, although they live in Belize, Guatemala, Nicaragua and the U.S., trace their origins to native Caribs Indians or Maroons (i.e., West Africans who were enslaved but escaped to the mountains creating self-sufficient communities) (Taylor, 2012).

9 A language derived from African, Indian and European Languages (Segura, 2010).

10 Sexualized behaviors are common in children who have experienced sexual abuse and these behaviors include "self-stimulation, sexual aggression toward peers, and imitations of adult sexual activity that are seen as age-inappropriate" (Wamser-Nanney, Sager, & Campbell, 2019, p. 37).

11 Although some states require adoptive homes be at 125% of the poverty level, many adoptive families are not. According to U. S. Department of Health and Human Services, Office of the Assistant Secretary for Planning and Evaluation (USDHHS-ASPE), in 2019, 100% of poverty for a family of 5 is $30,170, and 12% of the poverty level for this size family is $37,713.

12 In 2005, authorities found 11 adopted children with different types of disabilities (including Autism) in cages in the basement of their home in an Ohio town (https://www.nytimes.com/2005/09/13/us/11-children-are-found-locked-in-small-cages-in-an-ohio-home.html). The cages were less than 3.5 feet high. The children reported that they slept in the cages. The cages had alarms, but did not have blankets, mattresses or pillows inside.

13 Two other narrative assessments that incorporate both macro and micro structure analyses are the *Test of Narrative Language-2* (TNL-2, Gillam & Pearson, 2017), and the *Monitoring Indicators of Scholarly Language* (MISL, Gillam and Gillam, 2010).

Chapter 5
A Bilingual Child Diagnosed With Autism Spectrum Disorder (ASD)

Sheila Bridges-Bond
https://orcid.org/0000-0002-0122-3973
North Carolina Central University, USA

EXECUTIVE SUMMARY

Silvia and Antonio Juarez described their 4-year-old son Emanuel as often happy. Emanuel came from a bilingual home and spoke both Spanish and English. His favorite activities were reading and playing with his iPad over-and-over again. Reading was a favorite pasttime and something that the Juarez's felt he did well. While he was described as "loving to engage people," it was not clear that his efforts were successful nor was it clear that they were reciprocated. Briefly observing Emanuel's interaction with his parents, it was noted Emanuel used echolalic phrases and engaged in repetitive and restricted behaviors, toe walking, and finger flicking. These behaviors were noted to be unusual and warranted further evaluation. The Juarez's primary concern was regarding Emanuel's "talking and being able to hold a conversation." Through speech and language therapy, the family expected that Emanuel's communication skills would improve, and he would be able to participate in conversations and talk in sentences.

INTRODUCTION

According to ASHA's Code of Ethics, "…individuals who serve the ASD population should be specifically educated and appropriately trained to do so" (American Speech-Language-Hearing Association [ASHA], 2016, 2019a). To decrease diagnostic error attributed to over or under-diagnosis, cultural and linguistic variables reflecting the home and community environment must be considered in planning screenings and diagnostic testing. The selection of culturally and linguistically appropriate measures begins with identifying screening and assessment instruments that are psychometrically sound and/or sensitive to distinguishing differences from disorders (ASHA, 2019b). Culturally responsive screening procedures for differentiating Autism Spectrum Disorders (ASD) from other developmental disorders

DOI: 10.4018/978-1-7998-2261-5.ch005

and differences examine such behaviors in the context of cultural norms for eye gaze, joint attention, response to one's name, showing/pointing to desired items, nonverbal communication, pretend play, imitation, and language development (American Psychological Association [APA], 2013; ASHA, 2019a).

This chapter examines the above variables as critical factors for consideration in culturally responsive service delivery. Their relevance in service delivery is then illustrated in a case study of Emanuel, a simultaneous bilingual 4-year-old child with a suspected diagnosis of Autism Spectrum Disorder (ASD). The case study of Emanuel is significant in that it illustrates the complexities of culturally responsive service delivery addressing the following issues.

- Social and cultural variables
- Bilingual language assessment
- Bilingual service delivery
- Assessment and treatment of ASD
- Family-centered partnerships
- Interprofessional teaming/practice (IPP)

The case study concludes with a plan of care that is supportive of Emanuel's ASD and Spanish/English communication needs while engaging in family-centered services and interprofessional practice/teaming.

Autism

Autism Spectrum Disorder (ASD) is a neurodevelopmental disorder characterized by deficits in the following areas.

1. Social communication and social interaction (verbal and nonverbal)
2. Restricted repetitive, stereotypic behaviors, interests and activities
3. Inflexible adherence to routines
4. Restricted interests and activities
5. Hypo/Hypersensitivity to sensory input

(APA, 2013; ASHA, 2019a)

Prevalence of ASD

The U.S. Centers for Disease Control and Prevention (CDC) (2014) report a steady rise in the prevalence of ASD over the past 50 years. An examination of such factors as gender, race, and ethnicity finds great variability. Overall prevalence of ASD in the U.S. was reported by the CDC at 16.8 per 1,000 for the general 8-year-old population. Prevalence among males was reported to be 26.6 per 1,000 and 6.6 per 1,000 for females (CDC, 2019). Prevalence among non-Hispanic white children was reported at 17.2 per 1,000, while prevalence rates reported for racial and ethnic minorities, placed Hispanic children at a rate of 14.0 per 1,000 and non-Hispanic Black children at 16.0 per 1,000. Current data showing a rising rate of identification for non-Hispanic Blacks and Hispanic children may be attributed to reduced barriers to identification of children with ASD. Potential barriers include: 1) social stigma, 2) lack of access to healthcare services due to non-citizenship or low income and non-English primary language (CDC,

2019). These barriers contribute to under-identification and late diagnosis of ASD such that families have less opportunity to benefit from early intervention.

Heterogeneity and Core Features of ASD

The language and cognitive skills of individuals with ASD reflect a wide range of abilities and limitations, reflecting the heterogeneity of this population. One explanation of this heterogeneity can be found in the Dynamic Systems Theory (Kohnert, 2013). The Dynamic Systems Theory (DST) provides a model for understanding the emergent behavior in complex systems and the inherent connectivity and interaction of all systems and variables. DST explains the consequences of connectivity. Due to interactions across and within systems, change of one variable or subsystem will serve to impact other parts of that system. Another consequence is that outcomes cannot be precisely predicted due to an ever- present interaction. Language itself is a complex dynamic system, made up of multiple variables and subsystems that continuously interact with a multilayered environment characterized by culture, social, physical and acoustic systems. Language positively and negatively changes over time (Kohnert, 2013). This theory serves to explain the heterogeneity of language, bilingualism, culture, Autism Spectrum Disorders (ASD), and many other systems and variables as they interact and re-organize across time (Kohnert, 2013).

A core feature that remains the over-arching characteristic associated with ASD is impairment in social communication skills. Other core features are critical to the differential diagnosis of ASD from Social Communication Disorders and other language impairments (APA, 2013; ASHA, 2019a).

Screening and Evaluation of ASD

Screening procedures require ruling out hearing loss and its potential contribution to communication difficulty. Screening procedures also include norm referenced measures, parent interview, ethnographic interview, and systematic clinical observations (ASHA, 2019a).

Diagnosis is a process of discernment, distinguishing differences from disorders and determining constellations of behaviors critical in discerning one disorder from another. Social communication disorders in several ways mimic behaviors characteristic of ASD – evident in difficulty with social communication skills and pragmatics. Individuals with ASD most often engage in restrictive/repetitive behavioral patterns in addition to deficits in social communication/engagement. Yet, the restrictive behaviors are not characteristic of Social Communication Disorders but serve as core features of ASD (APA, 2013; ASHA, 2019a).

The role of the SLP in the assessment and diagnosis of ASD ideally is as a member of an interdisciplinary team that possess the expertise to diagnose ASD, distinguishing differences associated with cultural and language differences as well as from other medical conditions.

This medical definition now replaces an earlier definition where ASD along with Childhood Disintegrative Disorders, Rett Syndrome, and Pervasive Developmental Disorders-Not Otherwise Specified (PDD-NOS) were identified under the umbrella term Pervasive Developmental Disorders (APA, 2000). With the new DSM-V, PDD-NOS no longer exists, and instead, a diagnosis of Autism Spectrum Disorders (ASD) ranges across three levels of severity, indicative of the degree of support required to ameliorate social communication and restrictive and repetitive behaviors. Severity in these areas vary in context and may fluctuate with time (APA, 2013).

Not all norm referenced measures are responsive to the variability of cultural norms, so clinicians are cautioned in the selection and application of such measures. Acculturation and assimilation further contribute to variance in assessment outcomes and presentation of behaviors along with education, social economic status, language use, and test familiarity. Thus, case history information is vital for planning and making allowances for these and other variations (ASHA, 2019b).

The social function of communication defines its relevance across diverse contexts and interactants. Relationships may be tightly forged or destroyed as the result of communication exchanges "gone wrong". Parental bonding, reduction in school bullying and chastisement, educational opportunities, and career advancement are all impacted by perceived communicative competency and the effective use of appropriate social skills. Consequently, such factors as cultural competence, cultural humility, bilingualism and language of choice, language proficiency, and cultural and individual values define and direct service delivery.

Hispanic Bilinguals in the U.S.

Hispanic/Latinx populations span the globe, originating from various Spanish-speaking countries in Central and South America, the Caribbean and Europe (Spain) while reflecting a diverse racial heritage, ranging in hues of color and traditions. Historic countries of origin vary in their history, geography, politics, economics, education, health care systems, and social practices.

The major Hispanic ethnic groups in the U.S. represent Mexico, Puerto Rico, Cuba and El Salvador (Kayser, 2012). Their heterogeneity is further reflected in cultural values, beliefs, practices, identity, and language use. The largest concentration of Hispanic/Latinx populations in the U.S. are found across the four states of California, Texas, Florida, and New York (Kayser, 2012).

The Hispanic/Latinx population is the second largest racial/ethnic group behind the Caucasian population, reaching a total of nearly 59.9 million (Noe-Bustamente, 2019). Sixty percent of this population is of Mexican origin, followed by Puerto Ricans, Salvadorans, Cubans, Dominicans, Guatemalans, and Colombians (Noe-Bustamente, 2019).

Beyond country of origin, heterogeneity throughout the Hispanic/Latinx population in the U.S. is evident in social economic status (SES), such that consideration must be given to the intersection of race/ethnicity and SES in the U.S. SES impacts insurance and access to health care. Across racial and ethnic groups, Latinx children are reported to be the most uninsured (Flores, Abreu, & Tomany-Korman, 2006). Similarly, the intersection of social economic status and education require, further consideration. Educational attainment varies across Latinx ethnic groups with college degrees most often earned at a rate of 25% - 30% for Columbians, Peruvians and Cubans; contrasted with Mexicans, Guatemalans, and Salvadorans at 8.4% – 9.1% (Kayser, 2012).

As a result of poverty, a lack of access to healthcare and other services, there are differences in majority language (L2) proficiency that vary by nationality. Seventy percent of Latinxes' ages 5 and older speak English proficiently, yet English proficiency varies across bilingual communities in the U.S. South Americans have the largest percentage (66.8%) of children who speak English very well, while 43.1% of Mexicans and 41.0% of Central American children (ages 5 – 18 years) speak English less than well. Those of Caribbean (e.g., Puerto Rican, Cuban and Dominican) descent have the highest percentage of English only households (Kayser, 2012; Krogstad & Noe-Bustamente, 2019).

Social-Cultural Context of Bilingual Language Development

"Language is not simply a set of rules, but flexible systems of communication made up of the intertwining of the speaker's identity and the communication context" (Zentella, 2002, as cited by Hammer and Rodriguez, 2012, p. 31). Many variables play a role in bilingual language development. Most often cited are age of exposure and parental influence. However, many models of bilingual acquisition note that contributing variables are neither static nor one dimensional. Hammer and Rodriguez (2012) emphasize the social-cultural context in which language development occurs in order to understand the language acquisition of bilingual children. They enumerate several factors in the home environment that shape the bilingual child's language experience. Home language experience, acculturation, language value, social economic status, and cultural beliefs will be discussed.

Home Language Experience

Language patterns of use and proficiency may widely vary in households where more than one language is spoken (Iglesias & Rojas, 2012). When one or more parents/caregivers speak a language other than the majority language, the child's use of the minority language is found to exist along a continuum. The different conditions under which bilingualism is developed can be distinguished as simultaneous versus sequential language acquisition (Hammer & Rodriguez, 2012; Kohnert, 2013).

Simultaneous language acquisition is when a child is exposed to both languages early in life, typically at birth. Sequential language acquisition is when a child is exposed to one language much earlier than his/her exposure to the second language, typically after 3 years of age (Kohnert, 2012). The qualitative and quantitative differences in language exposure place these two bilingual (simultaneous and sequential) language learners at different points along the same continuum (Hammer & Rodriguez, 2012). Among the many factors influencing their positions along this continuum are age of L2 exposure and the differences in rate of language development.

Simultaneous and sequential bilingual learners differ in English and Spanish vocabulary and language comprehension in their early development. Sequential bilinguals are reported to have higher initial Spanish receptive vocabulary and language comprehension than simultaneous bilinguals. Yet, simultaneous bilingual learners have higher English receptive vocabulary and language comprehension. Rate of vocabulary acquisition differ as well. Sequential bilingual learners acquire English and Spanish vocabulary at a faster rate than their simultaneous bilingual counterparts (Hammer, Lawrence, & Micco, 2008). These differences change over time and are further influenced by the child's language use, maternal education, English proficiency, and generational status (Hammer et al., 2012).

In a multilingual household a variety of scenarios might occur reflecting each parent's level of language proficiency, frequency of use and context (e.g. both parents speak the minority and majority languages but with varying levels of proficiency and preferred context) (Iglesias & Rojas, 2012). As context changes, so does the content of the communication and the associated vocabulary. For instance, school vocabulary may be English, while home vocabulary may be Spanish or some combination thereof (Hammer & Rodriguez, 2012).

Minority language (L1) use is more often spoken by the children when it is the only language spoken by one parent or if spoken by both parents. Other variables include the prestige associated with the language and the gender of the parent speaking the minority language. More often maternal language use (e.g. English proficiency) is a predictor of the child's later language use (Hammer et al., 2012; Iglesias & Rojas, 2012).

Length of Residency and Acculturation

Acculturation, the cultural behavioral changes that may impact language, values, family traditions, roles, religious practices, etc., can occur as a result of the interplay between one's native culture and the majority culture, resulting in a blended biculture (Hyter & Salas-Provance, 2019; Ovando, 2008). The length of time that a child has resided in the U.S. is an aspect of acculturation that will also impact their language skills. For instance, it is anticipated that younger child immigrants are more likely to use English while the probability of becoming bilingual significantly declines each year of residency (Portes & Schauffer, 1994).

Often a progressive increase in acculturation is witnessed across family generations. This progressive increase in acculturation by 1st, 2nd and 3rd generation immigrants has been reported to simultaneously reflect a generational decline in use of the family's native language (L1). Telles and Ortiz (2008) found that Mexican American families evidenced a decline in Spanish proficiency by the 5th generation unlike many other Hispanic/Latinx families, who demonstrate an earlier bilingual to monolingual shift by the 3rd generation. A progressive generational decline in use of L1 reflects one of many changes attributed to acculturation.

Language Benefits and Value

There are many benefits (e.g. social, psychological, cognitive, and linguistic, etc.) to being bilingual. Benefits include:

- Greater sensitivity to semantic relationships and understanding of categories
- Better phonological awareness and reading ability
- Greater awareness of linguistic rules and structures
- Enhanced creativity and problem-solving ability
- Better academic outcomes
- Better community connection and sense of cultural identity
- Code switching ability
- Greater listening skills

(ASHA, 2019d; Hammer & Rodriquez, 2012; Ovando, 2008).

In societies where a child's home language is not valued or is stigmatized, the child is often at risk of losing their home language because the incentive to maintain one's home language is significantly reduced. To support minority languages, families and communities are encouraged to take action to implement strategies to protect and prevent attrition or language loss (Hammer & Rodriguez, 2012). In spite of the benefits of bilingualism just enumerated, many public schools do not provide support for maintaining a child's home language. This lack of bilingual support for school-aged Spanish-speaking children puts them at risk for falling behind academically as it typically requires 5 -7 years for children to acquire the language of academics, or Cognitive Academic Language Proficiency (CALP) (Hammer & Rodriguez, 2012; Kohnert, 2013; Roseberry-McKibbin, 2018).

The loss of connecting with one's family, ethnic history, cultural links, sense of community and self-identity reflect just some of the detrimental consequences of language attrition/language loss (Kohnert, 2013).

Socioeconomic Status (SES)

Critical to predicting a bilingual child's language proficiency, vocabulary growth, and literacy development is the family's socioeconomic status. Evidence suggests that SES may be one of the most critical variables in understanding child behavior and planning for a successful future (Roseberry-McKibbin, 2008).

Many low SES families experience poverty. Hispanics are overrepresented among this population. Representing 18.3 percent of the total population in 2017, Hispanics account for 27.2 percent of the population in poverty (Edwards, 2019). The potential negative effects of poverty are homelessness, increased illness, lower educational level of caregivers, fewer print and literacy resources in homes, lower level of oral language interaction between caregivers and children and a higher level of caregiver stress and depression (Roseberry-McKibbin, 2008). Lack of food and poor nutrition result in related birth defects, anemia, learning problems, lower test scores, and stunted physical growth (Roseberry-McKibbin, 2008).

Heads of families with more than a high school education are much higher among middle- and high-income families than it is among those in the low-income category (Simms, Fortuny & Henderson, 2009). Research examining the language and literacy development of monolingual children has shown that maternal education affects their development. Children of mothers with higher education were found to have larger vocabularies as well as more advanced language skills than children of mothers with less education (Hammer & Rodriquez, 2012; Paradis, Genesee, & Crago, 2011). These results were also found to be true for bilingual children, where a higher parental education was predictive of bilingual children's English vocabulary growth (Hammer & Rodriquez, 2012; Paradis, Genesee, & Crago, 2011).

Cultural Beliefs and Practices

A number of studies have examined how parents' cultural beliefs and values influence the environment in which they raise their children. Parents' beliefs guide the interactions and opportunities which support children's learning and language development.

Rodriguez and Olswang (2003) found that Mexican-American families believed that language development and impairment were the product of external (home environment, God/spirituality, home-school mismatch) or internal forces (medical condition, family history, heredity, bilingualism). Families were found to vary in the degree to which they believed they had influence over their child's language development and education. Families were reported to believe that what parents taught at home would be important to their children's school success.

Families who expected their children to speak Spanish in the home, preserving their native language and home ties, created opportunities to support this effort. Other families fully supported learning English while simultaneously maintaining their Spanish language and culture. In many of these instances being bilingual was held in high esteem. Families ensured that their children's English was supported in school while maintaining linguistic practices to support both languages (Hammer & Rodriquez, 2012).

Other family members, siblings, extended family as well as peers were found to be sources of influence particularly as children grew older and their social network moved from home to more diverse environments. In these instances, the community was found to have greater influence in determining the child's language preference (Iglesias & Rojas, 2012).

It should be noted that families may struggle with advocating for progressive acculturation while still maintaining traditional goals, values, and practices. It is important for practitioners to be sensitive to these conflicting beliefs and practices in establishing family-partnerships that are mutually beneficial and culturally responsive.

CASE STUDY OF EMANUEL

Background Information

Emanuel was 4;0 years old when he was referred to the university's inclusive preschool clinic that provided a combination of group and individual therapy services for children ages 2;0 years to 5;11 years from diverse cultural and language backgrounds. The referral came from Emanuel's parents Silvia and Antonio Juarez. They described Emanuel as a very happy child, who was a fast learner and enjoyed reading and iPad/tablet apps. Emanuel was bilingual, Spanish and English speaking, but most proficient in English. His parents were concerned that Emanuel did not use his Spanish nor his English skills to engage in conversation, ask the many questions that they witnessed in other children, nor negotiate sharing when approached by playmates.

Emanuel could read in both English and Spanish yet, he showed no interest in playing with his toys or with other children. Emanuel had received home schooling and attended a day care, but would soon be preparing to begin public school. The Juárezes had concerns about their son's limited expressive language and his lack of play and social skills. They felt that these skills would be critical to helping Emanuel to transition from home to public schooling as well as ensuring his academic success.

Questions for the Reader

1. What further information is needed to address the Juarezes concerns?
2. Do their concerns reflect a language difference or a disorder?

Discussion of Questions for the Reader

1. The Juarezes are concerned that Emanuel neither uses his Spanish nor his English to engage in conversation, communicate socially or engage in play in the ways they see other children communicate. They are also concerned about Emanuel's preparedness for school. It is important to know more about the Juarezes concerns: what have they witnessed in Emanuel's developmental history, home language exposure and use, as well as his day-to-day communication with adults and peers. Information gathering should begin with an ethnographic interview to learn more about the Juarezes' history, life experiences, values, traditions as well as day-to-day interactions.

2. There are some key cultural and linguistic considerations critical to differential diagnosis, distinguishing a language difference versus a language disorder. Emanuel's background must be considered regarding.
    - Hispanic/Latinx – race/ethnicity and cultural practices
    - Bilingual language development – Spanish and English languages
    - Language exposure – Initial exposure, amount, frequency and context

University Inclusive Preschool Clinic

The University Inclusive Preschool Clinic provided a broad range of services which included speech and language screenings, evaluations, group and individual therapy and parent consultation. Graduate clinicians providing direct services, specialized in working with culturally and linguistically diverse (CLD) families. Services were provided under the direct supervision of clinical faculty; the CLD Project director and the Bilingual Clinic director. The CLD project director presented with a moderate level of Spanish fluency while the Bilingual Clinic director was multilingual with native Spanish proficiency.

The clinic provided services for children from diverse language and cultural backgrounds and incorporated themes reflecting their diversity throughout the selection of toys, books, music, dramatic play, arts and crafts, and shared reading activities. The clinicians were provided iPad/tablet apps with Spanish lessons, translations and IPA transcription as well as interactive activities for the children. The clinic met two mornings a week. Evidence-based therapeutic group and individual activities targeted speech and language development as well as literacy, social, cognitive, fine and gross motor skills.

Emanuel was referred to the clinic by his parents and enrolled in the therapeutic inclusive preschool clinic the latter half of the semester. On his first day Emanuel signed the children's attendance sheet tracing the letters in his first name. Upon entering the room a clinician along with his father led him to the "Good Morning Circle" where Emanuel was welcomed by the other graduate clinicians and children. Emanuel did not acknowledge his peers nor the greetings from the clinicians until prompted by his father. He then joined the morning circle activity with the other children.

During Center Time, the children engaged in play with toys of their own choosing. Center Time supported the children's play skills and social development as they engaged in solitary, parallel or interactive imaginative and creative play. Social skill development targeted sharing, turn-taking, requesting, rejecting, etc. During this time Emanuel engaged in setting up and knocking down the bowling pins. When approached by another child, he independently shared the bowling pins for a short time and then withdrew.

During Circle Time, Emanuel identified the letter of the week, "F", and produced its corresponding phoneme /f/ without prompting. Emanuel was excited to see the picture of the firetruck and reported "F was for firetruck" and "firefighters put out fires".

During Arts and Crafts, Emanuel requested to play with the art supplies, but when he was shown a picture of the firefighter art activity, he pushed the supplies away and darted around the room. Emanuel was redirected many times throughout the activity. Once he returned to the art activity, he repeatedly tapped his fingers together, shook his hands, gazed up at the lights while jumping.

During Story Time, Emanuel spelled and read the word "Emergency" on the picture of the fire engine. He was invited to be the story time helper and with encouragement read the first three pages of the story book to the other children. Sensory activities were introduced during dramatic play and Emanuel laughed throughout. He particularly liked rolling down the hall on the rolling board and giggled when proprioceptive and vestibular movement were introduced. When the movement activities transitioned to social engagement, Emanuel once again began to dart around the room.

During Closing Time, Emanuel wandered to another area of the room where he came upon the bowling pins. This time he sat on the pins and bounced up and down while covering his ears with his hands. When his bouncing was interrupted, Emanuel was responsive to being redirected by the clinician and appeared to welcome standing up and walking around the room to the tune of the "Good bye" song.

Mr. Juarez was present throughout Emanuel's first day and stayed to observe his son. The supervising clinician took this opportunity to observe along-side Emanuel's father, discussed his concerns, their observations and engaged in conversation regarding Emanuel's daily routine, preferences, and communication patterns. Plans were made to assess Emanuel's social/pragmatic, and speech and language skills over the next 2 weeks as the clinicians became more familiar with Emanuel and as he became more acclimated to the program,

Questions for the Reader

1. How are the Juarezes' concerns consistent/inconsistent with Emanuel's behavior observed his first day attending the University Inclusive Preschool Clinic?
2. Does Emanuel demonstrate evidence of a communication disorder?
3. What are your recommendations at this point?

Discussion of Questions for the Reader

1. Emanuel engaged in the following behaviors, which were consistent with those described by his parents
    - Lack of social awareness, interest or social interaction with peers
    - Limited self-initiated verbal communication
    - Little interest in engaging in age appropriate solitary or interactive play
    - Difficulty complying with new routines
    - Brief interest in reading environmental signs, and word recognition

Emanuel was observed to engage in restricted and repetitive behaviors (toe walking, twirling, flapping, gazing, etc.) which were not described by his parents.

2. Emanuel demonstrated a constellation of behavior deficits in the following areas:
    - Social communication and social interaction
    - Repetitive and stereotypic behaviors, interests and activities
    - Restricted interests and activities
    - Hypo/Hyper sensitivity to sensory input
3. Emanuel's behavior deficits are suggestive of autism; however he would benefit from formal and informal culturally and linguistically appropriate screening measures to establish cultural differences versus communicative disorders.

Screening

Emanuel's communication needs posed a number of challenges for the clinicians charged with the delivery of evidence-based practice and culturally responsive services to the Juarez family. The following considerations guided the clinicians' planning for assessment and subsequent intervention.

- Family history and cultural background
- Cultural factors, values and family practices
- Language proficiency (pattern of use and preference)
- Spanish and English bilingual assessment (formal and informal assessment measures)
- Parent collaboration and goal setting
- Bilingual language intervention
- Pragmatic/social communication development
- Collaboration and partnership with related services
- Parent training, referral, and support services

Developmental History

Ms. and Mr. Juarez were 40 and 43 years of age respectively when Emanuel was born. Ms. Juarez reported that pre and perinatal development were normal during her pregnancy and Emanuel's birth was without any complications. Emanuel rolled over at 7 months, sat independently at 8 months and crawled at 12 months. Other motor milestones occurred later with standing at 15 months and walking at 18 months. While Emanuel was able to remove his clothes for toileting needs, daily dressing and undressing continued to be a struggle. At four years of age Emanuel appeared to be right hand dominant.

Emanuel was reported to say his first words at 15 months and two-word utterances at 2 ½ years. At the age of 4.0 he spoke frequently, but only expanded his utterances when reminded or encouraged. While his parents reported that they easily understood Emanuel, they indicated that other people somewhat understood him. Emanuel typically understood others and showed no indication of a hearing loss.

Emanuel's overall health was reported to be good, with no reported illnesses or conditions requiring hospitalization. Regular pediatric visits along with the recent hearing screening indicated hearing within normal limits.

Emanuel attended a day care program that promoted early learning and development. Reading, writing and early academics were emphasized at home along with preschool and developmental learning tablet apps and educational television programs.

Ethnographic Interview

Both parents played very active roles in Emanuel's life and participated in the ethnographic interview. An ethnographic interview removes the clinician from the role of interrogator, to the role of facilitator and listener. This style of interviewing utilizes open-ended questions, and avoids the use of yes no, dichotomous, leading, or why questions. Mr. and Ms. Juarez were encouraged to share information that they felt was relevant; their concerns for Emanuel, family history, priorities, values, life experiences, language use, etc.

Mr. Juárez's family history here in the US dated back three or more generations as his grandparents came to the U.S. from Mexico. They were the first of their family' young generation to migrate to the U.S. and it was some years later when other family members followed suit. As a young couple, his grandparents began building their lives and growing their family in Texas. They later relocated to NC, where his father and his father's siblings were raised and received their education. Mr. Juarez had lived in NC all of his life and over the years had gradually moved outside of the Mexican American community that had once been his home. While he was raised in a bilingual home, he saw that many of his younger siblings were now predominantly English speaking and spoke very little Spanish. Occasionally the family joined together for traditional holidays and celebrations. Mr. Juarez was committed to supporting the needs of the Hispanic-Latino businesses and worked with the Hispanic-Latino Chamber of Commerce.

Ms. Juarez was bilingual as well. Unlike her husband she learned Spanish in school and taught as an ESL high school teacher. The origin of her Mexican ancestry was somewhat vague as she had lived in NC all of her life and her ancestry reflected a long history of North Carolinians. Yet, she identified with her family heritage and insured that their son Emanuel would grow up in a bilingual Spanish-speaking household.

While Emanuel was described as predominantly English speaking, it was recognized that he was a simultaneous bilingual speaker, speaking both English and Spanish languages since early language development. During the day Emanuel attended a private day care center that was affiliated with the family's church. Ms. Juarez explained that she liked the day care center as it gave Emanuel the opportunity to build friendships, participate in community activities and develop his academic skills in anticipation of attending school the following year. Emanuel excelled in early literacy development with strengths in the areas of letter and sound recognition, phonological awareness, book orientation, and print knowledge. He particularly liked playing word games and other activities on his iPad tablet. While his tablet had served as an incentive to encourage Emanuel to participate, transition, and follow directions, it proved to be a source of frustration for him when he was required to part from it.

Mr. and Ms. Juarez found transitioning was difficult for Emanuel, when required to end an activity in which he was engaged, relinquish or share a toy, or join a new activity. Emanuel typically did not welcome play when invited in by his class mates, nor did he acknowledge or reciprocate this gesture. Ms. Juarez expressed concerns about Emanuel's limited use of sentences in both English and Spanish. She noted his use of one and two word phrases rather than more elaborate sentences, except when echolalic, repeating a rehearsed line or familiar phrase. Emanuel's parents also expressed concerns regarding his lack of response when called or when others attempted to get his attention. They were uncertain of his understanding, noting his inconsistency in following directions.

Communication Assessment

Speech and Hearing Screening

It was reported that Emanuel was recently examined by his pediatrician for his annual health check-up. Results verified that there were no health concerns, and both hearing and vision were within normal limits. Most recent dental visit reported that Emanuel's teeth were healthy, and this was in good agreement with the oral mechanism examination performed at the speech and hearing clinic. Oral structures were normal in appearance, structure, range of motion, and overall function. Speech was intelligible and voice and fluency were within normal limits for Emanuel's age and gender.

Administration of the PLS-5 Articulation Screener (Zimmerman, Steiner, & Pond, 2012) corroborated previous findings that Emanuel excelled in production of target speech sounds, producing all target phonemes in multiple word positions.

Home Questionnaire

The Juarezes reported that English was Emanuel's primary language, used at home, at his day care and in the community. Some Spanish was reported to be used at home and occasionally when visiting relatives. Much of Emanuel's days during the week were spent at his day care while weekends were spent at home with his parents. Emanuel was an only child and had limited interaction with children beyond his daycare and church. In these instances play with other children was typically parallel play, playing alongside other children without interacting or sharing toys. In some instances Emanuel would imitate other children at play, echoing their speech but without sharing or interacting with them.

Emanuel typically attended to his parents by smiling, talking, exchanging turns and joining them in play. Expressive vocabulary included naming animals, clothing, body parts, toys and food. Emanuel produced one to three word sentences, while supplementing communication with pointing, gestures and vocalizations. Emanuel recognized family members and identified them by name.

Diagnostic Evaluation

Case History, parent report and screening results suggested the need for further testing. Test selection included the following: *The Preschool Language Scale-5* (*PLS-5*) English Edition (Zimmerman, Steiner, & Pond, 2011) and the *Gilliam Autism Rating-2* (*GARS-2*) (Gilliam, 2006).

The PLS-5 English was selected due to its sensitivity to culturally and linguistically diverse children including bilingual Spanish speaking children. The PLS-5 is a comprehensive developmental language assessment for children ranging in age from birth to 7:11 years. Designed as a play based standardized, norm-referenced assessment instrument, it evaluates a variety of early play skills with items ranging from pre-verbal, interaction-based skills to emerging language and early literacy.

Standard scores include auditory comprehension (AC), expressive communication (EC) and total language score. Progress can be tracked using Growth Scale Values (GSV) to monitor skill development and school readiness.

At the time of its development (2011) the standardized population reflected the most current US Census figures for region, race/ethnicity, and level of caregiver education.

The PLS-5 is available in English and Spanish.

Emanuel received an AC standard score of 83, placing him in the 13th percentile with an age equivalent of 3:4 years. Strengths were in the area of making inferences, understanding analogies and understanding negative sentences, identifying colors, letters and body parts. Difficulty was noted in the areas of understanding quantitative concepts, spatial concepts and pronouns.

Emanuel received an EC standard score of 78, placing him in the 7th percentile with an age equivalent of 2:11years. Strengths were in the area of producing 4 – 5 word sentences, using the present progressive, plurals, and answering simple questions logically. Difficulty was noted in the areas of answering what and where questions, using possessives, prepositions, and personal pronouns.

Observation of Emanuel's test taking behavior during formal and informal assessment, participation in group and individual therapy activities as well as his ethnographic/case history report, provided evidence of several core features critical to the differential diagnosis of ASD. These included, 1) restricted and repetitive behaviors, and 2) impaired social communication, language and related cognitive skills. For a clearer understanding of these behaviors, the *Gilliam Autism Rating Scale 2nd Edition* was administered.

The *Gilliam Autism Rating Scale 2nd Edition* (GARS-2) (Gilliam, 2006) is a norm-referenced instrument designed to assist in the diagnosis and estimated severity of ASD in individuals 3 to 22 years of age. Population norms represent 1,107 people with ASD in 48 states across the United States. The three subtests, *Stereotyped Behavior, Communication, and Social Interaction* in addition to the GARS-2 Parent Interview assisted in determining the probability of ASD.

Emanuel was observed while engaged in play and during group and individual activities. A structured parent interview provided critical information for gathering diagnostically significant information. Emanuel received the following subtest scores.

Emanuel received a standard subtest score of 7 for *stereotyped behaviors*, characterized as restricted, repetitive, behaviors such as "flapping hands or fingers in front of face or at sides". A subtest score of 7 suggested a high probability of ASD. Emanuel received a subtest score of 10 for *communication,* with behaviors characterized as "repeating words out of context, repeating words or phrases over and over, and using pronouns inappropriately". A score of 10 was indicative of a "very likely probability of ASD". The subtest score for *social interaction,* was 5 characterized by "avoids eye contact and does certain things repetitively". A standard score of 5 indicated a possible probability of ASD. The sum standard score of 22 and an Autism Index of 83 (13% percentile) suggested a "possible probability of ASD".

Questions for the Reader

1. What additional information does an ethnographic interview provide that distinguishes it from a case history?
2. After reading Emanuel's communication assessment, determine whether the evaluation results reflect a definitive diagnosis of ASD.

Discussion of Questions to the Readers

1. Unlike a case history interview, the ethnographic interview relinquished the control from the clinician/interviewer and provided Emanuel's parents an open forum to tell their story, responding to open-ended questions, and commenting without judgement or expectations. This method of interviewing encouraged Emanuel's parents to share their concerns, life experiences, cultural values, traditions and expectations.
2. Emanuel's communication assessment report summarizes the informal assessment measures and standardized tests administered. Emanuel was observed to engage in restricted and repetitive behaviors, and impaired social communication, language and related cognitive skills that were suggestive of ASD. The *Gilliam Autism Rating Scale, 2nd Edition* (Gilliam, 2006) was administered. Subtest scores ranged from "high probability of ASD" for stereotyped behaviors ((flapping hands or fingers in front of his face) to "possible probability of ASD" for social communication. A sum standard score of 22 and an Autism Index of 83 (13% percentile) were suggestive of a "possible probability of ASD" indicating the need for further testing.

OUTCOMES

Overview of Data Gathering

A variety of assessment measures (standardized tests, ethnographic interview, naturalistic observation, and parent questionnaire) were used to help provide a comprehensive picture of Emanuel's communication needs and abilities. Ethnographic interviewing provided Emanuel's parents a forum to tell their story, share their views, life experiences, expectations, values, etc. The Juarezes, self-identified as being of Hispanic/Latinx ethnicity. Their heritage and life experiences were somewhat different from one another and they varied in their assimilation/acculturation to mainstream Middle American culture. Yet, both expressed a commitment to maintaining a bilingual home environment and ensuring that Emanuel was raised with the knowledge of family and traditions.

Emanuel was their only child so they lacked the experience of raising a child with whom they could compare Emanuel. However, as an ESL teacher, Ms. Juarez was familiar with both the challenges and the benefits of bilingualism.

Naturalistic observation provided insight into Emanuel's communication in everyday social settings within a context that evoked the functional dynamics of language use. Observing Emanuel's interaction with his parents, the clinicians, and the other children provided the opportunity to view him in diverse contexts. Emanuel excelled in reading, letter identification, print awareness, sight word vocabulary, print word and phonological awareness. However, play was sometimes consumed by repetitive, restricted behaviors which interfered with peer interaction and transitioning.

Parent Case History Interview

Case History forms, developmental questionnaires, test supplements (e.g., GARS-2 Parent Interview; Clinic Case History form) appear in a variety of formats: checklist, inventories, protocols, scales, etc. Utilizing a variety of report methods helped to create a more comprehensive picture and clearer understanding of Emanuel's behavior and his family's concerns, priorities, and needs.

Standardized assessments are measurements/instruments designed to determine the presence, absence, and/or severity of a disorder based on empirical design and psychometric measures establishing their validity and reliability. Culturally and linguistically appropriate standardized measures should provide population norms for the individuals being assessed. When populations or individuals are not well represented in the test sample population norms, scores may be invalid for diagnostic purposes and caution must be used in their interpretation.

Standardized measures may require modification and/or accommodation to provide descriptive information and comparative data concerning similarities and differences between the test sample population norm and individuals who may lie outside of the sample population.

Accommodations can involve changes or adjustments made to the client or testing environment to reduce barriers and/or increase access. For instance, it was noted Emanuel was unable to attend to testing for long periods of time, but performed at his best when scheduled breaks were provided with the opportunity to walk or engage in a preferred unrelated activity before resuming testing. Emanuel returned to testing, less distracted and more motivated. While modifications can refer to changes made in the test content, test materials or response mode or pattern of the client.

The *PLS-5 English Edition* was selected for Emanuel as the test administration and interpretation allowed for both accommodations and modifications for non-mainstream and special populations. Alternative responses are provided in the test manual for children with special needs (echolalia, sensory stimulation, lack of eye contact) as well as dialectal variations illustrating examples of English influenced by Spanish (Zimmerman, Steiner & Pond, 2011). It was noted that Emanuel's responses were consistently in English, without codeswitching nor language mixing. The examples of English influenced by Spanish provided in the PLS-5 test manual did not apply in this instance.

Modification in test administration must be documented in the diagnostic report. When test administration is modified, normed test scores are not reported as definitive diagnoses but rather provide descriptive information important to information gathering. It is important to note that these standard measures (PLS-5 and the GARS-5) have been standardized on monolingual English-speaking children and the test scores may not be directly translated to children with special needs, nor those from diverse language backgrounds. Test scores and tests results are viewed with caution and are not used independently for diagnostic purposes. Rather, both formal and informal assessment measures contributed to a clearer picture of Emanuel.

Questions for the Reader

1. What recommendations would you make based on the assessment results and the parent interview?
2. What goals would you recommend?
3. What other professionals would you select to serve with you on an interprofessional collaborative team?

Discussion of Questions for the Reader

1. Based on Emanuel's assessment results the following is recommended.
    a. Emanuel would benefit from a culturally responsive treatment model that supports both his cultural and communication needs.
    b. Establish a parent partnership with the Juarezes discussing their priorities, goals and aspirations for Emanuel.
    c. Emanuel is a simultaneous bilingual speaker. A culturally responsive bilingual assessment requires the evaluation of communication skills in both Spanish and English. The PLS-5 English and Spanish, allows a comparison of Emanuel's performance on equivalent measures, while combined scores will serve to provide greater representation of his total English-Spanish communication skills.
    d. Emanuel should be referred to TEAACH Autism Program to establish a diagnosis of ASD.
    e. Emanuel would benefit from communication services in both English and Spanish,
2. Treatment goals should support Emanuel's social communication, linguistic, and cognitive needs while honoring his family's priorities and cultural values.
    a. Demonstrate joint attention and acknowledgement of others (verbal and non-verbal exchange)
    b. Engage in social reciprocity and turn-taking
    c. Expand use of grammatical structures (locatives, pronouns, modifiers, possessives)
    d. Sequence story events during shared reading activity
    e. Regulate repetitive and stereotypic behaviors

3. Emanuel would benefit from an interprofessional collaborative team to support his social communication, sensory, and motor needs
    a. University's Inclusive Preschool Clinic
    b. Spanish/Bilingual Preschool Clinic
    c. TEACCH Program
    d. Occupational Therapist
    e. **Physical Therapist**

Recommendations

Emanuel's assessment findings suggested that a team evaluation to determine a diagnosis of ASD was warranted. Repetitive and restrictive behaviors included darting and walking on his toes and repeating words and phrases over and over again in and out of context. At times, Emanuel avoided looking at the speaker when being addressed, or when called by name, and seldom initiated conversation. Pronouns, including "I" were used inappropriately and play as well as conversation were seldom initiated with peers or adults. Most often Emanuel was happy and often laughed and giggled, at times responding affectionately to others and calling the clinicians and his peers by name.

Receptive and expressive language scores should be interpreted with caution, as the PLS-5 English Edition, reflects population norms for monolingual English speaking children. It is further cautioned that language differences may reflect discrepancy in language and cultural experiences that are consistent with developmental norms of bilingual children. Norm- and criterion-reference measures of English language skills indicated receptive and expressive language differences in the understanding and use of modifiers, quantifiers, descriptors, personal and possessive pronouns and locatives. Strengths were in the area of producing 4 – 5 word sentences, using the present progressive, plurals, and answering simple questions logically.

According to ethnographic interview, Emanuel resided in a bilingual home where both Spanish and English were spoken. While Emanuel was considered a simultaneous bilingual speaker, his dominant language was English. His parents had strongly communicated their commitment to maintain the language and practices of their Hispanic/Latinx culture, and it was their desire for Emanuel to further develop his Spanish speech and language skills. The university's bilingual clinic director participated in Emanuel's initial evaluation and supervised Emanuel's bilingual evaluation, to include the administration of the PLS-5 Spanish Edition for comparative purposes, thus gaining a comprehensive picture of Emanuel's bilingual communication skills. It was further recommended that Emanuel would participate in both the University's Inclusive Preschool and Bilingual Preschool clinics twice a week, where he would receive services in English as well as in Spanish.

The results of these findings were discussed with Emanuel's parents to ensure that they received culturally responsive family-centered services, a definitive diagnosis regarding ASD, and treatment that would be interdisciplinary and collaborative in nature. Family-centered service delivery models recognize the critical role that families play across the life span. The role played by families is essential to the successful planning and implementation of culturally responsive services. Family-centered practices recognize that family and individual values and beliefs will vary based on culture, background, personal preferences and individual variability (ASHA, 2019e).

For the Juarez family, family-centered practices included

- Building rapport and trust about their needs and interests;
- Identifying and valuing their family's values and views;
- Individualizing services that incorporated their family's needs and desires when making decisions;
- Planning interventions that would give careful consideration to their concerns and priorities, and
- Using items, materials and activities during evaluations and therapy sessions that were familiar and culturally relevant to their child and their family.

Referrals were made for further evaluation and interprofessional partnering (IPP). Criteria used for prescribing referrals included the following (Kirsch, 2017).

- Evidence-based practice
- Culturally responsive service delivery
- Bilingual services respectful of cultural as well as linguistic differences
- Family-Centered service delivery where family values, needs, and cultural practices were central to every aspect of service delivery.
- Interprofessional collaborative practice applying the values and principles of interprofessional team dynamics, committed to collaborative service delivery that was safe, timely, efficient, effective and equitable for Emanuel and his family.

A referral was made to the Interdisciplinary Treatment and Education of Autistic and Communication related handicapped CHildren (TEACCH) Center to schedule an interdisciplinary team evaluation; a) to address a suspected diagnosis of ASD, 2) to evaluate motor and sensory concerns regarding toe walking and proprioceptive and vestibular sensitivities, and 3) to assess fine motor skill development (especially noted for writing, cutting, coloring, and dressing).

Services were initiated with the University Inclusive Bilingual Preschool Clinic, 1) to complete a Bilingual Language Assessment, 2) to initiate biweekly group and individual therapy services, 3) to promote Spanish language development, and 4) to participate in the interprofessional partnership established across clinics and agencies.

Service delivery by the University Inclusive Preschool Clinic continued to meet biweekly, 1) to implement therapy services in partnership with the Bilingual Clinic, 2) to continue ongoing assessments, evaluating early literacy, and communication skills, 3) to participate in the interprofessional partnership established across clinics and agencies, and 4) to provide parent consultation and training to facilitate communication development at home.

The TEACCH team evaluation for Emanuel was conclusive and verified a diagnosis of autism. Services were initiated.

Treatment: Goals and Intervention

Communication competence is defined based on successful communication that incorporates cultural, linguistic and personal values and attributes. Treatment goals must take these factors into consideration along with family priorities while targeting core deficits in ASD (ASHA, 2019a, 2019f).

Emanuel's treatment goals were based on assessment data, targeted core deficits and focused on reciprocal communication across activities, environments, and communication partners. Therapy goals were established in the four core deficit areas: joint attention, social reciprocity, language and related cognitive skills, and behavioral and emotional regulation. These goals were also aligned with Emanuel's goals targeted in the Bilingual Clinic, as well as the concerns shared by his parents (ASHA, 2019g)

Goals for Joint Attention

- Acknowledge what others are indicating with their gaze and gestures by
  - Turning his head in response to a distal point, or
  - Shifting gaze in tandem with a communication partner, or
  - Giving something when a communication partner holds their hand out during free play with minimal clinician prompting.
- Expand use of communication functions (e.g., greeting, initiations, requests, etc.) during group therapy activities with minimal clinician prompting.

Goals for Social Reciprocity

- Maintain a joint engaged (Adamson, Bakeman, & Deckner, 2004) interaction by initiating, taking, and relinquishing turns for 3 minutes during a 30 minute treatment session with visual supports.

Goals for Language and Related Cognitive Skills

- Describe sequence of events in stories
- Identify and use increasing levels of sophisticated grammar including pronouns, possessives, modifiers, and locatives

Goals for Behavioral and Emotional Regulation

- Use language to maintain engagement within an activity (e.g. "first.... then")
- Request a break from a given activity

A range of intervention strategies were implemented to enhance Emanuel's communication, using developmental and behavioral approaches as determined by baseline measures and systematic progress monitoring. Group and individual therapy plans were designed to support Emanuel's communication objectives.

Progress Report

Mr. and Ms. Juarez reported that Emanuel had shown much improvement in making eye contact, greeting his peers, and generating multiword utterances. These improvements were also reported by his teacher. Emanuel was described as participating more in group and less often engaging in restrictive, repetitive behaviors. Also increased, were Emanuel's use of eye contact and self-initiated comments, requests, greetings, humorous commentaries and turn-taking during group activities.

Vocabulary objectives continued to target Emanuel's understanding and use of modifiers, spatial concepts, and descriptors. Spatial concepts were found to improve when Emanuel used locatives to describe where he was and what he was doing (e.g. "standing on the chair").

It was important to support Emanuel's dual languages across clinics. Spanish vocabulary and concepts along with Mexican-American culture were integrated in the University Inclusive Preschool Clinic through shared book reading, dramatic play, and weekly themes addressing diversity. These activities were supported by the Spanish-speaking bilingual graduate clinicians, Spanish-English story books and iPad/tablet apps.

Most beneficial over two years was the partnership across programs with Emanuel's parents. Goals and objectives along with strategies and rewards were implemented across programs as well as at home. Tangible rewards included star stickers and iPad/tablet time, along with timed physical/sensory breaks (e.g. walking, jumping, bouncing, etc.). When Mr. and Ms. Juarez found strategies that were successful at home, they would share these with the other team members to incorporate in our respective clinics.

In conclusion, a culturally responsive treatment model was key to providing the services that the Juarez family needed and warranted to support the needs of their son Emanuel. Utilizing an asset rather than a deficit model empowered the team to recognize the family's resources, talents and resilience that contributed to a successful treatment program. A bilingual approach assisted Emanuel in attaining the many benefits of bilingualism. This approach was not only necessary to perform a valid and reliable assessment of Emanuel's communication skills in both English and Spanish, but also supported the family's commitment to raise their son with a strong sense of cultural identity and connectedness with his home and community.

KEY POINTS

The following key points are critical to addressing the three guiding principles of evidence-based practice (ASHA, 2019c) in the delivery of high quality, family-centered services to culturally and linguistically diverse families.

1. Work collaboratively with the family throughout the service delivery process. Honor their roles, values, experiences, interests, and acknowledge their goals and expectations.
2. Engage in culturally responsive clinical practice and provide high quality clinical care grounded by scientific evidence
3. Collaborate with other professionals, sharing/exchanging clinical experiences and expertise through interprofessional practice and training.

REFERENCES

Adamson, L. B., Bakeman, R., & Deckner, D. F. (2004). The development of symbol-infused joint engagement. *Child Development*, *75*(4), 1171–1187. doi:10.1111/j.1467-8624.2004.00732.x PMID:15260871

American Psychiatric Association. (2000). Diagnostic and statistical manual of mental disorders, text revision. (DSM-IV-TR). Washington, DC: American Psychiatric Association.

American Psychiatric Association. (2013). *Diagnostic and statistical manual of mental disorders* (5th ed.). Washington, DC: American Psychiatric Association.

American Speech-Language-Hearing Association. (2016). *Code of ethics*. Retrieved from www.asha.org/policy

American Speech-Language-Hearing Association. (2019a). *Autism*. Retrieved from https://www.asha.org/practice-portal/clinical-topics/autism/

American Speech-Language-Hearing Association. (2019b). *Cultural competence*. Retrieved from https://www.asha.org/PRPSpecificTopic.aspx?folderid=8589935230&section=Overview

American Speech-Language-Hearing Association. (2019c). *Evidence-Based Practice* Retrieved from https://www.asha.org/research/ebp/evidence-based-practice/

American Speech-Language-Hearing Association. (2019d). *Advantages of being bilingual*. Retrieved from https://www.asha.org/public/speech/development/The-Advantages-of-Being-Bilingual/

American Speech-Language-Hearing Association. (2019e). *Bilingual service delivery*. Retrieved from https://www.asha.org/practice-portal/professional-issues/bilingual-service-delivery/

American Speech-Language-Hearing Association. (2019f). *Family centered practices*. Retrieved from https://www.asha.org/Practice-Portal/Clinical-Topics/Autism/Family-Centered-Practice/

American Speech-Language-Hearing Association. (2019g). *Sample intervention goals based on core challenges in Autism Spectrum Disorder*. Retrieved from https://www.asha.org/uploadedFiles/ASHA/Practice_Portal/Clinical_Topics/Autism/Sample%20Intervention%20Goals.pdf

Centers for Disease Control and Prevention (CDC). (2019). *Data & statistics on Autism Spectrum Disorders*. Retrieved from https://www.cdc.gov/ncbddd/autism/data.html

Edwards, A. (2019). Hispanic poverty rate hit an all-time low. Rate dropped to 18.3 percent, down 1.1. points from 2016. *U.S. Census Bureau*. Retrieved at https://www.census.gov/library/stories/2019/02/hispanic-poverty-rate-hit-an-all-time-low-in-2017.html

Gilliam, J. (2006). Gilliam Autism Rating Scale Second Edition GARS-2. Austin, TX: Pro-Ed.

Gutierrez-Clellen, C., & Kreiter, J. (2003). Understanding child bilingual acquisition using parent and teacher reports. *Applied Psycholinguistics*, *24*(2), 267–288. doi:10.1017/S0142716403000158

Hammer, C., Komaroff, E., Rodriguez, B., Lopez, L., Scarpino, S., & Goldstein, B. (2012). Predicting Spanish-English bilingual children's language abilities. *Journal of Speech, Language, and Hearing Research: JSLHR*, *55*(5), 1251–1264. doi:10.1044/1092-4388(2012/11-0016) PMID:22337497

Hammer, C., Lawrence, F., & Micco, A. (2008). Exposure to English before and after entry into Head Start: Bilingual children's receptive language growth in Spanish and English. *Journal of Bilingual Education and Bilingualism*, *11*(1), 30–56. doi:10.2167/beb376.0 PMID:26430382

Hammer, C., & Rodriguez, B. (2012). Bilingual language acquisition and the child socialization process. In B. Goldstein (Ed.), *Bilingual language development and disorders in Spanish-English speakers* (2nd ed.; pp. 31–46). Baltimore, MD: Paul H. Brookes.

Hammer, C., Rodriguez, B., Davidson, M., Lawrence, F., & Miccio, A. (2011). Changes in language usage of Puerto Rican mothers and their children. Do gender and timing of exposure to English matter? *Applied Psycholinguistics*, *32*(2), 275–297. doi:10.1017/S014271641000041X PMID:23258946

Huerta, M., Bishop, S., Duncan, A., Hus, V., & Lord, C. (2012). Application of DSM-5 criteria for autism spectrum disorder to three samples of children with DSM-IV diagnoses of pervasive developmental disorders. *The American Journal of Psychiatry*, *169*(10), 1056–1064. doi:10.1176/appi.ajp.2012.12020276 PMID:23032385

Hyter, Y., & Salas-Provance, M. (2019). Definitions. In Y. D. Hyter & M. B. Salas-Provance (Eds.), *Culturally responsive practices in speech, language, and hearing sciences* (pp. 15–38). San Diego, CA: Plural Publishing.

Iglesias, A., & Rojas, R. (2012). Bilingual language development of English language learners: Modeling the growth of two languages. In B. Goldstein (Ed.), *Bilingual language development and disorders in Spanish-English speakers* (2nd ed.; pp. 31–46). Baltimore, MD: Paul H. Brookes.

Kayser, H. (2012). Hispanic and Latino cultures in the United States and Latin America. In D. Battle (Ed.), *Communication disorders in multicultural and international populations* (4th ed.; pp. 102–118). St Louis, MO: Elsevier. doi:10.1016/B978-0-323-06699-0.00015-7

Kirsch, T. (2017). *IPE/IPP in academic and clinical curriculum*. Retrieved from https://caa.asha.org/news/ipeipp-in-academic-and-clinical-curriculum/

Kohnert, K. (2013). *Language disorders in bilingual children and adults* (2nd ed.). San Diego, CA: Plural Publishing.

Krogstad, J., & Noe-Bustamente. (2019). *7 facts for National Hispanic Heritage Month*. Retrieved from https://www.pewresearch.org/fact-tank/2019/10/14/facts-for-national-hispanic-heritage-month/

Noe-Bustamente, L. (2019). *Key facts about U.S. Hispanics and their diverse heritage*. Retrieved from https://www.pewresearch.org/fact-tank/2019/09/16/key-facts-about-u-s-hispanics/

Oller, D., & Eilers, R. (2002). *Language and literacy in bilingual children*. Tonawanda, NY: Multilingual Matters. doi:10.21832/9781853595721

Ovando, C. (2008). Acculturation. In J. M. Gonzalez (Ed.), *Encyclopedia of bilingual education* (pp. 9–10). Thousand Oaks, CA: Sage.

Paradis, J., Genesee, R., & Crago, M. (2011). *Dual language development & disorders* (2nd ed.). Baltimore, MD: Brookes Publishing.

Portes, A., & Rumbaut, R. (2001). *Legacies: The story of the immigrant second generation*. Berkeley, CA: University of California.

Rodriguez, B., & Olswang, L. (2003). Mexican-American and Anglo-American mothers' beliefs and values about child rearing, education, and language impairment. *American Journal of Speech-Language Pathology*, *12*(4), 452–462. doi:10.1044/1058-0360(2003/091) PMID:14658997

Roseberry-McKibbin, C. (2008). *Increasing language skills of students from low income backgrounds.* San Diego, CA: Plural Publishing.

Roseberry-McKibbin, C. (2018). *Multicultural students with special language needs: Practical strategies for assessment and intervention* (5th ed.). Oceanside, CA: Academic Communication Associates, Inc.

Simms, M. C., Fortuny, K., & Henderson, E. (2009). *The urban institute fact sheet racial and ethnic disparities among low income families.* Retrieved from https://www.urban.org/sites/default/files/publication/32976/411936-racial-and-ethnic-disparities-among-low-income-families.pdf

Snow, C. E., Burns, M. S., & Griffin, P. (1998). *Preventing reading difficulties in young children.* Washington, DC: National Academies.

Telles, E. F., & Ortiz, V. (2008). *Generations of exclusion: Mexican American assimilation and race.* New York, NY: Russel Sage Foundation.

U.S. Centers for Disease Control and Prevention (CDC). (2014). Autism and Developmental Disabilities Monitoring Network surveillance year 2010 principal investigators. Prevalence of autism spectrum disorders–Autism and Developmental Disabilities Monitoring Network, 11 sites, United States, 2010. *Morbidity and Mortality Weekly Report, 63*(SS02), 1–18. PMID:24402465

Zentella, A. (1997). *Growing up bilingual.* Malden, MA: Blackwell.

Zimmerman, I. L., Steiner, V. G., & Pond, R. E. (2011). Preschool Language Scales 5th Edition: Administration and Scoring Manual. Bloomington, MN, Pearson.

Zimmerman, I. L., Steiner, V. G., & Pond, R. E. (2012). Preschool Language Scales 5th Edition: Articulation Screener. Bloomington, MN, Pearson.

KEY TERMS AND DEFINITIONS

Acculturation: Reflects cultural behavioral changes that occur as a result of the interaction or cultural mixing between an individual's native culture and the dominant or majority culture. The consequence is a bicultural blending that potentially impacts, language, traditions, values, roles, beliefs, etc. (Hyter & Salas-Provance, 2019; Ovando, 2008).

Autism Spectrum Disorder (ASD): Is a neurodevelopmental disorder characterized by deficits in the following areas: social communication and social interaction (verbal and nonverbal communication); restricted repetitive, stereotypic behaviors, interests, and activities (e.g., speech, movement, object manipulation, etc.); inflexible adherence to routines; restricted interests and activities; hypo/hyper sensitivity to sensory input (APA, 2013; ASHA, 2019a).

Bilingualism: Is having the ability to engage in communication involving more than one language. Proficiency across languages may exist on a continuum, fluctuating according to age, time, language environment, communicative partner, setting, etc. The acquisition of a second language also exists along this continuum and is referred to as simultaneous or sequential bilingualism (ASHA, 2019e; Kohnert, 2013; Paradis, Genesee, & Crago, 2011). Simultaneous bilingualism reflects the introduction of two languages at the same time, at birth or soon thereafter (ASHA, 2019e; Kohnert, 2013; Paradis, Genesee, & Crago, 2011). Sequential bilingualism is the introduction of a second language after some level of proficiency has been developed in the primary or native language. This typically occurs after 3 years of age (ASHA, 2019e; Kohnert, 2013; Paradis, Genesee, & Crago, 2011).

Evidence-Based Practice: Reflects the guiding principles of high-quality health care and clinical practice and guides best practice in good decision making. In the clinical practice of speech-language pathology and audiology EBP is the integration of clinical expertise/expert opinion, external scientific evidence, and client/patient/caregiver perspectives (ASHA, 2019c; Kohnert, 2013).

Family-Centered Services: Give recognition to families across the lifespan for the essential role they play in service delivery. The values, beliefs, cultural practices, diverse experiences and perspectives that families bring are recognized and respected in culturally responsive quality health care (ASHA, 2019e).

Interprofessional Practice (IPP): Also known as interprofessional collaborative practice involves the partnership or teaming of healthcare, education and/or multidisciplinary service providers for the delivery of the highest quality comprehensive services across settings (Kirsch, 2019).

Chapter 6
Systems-Based Approaches to Speech-Language Pathology Service Delivery for School Age Children

RaMonda Horton
Midwestern University, USA

EXECUTIVE SUMMARY

This chapter will provide readers with an overview of how a systems-based approach can be used to understand the relationship between culture, environment, language, and disability. It will identify a useful model of ecology, culture, and development that can and should be considered in conjunction with the WHO-ICF framework to guide service delivery in school-based settings. This chapter will also provide an overview of systems-based approaches that can be used when working with children from traditionally marginalized backgrounds. Finally, a case study example will be used to provide guidance on the application of systems-based approaches to service delivery for children in school-based settings.

INTRODUCTION

The Need for Systems Based Approach in SLP Service Delivery to Children of Color

The goal of this chapter is to provide school based practitioners with a (w)holistic approach to communication development that will enable them to deliver culturally responsive speech-language pathology (SLP) services to children from traditionally marginalized backgrounds. This terminology is used intentionally to acknowledge that 1) cultural and linguistic diversity are identity markers that shape communication development that may or may not marginalize an individual (Matthew, Rodriguez, & Reeves, 2016) ; 2) marginalization is a systemic and structural process tied to social stratification based on identity markers such as race, ethnicity, socioeconomic status, and language (Adair, 2015); and 3)

DOI: 10.4018/978-1-7998-2261-5.ch006

there are historical, current, and accumulated inequities faced by certain groups of students in U.S. schools (Bowman, Comer, & Johns, 2018; Schneider, Martinez, & Owens, 2007).

Research indicates that cultural and linguistic differences have the potential to result in different norms and expectations for communication, cognitive, and reading development (Bedore et al., 2018; Whiteside-Mansell, Bradley, & McKelvey, 2009). These differences can impact how speech-language pathologists assess and treat disabilities. IDEA (2004) outlines a number of regulations regarding the evaluation and determination of disability. In particular, section 300.304 establishes that evaluation procedures should include a diversity of assessment tools and strategies. Evaluation procedures and the selection of assessment tools and strategies need to be "non-discriminatory" and administered in the child's native language. Furthermore, for any disability category, eligibility decisions made by the team must demonstrate that determinations are not based on "lack of appropriate instruction or "limited English proficiency" (§300.306b).

Tangentially, there is also a growing body of research indicating that a number of systemic and structural factors play a significant role in communication, cognitive, and reading outcomes (Feliciano, 2018; Gonzalez, Stein, Kiang, & Cupito, 2014; Quintana & Mahgoub, 2016). Furthermore, IDEA (2004) outlines additional exclusionary criteria for the category of specific learning disability (§300.8). Speech-language pathologists may be primary or related service providers for children with learning disabilities given the category's emphasis on oral and written expression, listening comprehension, and reading comprehension. Special education teams must demonstrate that a child's difficulties are not the result of another disability, cultural factors, language proficiency, or environmental/socio-economic disadvantage (§300.309). However, there has been very little discussion of the latter in regard to assessment and intervention approaches. School based practitioners represent more than half of our profession who serve pediatric populations. These SLPs should be aware of the type of socio-cultural and socio-political factors that have the potential to impact speech, language, and communication behaviors necessary for learning. Consider the following scenario:

Jeff is 5-year-old boy from Jamaica. Jeff's family migrated to Tampa, FL last year. Jeff and his 10-year-old sister speak English but their mother usually speaks to them using English or her native Jamaican Patois. Jeff's father is not in the US. The family has a few extended family members in the area that they are living with until the Mother is able to find permanent employment and housing. At this time, Jeff's kindergarten class has been staffed by three long-term substitutes and one parent volunteer. The parent volunteer is concerned that Jeff does not play with other peers and cannot do his work. She is also concerned that when she has observed him making requests and attempting to communicate that she is never sure of what he is saying. The current teacher indicates that Jeff does not talk very much but that he seems to understand classroom directions "just fine." The first quarter of the school year has ended. Jeff's attendance records indicate that he missed at least two days per week and arrived tardy on more than 50% of those days in attendance. You are the full time speech-language pathologist at Jeff's school. Your LEA representative and the MTSS coordinator would like to meet with you to discuss a plan of action for trying to determine if Jeff has any significant communication issues that are impacting his learning.

Speech-language pathologists working in school-based settings are presented with similar scenarios in the day-to-day management of caseloads that are far too large and complex. There are a number of socio-cultural and environmental variables that will need to be taken into consideration as the SLP and her team begins to think about the screening and assessment process for Jeff. Inadequate planning can result in the continuation of poor intervention efforts that may not be helping. Low levels of cultural competence on the part of the professionals involved also may result in treatment efforts which produce additional harm/stress to the five-year old boy and family in this situation. Traditional approaches to assessment and intervention offer little guidance in how to consider the unique experiences of children who are from culturally and linguistically diverse backgrounds and who also may be more likely to experience marginalization. However, alternative frameworks aligned with systems based approaches (SBAs) may offer a more culturally responsive, ecologically valid, and effective paradigm for assessing and treating communication disorders.

SBAS FOR UNDERSTANDING DEVELOPMENTAL COMPETENCIES AND DISABILITY IN CHILDREN FROM TRADITIONALLY MARGINALIZED BACKGROUNDS

SBAs are guided and informed by systems theory. Systems theories emerged from the natural sciences and math disciplines as a heuristic for describing how separate and multiple components and processes interact with one another to achieve a particular goal or function (Johnson, Miller, & Horwowitz, 2010). Systems theories assume that individual and even minor changes in components or interactions can result in changes in how an entire system operates. Systems theories have been especially useful in understanding how unique pathways of development can lead to individual variation that results in similar and diverse developmental outcomes among children (Thelen & Smith, 1994; Smith & Thelen, 2003).

One systems-based theory that has significant implications for understanding, preventing, and treating developmental communication difficulties is Bronfenbrenner's Ecological Systems Model (1994). This theory asserts that development is influenced by multiple and nested environmental systems that are interacting with each other over the course of a child's life. Three of the more frequently discussed environments include the micro, meso, and macrosystems. The microsystem is comprised of those individuals or institutions that have direct interaction with the child, whereas interactions between those individuals or institutions in the microsystem comprise the mesosystem. The macro system is the environment which mediates and influences what can happen within the other systems, and as a result this can be seen as directly impacting the context of a child's development. Societal values, ideology, and policy are examples of macro contextual influences (Bronfenbrenner, 1994). Each of these environmental systems are not under the child's control. They interact with one another in such a way that they have the potential to change the context in which development occurs, thereby changing individual outcomes. Ecologically-based systems models are especially useful to understanding not only the relationship between development and environment, but also the role of society in creating contexts and environments that impact how an individual is able to access, participate, and benefit from opportunities in their daily lives.

Given this greater understanding of the relationship between development and maturation, environment, and social systems, there has also been a shift in how disability is conceptualized. Currently, the World Health Organization (WHO) promotes a biopsychosocial model that emphasizes the importance of understanding the types of biological, individual, and social factors that shape a disability (2001;2013). This model incorporates some of the theoretical underpinnings of Bronfenbrenner's model. Over the past decade, there has been an increased focus on the importance of using the WHO-International Classification of Functioning, Disability, and Health (ICF) framework to guide decision-making about service delivery (Ma, Threats, & Worrall, 2008; Threats, 2010). However, the majority of literature concerning WHO-ICF framework focuses rather heavily on adults or healthcare settings even though the World Health Organization has released specialized guidance on implementing the ICF framework with children and youth (WHO-ICF-CY, 2007). There continues to be a limited amount of information on implementing WHO-ICF framework in U.S. school-based contexts with child populations (McNeily, 2018; Westby & Washington, 2017). Additionally, there are only a few of these sources which address important issues related to cultural differences and culturally responsive service delivery (Fannin, 2016; Harris & Fleming, 2009).

The literature that does explore the implementation of the WHO-ICF-CY framework in school-based settings provides little guidance on how to address culture beyond the individual level. There is limited information available on approaches and strategies that can be used to evaluate and address the types of social and systemic environmental factors that might be unique for families and children from traditionally marginalized groups in the United States. This is especially concerning for three primary reasons. First, children of color and their families continue to face inequities in special education service provision and placement decisions affecting children's access to the general curriculum (Losen, Hodson, Ee, & Martinez, 2014; Rosenbloom & Way, 2004; Sciuchetti, 2017; Voulgarides, 2018). Secondly, there is a large body of research that indicates that children of color attend schools in which they will be exposed to personal and structural discrimination based upon their race, class, language, or immigrant status (Adair, 2015; Brittian & Gray, 2014; Hunter, 2016). Finally, there is a growing body of evidence indicating that African-American and Latinx student populations and those with disabilities are more likely to experience adverse childhood experiences (ACEs) as they are disproportionately affected by poverty and conditions associated with poverty (Maguire-Jack, Lanier, & Lombardi, 2019; Zeng & Hu, 2018). In order to effectively provide school based services, which incorporate the WHO-framework, there continues to be a need for greater understanding of the types of contextual factors that can impact activities and participation for children from traditionally marginalized backgrounds.

The Integrative Model (INT) of child development (Garcia-Coll et al., 1996) is an ecological systems model, which provides a complementary framework for addressing socio-cultural and socio-political dimensions that have not been articulated in recent discussions of WHO-ICF–CY environmental/personal factors and school-based context. In particular, the Integrative Model (INT) of child development (Garcia-Coll et al., 1996) offers a description of the ways in which social and economic systems promote segregation, creating physical, psychological, social, and economic environments/contexts that are specific and unique to children of color in the U.S. According to the INT Model, these mediate the trajectory of child development. The INT Model also provides a much needed, non-deficit oriented, strengths-based approach to research and practice concerned with prevention and intervention efforts targeted towards children of color (Garcia-Coll et al., 1998; Marks & Garcia-Coll, 2018; Perez-Brena, Rivas, Toomey, & Umana-Taylor, 2018).

Integrative (INT) Model of Developmental Competences in Minority Children: Reconceptualization of Risk Factors and Explanation of Adaptive Culture

The INT model was developed as an extension and alternative to the difference model for understanding the relationship between socio-cultural factors and young children developmental competencies (Garcia-Coll, et al., 1996; Marks & Garcia-Coll, 2018). It has now been used in more than 1350 studies in a variety of fields to understand developmental trajectories and outcomes for children from traditionally marginalized backgrounds (Prez-Brena, Rivas-Drake, Toomey, & Umana-Taylor, 2018). Developmental

Figure 1. Integrative model

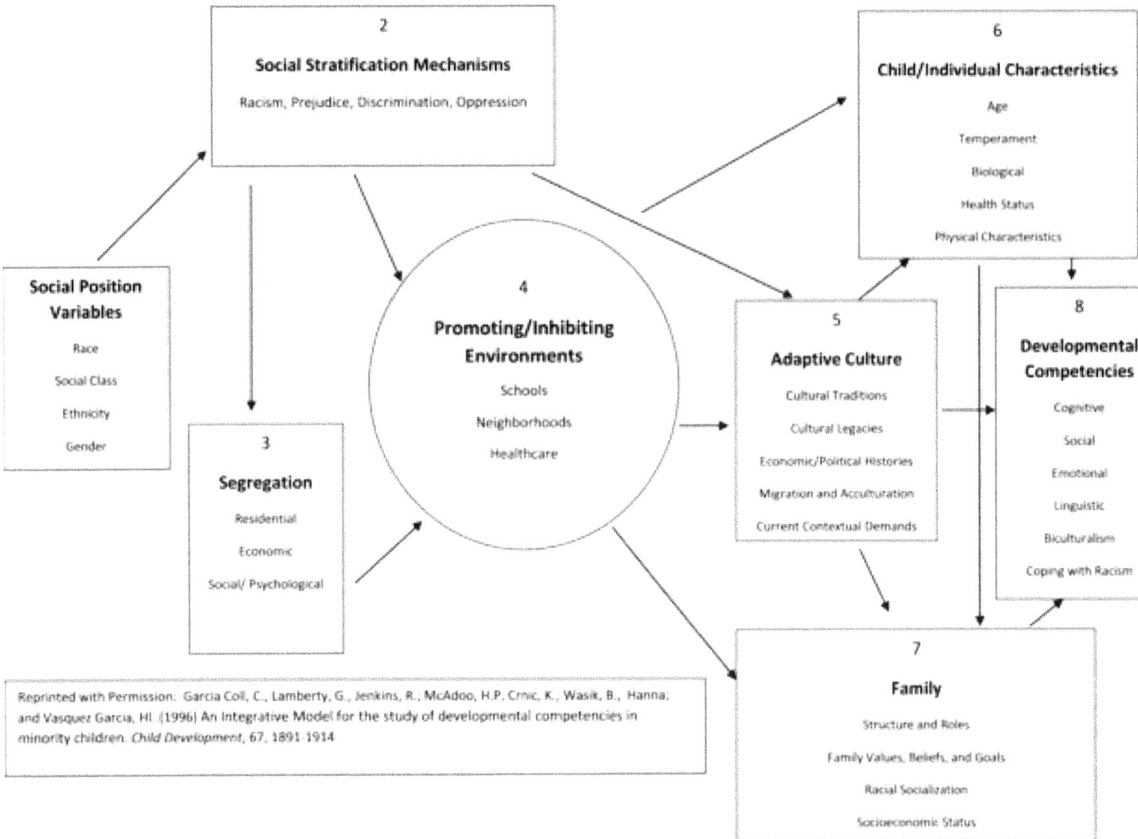

competencies identified in the model include outcomes for cognition, language, social, and emotional functioning to name a few. Historically, difference models of research, assessment, and intervention focused on describing and understanding the behaviors, beliefs, and attitudes of specific cultural groups. Within a difference paradigm, assessment and treatment frameworks should use cultural and community norms to determine expectations for typical and atypical behavior and priorities for intervention targets. The INT model extends the difference model, by recognizing that the environmental contexts of children of color create unique situations and experiences that mediate their development, thereby affecting outcomes and competencies. As such, it is comprised of macro, meso, and micro systems that are described as eight primary components influencing the development of children of color: 1) social position variables (race/ethnicity/gender), 2) social stratification mechanisms (racism/classicism/prejudice/discrimination/oppression)-macro, 3) segregation, 4) promoting/inhibiting environments-micro, 5) adaptive culture-meso, 6) child characteristics, 7) family-micro, and 8) developmental competencies. The model and example of factors for each component appears in Figure 1.

The INT model recognizes that children of color and their families are more likely to experience the effects of institutionalized and systemic inequitable practices that can result in not just residential segregation but also economic, social, and psychological (i.e., marginalization). Additionally, the model posits that developmental competencies emerge as a direct result of the interactions of factors four through seven which are wholly influenced by the first three factors. The INT model has been important in extending society's understanding of the relationship between child outcomes, traditional socio-cultural factors (race, SES, etc.) and mechanisms of social stratification not previously discussed (exposure to racism/discrimination, segregation and marginalization). Promoting and inhibiting environments are not merely physical spaces but also a set of systems that can be nested within one another that may protect children from or put children at risk for experiencing delays or poor developmental outcomes. For example, school can be a promoting or inhibiting environment. As an environment, that means that the context of schooling can be viewed as having multiple systems. For a child with a potential disability, these systems not only impact their academic and social outcomes, but also their opportunity, access, and level of participation in their environments (Ruppar, Allcock, & Gonsier-Gerdin, 2017).

However, what is perhaps most notable about the model and its wide and frequent use in the field of child development, is its conceptualization of adaptive culture (Prez-Brena, Rivas-Drake, Toomey, & Umana-Taylor, 2018). Garcia-Coll et al. (1996) described the adaptive culture as a phenomenon created in response to social stratification mechanisms (racism prejudice, discrimination) and promoting/inhibiting environments. Adaptive culture is defined as a system of "goals, values, and attitudes" that differ from mainstream culture (Garcia-Coll et al., 1996, p. 1904). The INT model highlighted the importance of identifying and understanding adaptive culture, and recognizing it as an important component that impacts individual child characteristics, family functioning, and developmental competencies in children of color.

Questions for the Reader

Review the earlier background information previously provided about Jeff. Using Garcia-Coll et al.'s INT model in Figure 1 name at least three factors that might be impacting the ecological context of Jeff's language and communication development. What sociocultural and sociopolitical contexts does the scenario raise from a systems based approach to examining Jeff's language competency? What additional information would you like to have?

Assessment of Childhood Language and Social Communication Disorders

The WHO-ICF-CY framework for assessment recommends that practitioners complete evaluation of body structures/function, activities, participation, and contextual factors related to environment and personal factors (2001; 2007). The CY version (WHO-2007) incorporates considerations for:

1. The impact of family systems on child functioning;
2. The conceptualization of developmental delay as an indicator of severity in the emergence of the above framework components (i.e., structure and functions).
3. The unique, dynamic, and complex nature of child participation
4. Environmental factors unique to children

The WHO framework also provides a universal classification system that can be used to describe and qualify an individual's ability to function across a variety of domains, level of disability, and the impact of the disability on daily access and participation. Guidance on how to use the classification system is available in the ICF-CY manual (WHO, 2007). A tutorial on the use of the coding conventions for describing communication disorders is beyond the scope of this chapter but has been described in other

Table 1. Comparison of WHO-ICF-CY framework with Garcia-Coll et al.'s (1996) Integrative Model

WHO-ICF-CY	Integrative (INT) Model
Body Structures and Functions	Child Characteristics
Activities/Participation	Developmental Competencies
Environment	Segregation Promoting/Inhibiting Environment/ Adaptive Culture Family
Personal Factors	Social Position Variables Social Stratification Mechanisms

resources (Fannin, 2016; Westby & Washington, 2017). However, a broad based approach to applying the framework for identifying key pieces of information, while incorporating tenets of the INT model will be discussed with examples of several codes.

Traditionally, within the context of child language development and impairment it has been recommended that SLPs focus the assessment planning on the use of procedures and strategies which allow SLPs to gain a comprehensive description of all modalities and areas of speech, language, and communication. For example, Paul and Norbury (2012) recommend that assessment include measures of form, content, and use. Assessment for the area of language form would include norm-referenced and criterion referenced measures to examine a child's syntax, morphology, and phonology. Whereas, assessment for the area of content and use would include norm-referenced and criterion referenced measures to evaluate semantic and pragmatic aspects of language. Evaluation of other areas likely to impact communicative functioning would include hearing, oral motor performance, cognition, and social skills and social environment (Paul & Norbury, 2012). Assessment planning for children from traditionally marginalized backgrounds using an SBA would merit the inclusion of evaluation procedures and strategies which allow for the examination of ecological context and factors relevant to promoting/inhibiting environment, adaptive culture, and family factors consistent with the INT model. Additionally, the data collected would need to be interpreted with consideration of socio-ecological factors. Table 1 provides an overview of how the INT model components can complement the WHO-ICF-CY framework.

Questions for the Reader

Review the rest of the case study containing traditional assessment findings for Jeff. Use Table two to see if you can match information from the assessment to various components of the WHO ICF-CY framework and the INT Model. More specifically, are you able to identify promoting/inhibiting environments? Adaptive culture? Family structure and roles? Child Characteristics? What additional information would you like to have? You should then refer to Appendix A to examine how the traditional assessment findings provide key pieces of information that can be linked to the INT-Model and WHO-ICF-CY framework.

Table 2. Blank assessment findings for Jeff-Traditional assessment procedures/strategies

Procedure/Strategy	*WHO-ICF-CY Framework*	*Information Available from Case Study Report*	*Integrative (INT) Model*
Referral and Background Information, Educational, History, and MTSS Data	Activities and Participation		Social Position Child Characteristics Developmental Competencies
Medical History Developmental Questionnaire	Structures and Functions		Child Characteristics
Hearing/Vision	Functions		Child Characteristics
Oral Motor	Structures and Functions		Child Characteristics
Norm and Criterion Referenced Tests (Collateral Areas)	Functions Activities and Participation		Developmental Competencies (Cognitive, Social, Emotional)
Norm Referenced Tests (Form, Content, Use)	Functions		Developmental Competencies (Language)
Criterion Referenced Procedures (Form, Content, Use)	Activities/Participation		Child Characteristics Developmental Competencies (Language)

CASE STUDY-TRADITIONAL ASSESSMENT FINDINGS

Referral and Background Information, Educational History, MTSS Data

Jeff Caldwell (Age: 5:10). Last year, Jeff attended the local Head Start program and has recently entered kindergarten. During his time at the local Head Start, his teachers expressed some concern about how much he communicates and understands. Jeff's mother thought that "someone checked on his communication but didn't find anything wrong". His mother also indicated that she and other family members understand him and that he communicates with them. Jeff's mother also reports that both of her children are a having a difficult time adjusting to their new life. She explains that they have to get up early to catch the bus and get to school. She usually drops the daughter off first and then Jeff. Once mom drops Jeff off, she is usually spending her day trying to find work and a permanent place for them to stay. Jeff attended his previous Head Start for six months but prior to that he attended three different preschools in the span of one year. The Head Start program reports that a special education referral was initiated for Jeff but that he was not enrolled in the summer program. As a result, the team was unable to contact parents via multiple methods to obtain consent for an evaluation. MTSS Data was not available.

Medical Records and Developmental History Questionnaire

There are no medical records available. The school's standard form was filled out by the mom with the assistance of the school social worker. It was reported that English and Jamaican Patois are spoken at home. Jeff's immediate family (Mother and sister) have been living in different places since they moved to the US when Jeff was three years old. Jeff's mother is divorced from his father, who mother reports was very involved with Jeff' s care until she left Jamaica. Mom reported that she experienced a normal pregnancy and delivery. She also noted that Jeff is in good health. He is not sick very often but he "had to get tubes in his ears when he was three." Jeff is not taking any medications, has never received counseling, developmental therapy, or early intervention services. Jeff's mother reported that there is no family history of learning, emotional, or mental disability. The checklist also indicated that milestones for all areas development were achieved in a typical fashion, except for communication. He did not talk until the age of two. Language proficiency questionnaire indicates English as primary language, with a Jamaican patois also used in the home. The family's current income places them well below poverty levels.

SCREENING AND EVALUATION OF COLLATERAL AREAS

Cognitive and Other Collateral Areas (Per School Psychologist Report)

The school psychologist administered the Differential Abilities Scale Second Edition-Early Years (DAS-II; Elliot, 2007). Given concerns about language proficiency, a non-verbal composite was used to examine cognitive ability. For children, younger than 6 years old, the nonverbal composite examines copying, pattern construction, and picture similarities. Jeff achieved a nonverbal composite standard score of 108. This is considered to be in the normal range and his performance is comparable to typically developing peers in the same age range. A two-day observation period was used to gather data for the Childhood Autism Rating Scale, 2nd Edition (CARS-2; Schopler, Van Bourgondien, Wellman, & Love, 2010). It was reported that Jeff demonstrates mild difficulties with peer interactions, but little to no symptoms of Autism. The Adaptive Behavior Assessment System-III (ABAS-II; Harrison & Oakland, 2015) which examines adaptive behavior including social and functional skills was administered. Jeff received a composite score of 89 and 95, based upon teacher and parent report. For conceptual and practical composites, all scores for teacher and mother were above 90. The social composite was his lowest area at 80 for his teacher, and 92 for his mother. Scores of 90 or above would mean that Jeff is functioning at or above the typical range for his same age peers.

Vision: Screening conducted by school nurse. Jeff passed and there are no difficulties at the present time.

Hearing: Bilateral pure-tone audiometric screening using ASHA guidelines indicated that Jeff passed the hearing screening for all required frequencies in both ears.

Oral Motor: The oral motor screening revealed no abnormalities in structure or function.

Voice and Fluency Screening: Observations of vocal quality and resonance during the collection of Jeff's spontaneous speech sample revealed no concerns. There were no noticeable disfluencies in Jeff's speech; however, he did demonstrate hyper-rate of speech.

Behavioral Observations: During the evaluation process Jeff appeared shy and reserved. It was noted that he seemed very lethargic. Attempts were made to engage Jeff in a conversational interview for the purposes of language sample analysis, but these attempts were not successful in generating sufficient and productive language. He did not ask questions or initiate topics outside of the testing context. Jeff easily completed tasks associated with standardized test administration. When asked about a favorite TV show, he became a bit more animated and was able to provide a narrative retell of the last episode of PAW PATROL.

Table 3. Jeff's results on the clinical evaluation of language fundamentals-5th edition (CELF-5; Wiig, Semel, & Secord, 2013)

	Composite Language Index	Percentile Rank
Receptive Language	87	24
Expressive	83	13
Content	84	14
Structure	82	12
Core	82	12

Norm Referenced and Criterion Referenced Procedures

Speech: The Goldman Fristoe Test of Aritculation-3 (GFTA-3; Goldman & Fristoe, 2015) was administered. Jeff achieved a standard score of 98 and on the Sounds in Words (45th percentile) and a standard score of 90 on the Sounds in Sentences (25th percentile), with an intelligibility rating of 90%. Error analysis revealed stopping of fricatives (th) and reduction of the following consonant clusters in the final position (nd, ld, nt) and /g/. However, Jeff's speech inventory contained all of the developmentally appropriate consonant sounds for English. "Errors" are consistent with dialect/vernacular (Patois).

Language: The Receptive One Word Picture Vocabulary Test-4th Edition (ROWPVT-4; Martin & Brownell, 2011) was administered and Jeff achieved a standard score of 97. The Expressive One Word Picture Vocabulary Test- 4th Edition (EOWPVT-4; Martin and Brownell, 2011) was administered and Jeff achieved a standard score of 97. Expressive and receptive vocabulary performance are considered to be similar to his same aged peers.

The Children's Communication Checklist-2 (CCC-2; Bishop, 2006) was completed by his mother indicated that he obtained a general composite standard score of 70. He demonstrated significant deficits (less than 15th%ile) in the area of coherent discourse, initiations, context, and social relations. Creaghead's Peanut Butter Protocol Pragmatic Assessment (Creaghead & Marguilies, 1982) revealed that he was able to greet, request objects, comment on objects, and actions, make choices and attend to events. However, he struggled with initiating, changing, and maintaining topic during conversation. He did not ask questions, request clarification, or predict what should happen next.

Language sample analysis was used to examine Jeff's connected discourse. A narrative language sample was collected and evaluated using protocols and procedures outlined in the Systematic Analysis of Language Transcripts (SALT) manual (Miller, Andriacchi, & Nockerts, 2012). When compared to other kids in the database Jeff demonstrated the following:

Jeff produced a combination of simple, compound, and complex sentences. He demonstrated use of the all 14 morphemes with at least 80% accuracy; some language differences noted. The sample revealed that he was able to understand and respond appropriately to wh-questions about the episode. His retelling of the episode also contained a clear beginning, middle, and end. Key characters were identified, and he discussed actions taken by the characters. Jeff seemed more comfortable talking and providing information in a narrative format. However, he struggled with answering spontaneous questions.

Table 4. SALT analysis of Jeff's narrative language sample

Measure	Student Performance	Database Performance *Narrative Sample (Student Self Select)*	Standard Deviation
MLU-W	4.2	4.5	.28
No. complete words	350	372	.15
Number of Diff. Words	280	289	.00

Discussion of the Questions for the Reader

As shown in Appendix A, the traditional assessment findings provide key pieces of information that can be linked to the WHO-ICF-CY framework. The background and case history gathered from medical or educational records can provide the clinician with information related to what specific body structures/function may be involved with the potential communication difficulties. A thorough review of a student's school records, and the reason and source of the referral can also provide information on child characteristics and current performance levels in the area of language, cognitive, social, and academic outcomes. Norm referenced/standardized tools examining speech intelligibility, expressive and receptive language, and possibly fluency and voice can also be useful for informing perspectives on the type of impairments in body functions or structures and identify activity limitations (Westby & Washington, 2017). It is also recommended that the clinician utilize language sampling analysis procedures to analyze the quantity and quality of connected discourse. Information from language sampling procedures can also inform the SLPs findings related to activity and participation (Washington, 2007; Westby, 2007). However, the traditional assessment procedures and data provide limited information if any, on key socioecological contexts outlined in the components of the INT model or a comprehensive description of contextual factors (environmental and personal) discussed in the WHO-ICF-CY framework.

ETHNOGRAPHY AND INTERPROFESSIONAL COLLABORATION AS ADDITIONAL AND NON-TRADITIONAL TOOLS AND STRATEGIES FOR GATHERING INFORMATION ON SOCIO-ECOLOGICAL FACTORS FOR CHILDREN OF COLOR

Ethnography

Non-traditional strategies and approaches will be more useful in the collection of data that describes the socio-ecological context of Jeff's language and communication development. SLPs should have knowledge on how to use ethnographic strategies and procedures such as semi structured interviews, surveys and checklists, and observations to gather qualitative data that will help in understanding their client and families' sociocultural ecology and environment (Brice, 2002; Hays, 2001; Langdon, 2008). For example, semi structured interviews gather information about cultural and linguistic differences, family beliefs, and language proficiency of their family and students for the purposes of assessing participation and environmental factors within the WHO-ICF framework (WHO-2001; 2007). Roseberry-McKibbin (2014) recommends that students, parents, and teachers be used as informants. Ethnographic interviews can also be designed to assess components aligned with the INT model (Promoting/Inhibiting Environment; Adaptive Culture, and Family) when queries focus on understanding and identifying, the structure and contexts of a client's cultural reality (daily routines and stressors); cultural norms (behaviors and practices), and cultural congruence (views and beliefs) (Comos-Diaz, 2012; Hays 2016; Hwang, 2006).

Interviews and checklists on acculturation can be gathered and completed with students and parents as informants so that they can provide insight on how a child and their family may be adjusting to a new culture and/or environment. Collier, Brice, and Oades-Sese (2007) notes that there are certain psychological side effects of acculturation that can mimic symptoms of disability, including but not limited to refusal to communicate, withdrawal, and confusion. SLPs and other special educators will need to understand and recognize how the acculturation process may impact social and academic learning behaviors. The Acculturation Quick Screen-Third Edition (AQS-III; Collier, 2016) is a useful tool that may assist special education team members in documenting and characterizing a student's level of acculturation for initial evaluation purposes but also for instructional planning and programming. This tool examines factors such as the student's time in the U.S., rate of attendance, cultural identity, English language instruction, Native and English Language Proficiency, and school language composition of student population. It helps school personnel develop of a profile of student needs based on level of acculturation. Levels of acculturation are divided into six categories and can range from significantly less acculturated to highly acculturated. It has also been recommended that clinicians use tools such as culturagrams to guide the content of semi-structured interview questions that focuses on information about relocations, cultural transitions, and sociocultural contexts for acculturation (Comos-Diaz, 2012). Culturagrams are visual tools which allow family members and clinicians to identify family composition, structure, roles; trauma, education/work values, languages spoken and experience; and reason for transition, time in community, spiritual practices and beliefs.

Formal observations in which the SLP observes student, teachers, peers, and parents across multiple settings are also recommended for gathering important socio-cultural information (Brice, 2002; Langdon, 2008). These will provide information that should help the SLP understand a child's activity limitations and level of participation within the WHO-ICF-CY framework. Observations of physical space can also provide information on environmental factors. Simultaneously, they will also provide a rich source of data for describing promoting and inhibiting environments.

Interprofessional Collaboration

Interprofessional collaborative practice has been widely promoted by WHO and ASHA as a strategy that can help improve the health outcomes, educational programming, and decision-making process for individuals with disabilities (Ludwig & Kerins, 2019). Therefore, it is also recommended that the SLP work collaboratively with the school social workers and/or counselors to gather additional socioecological information that helps identify and clarify family stressors and functioning. School-based social workers are trained to assess and evaluate ecological systems of the student to identify potential areas of need that can impact child outcomes across a variety of areas, including social, behavioral, and academic (National Association of Social Workers, 2012). Additionally, school counselors interact with students in different ways than classroom teachers and the SLP. Most school counselors are tasked with providing support for students who have experienced or may be experiencing ACE or trauma (American School Counselor Association, 2019). School counselors and social workers specialize in trauma informed interventions and can provide the SLP with information with how adverse and traumatic experiences might impact

Table 5. Blank assessment findings for Jeff-Additional and non-traditional procedures/strategies

Procedure/Strategy	WHO-ICF-CY Framework	Information Available from Case Study Report	Integrative (INT) Model
Parent Interview	Activities/Participation Environment Personal Factors		Social Position Social stratification mechanisms Promoting/Inhibiting Environment Adaptive Culture Family Child Characteristics Developmental Competencies
Teacher Interview	Activities/Participation Environment		Promoting/Inhibiting Environments Developmental Competencies
Observation of Daily Routines	Activities/Participation Environment		Segregation Promoting/Inhibiting Environments Adaptive Culture Family
Data from Interprofessional collaboration	Activities/Participation Personal Factors		Social position Social stratification Segregation Adaptive Culture

a child's academic and social function (Santiago, Raviv, & Jaycox, 2018). Such information should be used to accurately interpret assessment findings for speech and language difficulties.

Additional Questions for the Reader

Review the additional information containing assessment findings from interviews, observations, and interprofessional collaboration for Jeff and his family. Next use Table three to see if you can match information obtained from the additional and non-traditional assessment procedures to various components of the ICF-WHO framework and the INT Model. More specifically, are you able to identify promoting/inhibiting environments? Adaptive culture? Family structure and roles? You should then refer to Appendix B to examine how the additional and non-traditional assessment findings provide key pieces of information that can be linked to the WHO-ICF-CY framework.

CASE STUDY-ADDITIONAL AND NON-TRADITIONAL ASSESSMENT STRATEGIES

Data Obtained from Ethnographic Procedures

Ms. Caldwell expressed some concern about Jeff's communication since he didn't speak until he was two years old. She noted that once he began talking, it was not just words but sentences. She thought that everything was fine but that he seemed to shut down when they had to move to Florida. Prior to moving to Florida, Jeff was enrolled in an early childhood program and his teachers were always pleased with his performance. Mom reports that one of Jeff's strengths is he is a quiet child who seldom causes trouble. She also indicated that she worries that he will not outgrow his shyness or make friends easily. Ms. Caldwell indicated that Jeff and his sister learned English since that is what was taught at school. Mom uses English and the Patois at home.

Teacher Interviews

The current classroom teacher (substitute) and the parent volunteer completed checklists and answered questions. His current kindergarten teacher says he is quiet and does not bother anyone. The parent volunteer noted that he did not participate in classroom activities nor did he use language to request basic items. His teacher reports that he seldom communicates and has difficulty relating to peers. His responses during daily interactions are short and he rarely shares information about important events, likes, dislikes, and family. Jeff has not developed relationships with any of his peers. He does not greet peers in the morning and ignores them when they attempt to directly interact with him. His teacher reports that, "it just seems like he can't be bothered." The current substitute teacher indicated that she has been in the classroom for three weeks. Several attempts made to contact previous teachers were not successful. The parent volunteer has worked in the classroom on Tuesdays and Thursdays since the beginning of the year.

Observations

Jeff was observed in his classroom setting for approximately two hours, including the portion of class reserved for Reading and English Language Arts. He was also observed during his art class. In the general education classroom, Jeff did respond to direct questions. He was able to follow simple and multi-step oral directions given by his classroom teacher. But he did require some additional prompting and scaffolding to complete classroom tasks with more complex oral directions. Jeff did not participate in circle time activities and discussion even when prompted by the teacher to share specific information. When given free time and the opportunity to play, Jeff would stand near a group of peers and watch them play for a bit. After observing he would either take a peer's toy or go off into a separate area to play by himself. During art, Jeff struggled to complete the craft activity that the class was working on for the period. He did not seek out assistance, clarification, or help to progress through the steps. When prompted with, "What should we do next?" He stated, "I don't know." When provided with additional prompting and encouragement to ask the teacher for help, Jeff raised his hand. Once the teacher arrived, he simply gestured to his materials.

Observations of Physical and Instructional Environment

The general classroom environment was organized into different sections for classroom activities. Jeff is one of 23 students in the classroom. Student desks are organized to face the white-board. Jeff's seat is in the next to the last row, away from the board. The classroom walls and bulletin boards were bare, with the exception of PBIS posters and a welcome board with all of the students' names. During the observation period it was noted that the teacher was focused on behavior management for other classroom students. Circle time activities seemed to provide the most routine and structure for all of the children in the classroom. ELA instruction was divided between worksheets and computer activities. When the teacher gave instructions or directions, they were long with only one check for student comprehension.

Data Obtained from Interprofessional Collaboration

An excerpt from the school social worker's report indicated the following:

Ms. Caldwell (mother) is a 28-year-old, college educated, divorced mother who grew up in Kingston, Jamaica and lived there until 18 months ago. She has a college degree in tourism and hospitality. She moved the family here in order to be closer to her "boyfriend"/fiancé. Upon first arriving in the U.S. she lived with her boyfriend. However, several incidents of domestic abuse required that she leave the relationship and find a new place to live. When asked if the children, witnessed any of these incidents she replied that they were involved with one. Initially, after ending the relationship, she and her two children lived in several area shelters until they could get moved in with family members. Over the last six months she and the children have been living with an aunt and cousins in a three-bedroom apartment. Ms. Caldwell and the children share one of the rooms. She currently relies on public transportation to get around the city. Ms. Caldwell also expressed some frustration with some of the people and negative attitudes that she has encountered while searching for employment and permanent housing related to her immigration status and language differences. She feels bad and thinks that maybe they should have stayed in Kingston.

After reviewing the information, the SLP should speak with the social worker to further clarify level of acculturation for the family and how the previously mentioned events and the timeline of events might interact with observed or non-observed social communication behaviors. A conversation with the social worker can also reveal patterns, inconsistences, on new details in information provided by those who interact with the child. For example, the social worker shared the following with the SLP and other team members in her case management

Ms. Caldwell reports that Jeff does not have any friends. Jeff's primary interactions are with mom, his sister, and the aunt. Jeff does not play with his same age cousins who live in the same residence. Ms. Caldwell notes that her aunt has been able to assume responsibility for making sure that all of the children stick to an afterschool routine of homework and chores. Jeff's 10-year-old sister usually helps him complete his chores and reads to him. The family generally does not engage in any community or after school activities beyond church. They all go to Wednesday evening studies and Sunday morning services. The aunt has taken all of the children to Saturday youth ministry on a consistent basis. Ms.

Caldwell has not observed Jeff engaging in any aggressive or violent behaviors. She does not believe that Jeff has any attention issues. She is worried that, "he's not happy like he was before we moved here."

The social worker indicated that Jeff's aunt has caregiving responsibilities. The aunt's input can provide important and relevant information about communication difficulties and opportunities. The SLP and social worker collaborated with Jeff's aunt, Mother, and school personnel to complete the Acculturation Quick Screener-III (Collier, 2016). It was determined that Jeff was in the third category, middle range, referred to as "In Transition". Collier (2016) notes that students at this stage are still in the process of adapting to the unfamiliar culture. Students at this stage are likely to still be experiencing some level of cultural shock and stress that accompanies the process of acculturation.

Outcomes

The speech-language pathologist has considered all of the information gathered. In her report findings she indicates that at this time Jeff demonstrates receptive and expressive language skills are consistent or nearly consistent with his same age peers. However, she also expressed concern about Jeff's social communication skills. Criterion referenced measures, parent report, interviews, and observations indicate that Jeff does not use his language to socialize and interact with peers, or to meet his academic needs. However, she notes that there are a number of school and home factors that have impacted or may continue to impact his development of social skills and use of language to interact and participate in daily activities. The SLP noted that Jeff has faced a significant amount of transitions over the last two years. The Caldwell family's move to the U.S. from Jamaica means that they are immigrants in a new society. Cultural expectations and norms for communication beyond the use of the English language do exist. The family is experiencing a set of unfamiliar circumstances. He and his family have also been exposed to accumulated stress and trauma which can have an impact on communication development and performance. Jeff attends a school where long term substitutes have rotated in and out of his classroom. This has made it difficult for him to receive consistent, quality, evidence-based instruction. The SLP has recommended that Jeff receive services to address social communication issues. Both the SLP and the school Social Worker believe that it will be important to enhance and facilitate supports from outside of the school environment. They also believe that it will be necessary to develop a core set of integrated IEP targets that can be addressed by the SLP and school counselor.

Based on all of the information obtained, Jeff's IEP goals will be focused on using his existing language skills to increase his interactions with adults and peers in his environment, and participation in daily school activities and routines. The SLP will use a push-in collaborative model to help school personnel create opportunities for Jeff to do the following:

1. Demonstrate age appropriate peer entry into play;
2. Engage in extended conversations with peers;
3. Ask and respond to questions.

The school counselor and SLP will also help facilitate school personnel's implementation of the several instructional strategies to assist with Jeff's process of acculturation to the classroom and school climate. These approaches will include the use of cross cultural communication strategies; context embedded instruction; and advanced organizers for beginning lessons (KWL-**K**now, **W**ant to Know,

Learn); as recommended by Collier (2016). The School Counselor will enroll Jeff into the kindergarten social skills group sessions that she leads twice a week. During these groups she will teach students how to self-monitor and reinforce socially appropriate behaviors and utilize role play scenarios to help Jeff develop problem solving skills (Collier, 2016). Rubrics and data collection forms to track Jeff's progress will be completed by classroom personnel, the SLP, and the school counselor.

In order to remain consistent with a systems based approach that considers components of the WHO-ICF and INT model the team should also incorporate principles of family centeredness (Dunst & Trivette, 2009) and trauma informed frameworks (Romero, Robertson, & Warner, 2018). The school social worker will work with classroom teachers and aides. It is recommended that all school personnel be provided with training to facilitate their understanding of Jeff's socio-emotional responses to daily stresses that he may encounter prior to arriving at school and triggers that may result in his withdrawal or other internalizing behaviors throughout the school day (Romero, Robertson, & Warner, 2018). The school social worker will also serve as a resource and bridge between the classroom teacher and family to help address attendance issues. The school social worker will work with Jeff's mom and aunt to coordinate resources, services, and supports to assist the family with employment, housing, and transportation issues.

KEY POINTS

SBAs facilitate practitioner sensitivity, awareness, and responsiveness to greater ecological contexts for development and maturation. As such, there is a greater likelihood that service delivery will improve outcomes beyond the individual child level. Through SBAs such as the Integrative Model (Garcia-Coll et al., 1996) and the WHO ICF-CY framework (2007), sociocultural and sociopolitical contexts of potential disability can be comprehensively evaluated and considered during intervention contexts. Implementation of tools and strategies aligned with SBAs makes it possible for the SLP is able to facilitate greater access, increased opportunities, and more participation in society for the child and family dealing with a disability.

REFERENCES

Adair, J. K. (2015). *The impact of discrimination on the early schooling experiences of children from immigrant families*. Migration Policy Institute. Available at http://www.migrationpolicy.org

American Psychological Association. (2017). *Multicultural guidelines: An ecological approach to context, identity, and intersectionality*. Retrieved from http://www.apa.org/about/policy/multicultural-guidelines.pdf

American School Counselor Association. (2019). *ASCA School Counselor Professional Standards & Competencies*. Alexandria, VA: Author.

Bedore, L., Pena, E., Anaya, J., Nieto, R., Lugo-Neris, M., & Baron, A. (2018). Production of English grammatical forms by English language learners. *Language, Speech, and Hearing Services in Schools*, *49*(2), 277–291. doi:10.1044/2017_LSHSS-17-0027 PMID:29621806

Bishop, D. V. M. (2006). *The Children's Communication Checklist* (2nd ed.). San Antonio, TX: Psychological Corporation.

Bowman, B., Comer, J., & Johns, D. (2018). Addressing the African-American achievement gap: Three leading educators issue a call to action. *Young Children, 73*(2). Retrieved from https://www.naeyc.org/resources/pubs/yc/may2018/achievement-gap

Brice, A. (2002). *The Hispanic child: Speech, language culture, and education*. Boston, MA: Pearson Education.

Brittian, A. S., & Gray, D. L. (2014). African American students' perceptions of differential treatment in learning environments: Examining the moderating role of peer support, connection to heritage, and discrimination efficacy. *Journal of Education, 194*(1), 1–9. doi:10.1177/002205741419400103

Bronfenbrenner, U. (1994). Ecological models of human development. In International Encyclopedia of Education (2nd ed.; vol. 3). Oxford, UK: Elsevier.

Collier, C. (2016). Acculturation Quick Screen-Third Edition (AQS-III). Administration Manual and Scoring Form. Cross Cultural Developmental Education Services.

Collier, C., Brice, A. E., & Oades-Sese, G. V. (2007). Assessment of acculturation. In G. B. Esquivel, E. C. Lopez, & S. Nahari (Eds.), *Handbook of multicultural school psychology: An interdisciplinary perspective* (pp. 353–380). Mahwah, NJ: Lawrence Erlbaum Associates.

Comos-Diaz, L. (2012). *Multicultural care: A clinician's guide to cultural competence*. Washington, DC: American Psychological Association. doi:10.1037/13491-000

Creaghead, N. & Marguilies, C. (1982). Evaluating pragmatic skills of verbal and nonverbal children. *Communicative Disorders: A Journal for Continuing Education, 7*, 73-86.

Dunst, C., & Trivette, C. (2009). Capacity building family systems intervention practices. *Journal of Family Social Work, 12*(2), 119–143. doi:10.1080/10522150802713322

Elliot, C. D. (2007). *Differential abilities scales* (2nd ed.). San Antonio, TX: The Psychological Corporation.

Fannin, D. (2016). The intersection of culture and ICF-CY personal and environmental factors for alternative and augmentative communication. *Perspectives of the ASHA Special Interest Groups, SIG 12, 1*(3), 63-82.

Feliciano, C. (2018). How family, immigrant group, and school contexts shape ethnic educational disparities. *Ethnic and Racial Studies, 41*(2), 189–209. doi:10.1080/01419870.2017.1355974

Garcia-Coll, C., Lamberty, C., Jenkins, R., MacAdoo, H., Crnic, K., Wasik, B., & Vasquesz, G. (1996). An Integrative Model for the study of developmental competencies in minority children. *Child Development, 67*(5), 1891–1914. doi:10.2307/1131600 PMID:9022222

Goldman, R., & Fristoe, M. (2015). *Goldman Fristoe Test of Articulation* (3rd ed.). Bloomington, MN: PsychCorp.

Gonzalez, L., Stein, G., Kiang, L., & Cupito, A. (2014). The impact of discrimination and support on developmental competencies in Latino adolescents. *Journal of Latina/o Psychology*, *2*(2), 79–91. doi:10.1037/lat0000014

Harris, J., & Fleming, V. (2009). Toward model-driven interventions for African-Americans with cognitive-communicative disorders. *Seminars in Speech and Language*, *30*(3), 207–216. doi:10.1055-0029-1225957 PMID:19711238

Harrison, P. L., & Oakland, T. (2015). *Adaptive Behavior Assessment System* (3rd ed.). Torrance, CA: Western Psychological Services.

Hays, P. A. (2001). Sorting things out: Culturally responsive assessment. In *Addressing cultural complexities in practice: A framework for clinicians and counselors* (pp. 89–109). Washington, DC: American Psychological Association; doi:10.1037/10411-006

Hays, P. A. (2016). Conducting a culturally responsive assessment. In *Addressing cultural complexities in practice: Assessment, diagnosis, and therapy* (3rd ed.; pp. 127–160). Washington, DC: American Psychological Association; doi:10.1037/14801-007

Hunter, M. (2016). Colorism in the classroom: How skin tone stratifies African American and Latina/o Students. *Theory into Practice*, *55*(1), 54–61. doi:10.1080/00405841.2016.1119019

Hwang, W. (2006). The psychotherapy adaptation and modification framework: Application to Asian Americans. *The American Psychologist*, *61*(7), 702–715. doi:10.1037/0003-066X.61.7.702 PMID:17032070

IDEA-2004, Individuals with Disabilities Education Act, 20 U.S.C. § 1400 (2004).

Johnson, J. K., Miller, S. H., & Horowitz, S. D. (2008). Systems-Based Practice: Improving the safety and quality of patient care by recognizing and improving the systems in which we work. In *Advances in patient safety: New directions and alternative approaches (Vol. 2: Culture and Redesign)*. Rockville, MD: Agency for Healthcare Research and Quality (US). Available from https://www.ncbi.nlm.nih.gov/books/NBK43731

Langdon, H. (2008). *Assessment and intervention for communication disorders in culturally and linguistically diverse populations*. Clifton Park, NY: Thomson Delmar.

Losen, D., Hodson, C., Ee, J., & Martinez, T. (2014). Disturbing inequities: Exploring the relationship between racial disparities in special education identification and discipline. *The Journal of Applied Research on Children*, *5*(2). Retrieved from https://digitalcommons.library.tmc.edu/childrenatrisk/vol5/iss2/15/

Ludwig, D., & Kerins, M (2019). Interprofessional education: Application of interprofessional education collaborative core competencies to school settings. *Perspectives of the ASHA Special Interest Groups, SIG 2, 1*(3), 1-6.

Ma, E., Threats, T., & Worrall, L. (2008). An introduction to the International Classification of Functioning, Disability, and Health for speech-language pathology. *International Journal of Speech-Language Pathology*, *10*(1-2), 2–8. doi:10.1080/14417040701772612

Maguire-Jack, K., Lanier, P., & Lombardi, B. (2019). Investigating racial differences in clusters of adverse childhood experiences. *The American Journal of Orthopsychiatry*; Advance online publication. doi:10.1037/ort0000405 PMID:30816722

Marks, A., & Garcia-Coll, C. (2018, December). (201). Education and developmental competencies of ethnic minority children: Recent theoretical and methodological advances. *Developmental Review*, *50*, 90–98. doi:10.1016/j.dr.2018.05.004

Martin, N., & Brownell, R. (2011). *Expressive One Word Picture Vocabulary Test* (4th ed.). Novato, CA: Academic Therapy Publications.

Matthew, D. B., Rodrigue, E., & Reeves, R. V. (2016). *Time for justice: Tackling race inequalities in health and housing. Report.* Washington, DC: Brookings. Retrieved from https://www.brookings.edu/research/time-for-justice-tackling-race-inequalities-in-health-and-housing/

McNeiley, L. (2018). Using the International Classification of Functioning, Disability, and Health framework to achieve interprofessional functional outcomes for young children: A speech-language pathology perspective. *Pediatric Clinics of North America*, *65*(1), 125–134. doi:10.1016/j.pcl.2017.08.025 PMID:29173712

Miller, J. F., Andriacchi, K., & Nockerts, A. (2012). *Assessing Language Production Using SALT Software: A Clinician's Guide to Language Sample Analysis*. Middleton, WI: Salt Software, LLC.

National Association of Social Workers. (2012). *NASW Standards for School Social Work Services*. Available at https://www.socialworkers.org/LinkClick.aspx?fileticket=1Ze4-9Os7E%3D&portalid=0

Paul, R., & Norbury, C. (2012). *Language disorders from infancy through Adolescence* (5th ed.). St. Louis, MO: Elsevier Mosby.

Perez-Brena, N., Rivas-Drake, D., Toomey, R., & Umana-Taylor, A. (2018). Contributions of the integrative model for the study of developmental competencies in minority children: What have we learned about adaptive culture. *The American Psychologist*, *73*(6), 713–726. doi:10.1037/amp0000292 PMID:30188161

Quintana, S. M., & Mahgoub, L. (2016). Ethnic and racial disparities in education: Psychology's role in understanding and reducing disparities. *Theory into Practice*, *55*(2), 94–103. doi:10.1080/00405841.2016.1148985

Romero, V., Robertson, R., & Warner, A. (2018). *Building resilience in students impacted by adverse childhood experiences: A whole staff approach*. London, UK: Sage Publications.

Roseberry-McKibbin, C. (2014). *Multicultural students with special language needs: Practical strategies for assessment and intervention* (4th ed.). Oceanside, CA: Academic Communication Associates.

Rosenbloom, S. R., & Way, N. (2004). Experiences of discrimination among African American, Asian American, and Latino adolescents in an urban high school. *Youth & Society*, *35*(4), 420–451. doi:10.1177/0044118X03261479

Ruppar, A., Allcock, H., & Gonsier-Gerdin, J. (2017). Ecological factors affecting access to general education content and contexts for students with significant disabilities. *Remedial and Special Education*, *38*(1), 53–63. doi:10.1177/0741932516646856

Santiago, C., Raviv, T., & Jaycox, L. (2018). *Creating healing school communities: School based interventions for students exposed to trauma*. Washington, DC: American Psychological Association. doi:10.1037/0000072-000

Schneider, B., Martinez, S., & Owens. (2007). Barriers to educational opportunities for Hispanics in the United States. In *Hispanics and the Future of America*. Washington, DC: National Academies Press. Available from https//:www.ncbi.nlm.nih.gov/books/NBK19909

Schopler, E., Van Bourgondien, M. E., Wellman, G. J., & Love, S. R. (2010). *Childhood Autism Rating Scale* (2nd ed.). Los Angeles, CA: Western Psychological Services.

Sciuchetti, M. B. (2017). Addressing inequity in special education: An integrated framework for culturally responsive social emotional practice. *Psychology in the Schools, 54*(10), 1245–1251. doi:10.1002/pits.22073

Smith, L., & Thelen, E. (2003). Development as a dynamic system. *Trends in Cognitive Sciences, 7*(8), 343–34. doi:10.1016/S1364-6613(03)00156-6 PMID:12907229

Thelen, E., & Smith, L. (1994). *A dynamic systems approach to the development of cognition and action*. Cambridge, MA: MIT Press.

Threats, T. (2010). The ICF and speech-language pathology: Aspiring to a fuller realization of ethical and moral issues. *International Journal of Speech-Language Pathology, 12*(2), 87–93. doi:10.3109/17549500903568476 PMID:20420350

Voulgarides, C. K. (2018). *Does compliance matter in special education? IDEA and the hidden inequities of practice. In Disability, Culture, and Equity Series* (pp. 31–49). New York, NY: Teachers College Press.

Washington, K. (2007). Using the ICF within speech-language pathology: Application to developmental language impairment. *International Journal of Speech-Language Pathology, 9*(3), 242–255. doi:10.1080/14417040701261525

Westby, C., & Washington, K. (2017). Using the International Classification of Functioning, Disability and Health in assessment and intervention of school-aged children with language impairments. *Language, Speech, and Hearing Services in Schools, 48*(3), 137–152. doi:10.1044/2017_LSHSS-16-0037 PMID:28630972

Whiteside-Mansell, L., Bradley, R., & McKelvey, L. (2009). Parenting and preschool child development: Examination of three low-income cultural groups. *Journal of Child and Family Studies, 18*(1), 48–60. doi:10.100710826-008-9206-1

Wiig, E. H., Semel, E., & Secord, W. A. (2013). *Clinical Evaluation of Language Fundamentals* (5th ed.). Bloomington, MN: NCS Pearson.

World Health Organization. (2001). *International Classification of Functioning, Disability, and Health*. Geneva, Switzerland: World Health Organization.

World Health Organization. (2007). *International Classification of Functioning, Disability, and Health, Children and Youth Version*. Geneva, Switzerland: WHO Press.

World Health Organization. (2013). *How to use the ICF: A practical manual for using the International Classification of Functioning, Disability and Health (ICF). Exposure draft for comment. October 2013.* Geneva, Switzerland: WHO Press.

Zheng, S., & Hu, X. (2018). Parents reporting adverse childhood experiences among young children with disabilities: Informing systems transformation. *Topics in Early Childhood Special Education, 38*(3), 162–173. doi:10.1177/0271121418790674

KEY TERMS AND DEFINITIONS

Cultural Competence: Awareness, knowledge, and skills necessary for interacting and communicating with individuals from diverse cultural backgrounds.

Culturally Responsive: Ideology and practices which prioritizes the consideration of culture when providing services to individuals.

Ecological Validity: Contextualized, naturalistic, and representative or applicable to real life situations.

Integrative Model: Model of minority child development which describes how social and economic systems create unique environmental contexts that mediate developmental outcomes for children of color in the U.S.

Marginalization: Systemic and structural process of psychological distance from mainstream culture.

Non-Discriminatory: Practices which do no not devalue or penalize cultural patterns or behaviors.

Service Delivery: Prevention, assessment, or treatment practices provided to client.

Systems Theory: Framework of describing how smaller, multiple units and components work together to create a larger system that is designed to carry out a particular function or meet a certain goal.

WHO-ICF-CY: World Health Organization, International Classification of Functioning, Disability, and Health for Children and Youth.

APPENDIX A. ANSWER KEY TRADITIONAL ASSESSMENT FINDINGS FOR JEFF

Table 7. Answer key additional and non-traditional assessment findings

	WHO-ICF-CY Category and Code Example	Case Study Information Available	Integrative (INT) Model Component
Parent Interview	**Activities and Participation** d710.2 Environment Personal Factors	Shy personality and does not cause trouble as described by mom. Does not make friends easily. Communication at home involves English and Jamaican Patois	Social Position and stratification Child Characteristics Promoting/Inhibiting Environment/ Adaptive Culture Family
Teacher Interview	**Activities and Participation** d71040.2 (initiating social interactions) d71041.2 (maintaining social interactions) d7200.3 (forming relationships)	Does not participate in classroom activities, or use language to request basic items. Difficulty relating to peers. No peer relationships.	Promoting/Inhibiting Environments
Observation of Daily Routines	**Activities and Participation** d2100.0 and d2104.0 (undertaking and completing a simple task) d2100.0 (undertaking a complex task) d2103.3 (undertaking a single task in a group) d3504.3 (conversing with many people d2502. 3 (managing behaviors appropriately for approaching persons/situation) d132.2 (acquiring information) **Environment** e330.4 (support and relationship by people in positions of authority) e5850.2 (Education and Training) e5853 (Special Education and Training)	Easily follows simple and multi-step directions. Does not participate in circle time activities or respond to prompts to share information. Problems with entering into peer play. Does not seek out additional assistance, clarification, or help when he does not understand what to do to complete some activities. High teacher turnover for his classroom Jeff's seat is in the next to the last row, away from the board. The classroom walls and bulletin boards were bare. Teacher was more focused on behavior management for other classroom student's ELA instruction was divided between worksheets and computer activities. When the teacher gave instructions or directions, they were long with only one check for student comprehension.	Promoting/Inhibiting Environments
Data gathered from Interprofessional Collaboration	**Activities and Participation** d910.3 (community life) d9300.0 (organized religion) **Environment** e310.+3 (Support and relationship Immediate family) e315.+3 (Support and relationship extended family) **Personal Factors**	No additional after school activities, beyond church. Participation in youth ministry. Mom and sister still operate as a family unit. Aunt involved in day to day child care. Church family provides emotional and spiritual support. Living with extended family. Mom is searching for employment and permanent housing. High mobility. Negative attitudes about immigrant status and language differences. Mother has college degree. History of domestic abuse. Mom discouraged. Mom's socio-emotional well-being is at risk. Jeff is at the "In transition" stage of acculturation as described by his AQS-III profile.	Degree of marginalization/segregation Promoting/Inhibiting Environments Adaptive Culture
Home Language and Language Proficiency	**Personal Factors**	High mobility Immigrant Poverty English as Primary Language, Jamaican Patois	Social position and stratification Marginalization/segregation Adaptive Culture

APPENDIX B

Table 6.

	WHO-ICF-CY Category and Code Example	Case Study Information Available	Integrative (INT) Model Component
Referral and Background Information, Educational, History, and MTSS Data	**Environment** e5850 (Education and Training) e5853 (Special Education and Training)	Kindergarten student Initial referral in preschool, no follow up No MTSS Data	Child Characteristics Developmental Competencies
Medical History	**Structures** s250.7 (qualitative change in structure of middle ear)	Normal Pregnancy and Developmental Milestones (except communication) PE Tubes	Child Characteristics
Hearing/Vision	**Functions** b2100.0 (acuity of vision) b2300.0 (sound detection)	Normal Screening for both ears and eyes	Child Characteristics
Oral Motor	**Structures** s3200.0 (teeth) s3202. 0 (palate) s3203.0 (tongue) s3204.0 (lips)	Normal screening	Child Characteristics
Norm Referenced Tests (Collateral Areas of Cognition and Adaptive Behavior)	**Functions** b163.0 (Basic cognitive functions)	School Psychologist Report: Normal Cognition-DAS-II scores CARS-II mild difficulties with peer interaction, little to no symptoms of ASD Social composite of ABAS-II-teacher was below norms	Developmental Competencies (Cognitive, Social, Emotional)
Norm Referenced Tests (Language Form, Content, Use)	**Functions** b16700.0 (Reception of spoken language). b16710.1 (Expression of spoken language) b320.0 (Articulation function)	Normal Vocabulary as indicated by ROWPVT-IV and EOWPVT-IV Within norms on CELF-5 Receptive Composite Slightly below norms for CELF-5 composites: Core Expressive, Content, and Structure CCC-2 general composite standard score below norms, significant deficits in coherent discourse, initiations, context and social relations Speech Intelligibility judged to be WNL as indicated by GFTA-3, detected errors consistent with home vernacular	Developmental Competencies (Language)
Criterion Reference Procedures (Language Form, Content, Use)	**Functions** b3302.1 (Speed of speech) b3100.0 and b3101.0 (Production of voice and voice quality) **Activities and Participation** d132.2 (acquiring information) d1631.1 (speculating) d3500.2 (starting conversation) d3501.2 (sustaining conversation) d3503.2 (Conversing with one person)	Hyper rate of speech observed. Voice quality judged to be normal. Peanut Butter Protocol Pragmatic assessment revealed difficulty with initiating, changing, and maintaining topic, asking questions, requesting clarification, and making predictions. Attempts to engage Jeff in conversational interview were unsuccessful. Narrative performance using SALT reference database indicated that he performed within norms. Produced a combination of sentence types. Narrative retell revealed strengths, but he struggled to respond to spontaneous questions.	Child Characteristics Developmental Competencies (Language)

Chapter 7
Working With a Culturally and Linguistically Diverse Individual With Specific Learning Disability

Ruixia Yan
North Carolina Central University, USA

EXECUTIVE SUMMARY

With the constantly rising multilingualism in the United States, cultural and linguistic diversity is gradually becoming more and more present at schools throughout the country. Therefore, there is a critical need for resources to support speech-language pathologists (SLPs) to work with culturally and linguistically diverse (CLD) clients. This case study examines a CLD client with a diagnosis of specific learning disability (SLD). SLD is a disorder characterized by one or more significant impairments in reading, spelling, writing, or arithmetical skills, which are not the direct result of other disorders or inadequate schooling. This chapter discusses approaches to appropriately assess the client's language skills and provides intervention suggestions to account for the CLD nature of the client and her SLD.

INTRODUCTION

The number of culturally and linguistically diverse (CLD) students has been growing significantly in recent years (Counts, Katsiyannis, & Whitford, 2018). With this quick growth comes an equally critical need for accurate evaluation, effective treatment in speech-language pathology as well as other related services for CLD students in the school system. There is a significant need for resources to support speech-language pathologists (SLPs) to work with CLD clients. Research indicates that specific learning disability (SLD) accounts for 50% of all identified disabilities among CLD populations (Langdon, 2008). SLD is a disorder characterized by one or more significant impairments in reading, spelling, writing, or mathematical skills, which are not the direct result of other disorders or inadequate schooling. This chapter focuses on Nancy, a CLD student with the diagnosis of SLD. The study discusses approaches and strategies to provide appropriate language services for Nancy.

DOI: 10.4018/978-1-7998-2261-5.ch007

CLD Issues in Communication Disorders

Currently 7,099 languages are spoken in the world (Simons & Fennig, 2017). The use of a language other than English at home is at an all-time high (Simons & Fennig, 2017), and is estimated to continue to increase, particularly in languages such as Spanish, Chinese, Portuguese, and Russian (Rumbaut & Massey, 2013). According to the 2010 American Community Survey (as cites in Rumbaut & Massey, 2013), 20.3% of the U.S. residents reported that they spoke a non-English language at home. It was noted that the percentage of the population who spoke only English by decade between 1980 and 2010 decreased from 89.1% to 79.7% (Rumbaut & Massey, 2013). In 2016, 22% of the children in U.S. spoke a language other than English at home (Kids Count Data Center [KCDC], 2018), and this number increased to 23% in 2017 (KCDC, 2019). According to Migration Policy Institute (2016), CLD students have increased more than 50% over the past decade, and this trend is expected to continue into the next decade. With the rapid multicultural, multiracial, and multilingual growth at schools, classroom teachers and SLPs have a critical role to play in identifying and meeting the needs of all students, including CLD students' language development and abilities. With this extreme growth in multilingualism comes an equally extreme need for accurate evaluation and effective treatment for CLD children in the school system. SLPs have to adjust to a variety of populations with different cultural and linguistic backgrounds instead of relying on "one-size-fits-all paradigm" (Centeno, 2015; Langdon, 2008, 2015; Levey et al., 2013; Ooi & Wong, 2012).

Specific Learning Disabilities (SLD)

Learning disabilities (LD) refers to a heterogeneous group of neurological disorders which cause significant difficulties with listening, speaking, reading, writing, reasoning, or mathematical skills (Ali et al., 2017). That is, LD influences an individual's ability to efficiently process, maintain, or convey information while communicating with the other people (Sharfi & Rosenblum, 2014). Two subgroups of LD are commonly identified, non-specific and specific. Non-specific LD are caused by problems with visual and/or auditory processing, and/or the processing speed. Specific LD (SLD) is a category that includes conditions such as imperfect abilities to listen, think, speak, read, write, spell, or do mathematical calculations (Backhouse & Morris, 2005; Banai & Ahissar, 2006; Casalis, Cole, & Sopo, 2004; Geary & Hoard, 2001; Schultz, Simpson, & Lynch, 2012). Although different researchers may have different classifications of SLD, and some researchers claim that SLD can be different across various individuals (Clark & Uhry, 1995; Myers & Hammill, 1976), the most commonly used classification of SLD is: (1) Dyslexia - difficulties in reading, spelling and writing (including changing the order of letters and pronunciation; (2) Dyscalculia - problems calculating numbers or understanding mathematical concepts; and (3) Dysgraphia – problems with hand writing such as illegible writing. That is, the general characteristics and signs of SLD include language and math. According to studies conducted in different parts of world, the prevalence of specific reading disorder is 4% of the school-age population and the prevalence of specific spelling disorder is almost the same, while the prevalence of specific disorder of mathematical skills is 6% of the school-age population (Fletcher & Miciak, 2017). Although the number of students classified with SLD grew steadily from 1975 until 2000 at which time they began to decline since 2000 (Cortiella, 2011), SLD continues to be the largest of the eligibility classifications under the Individuals with Disabilities Education Act (IDEA; Zirkel, 2018).

In comparison to their age group, individuals with SLD have poor reading, writing, and mathematical skills in their learning processes. Fletcher et al. (2011) indicate that children with SLD have difficulties reaching pre-defined learning objectives. Poor academic performance of the students with SLD at schools may even cause them to drop out. Children with SLD face socio-emotional problems as a result of their academic challenges (Haft et al., 2019). In comparison to typically developing children, children with SLD experience poorer emotional well-being, lower self-esteem and satisfaction in their relationships with family and friends (Ginieri-Coccossis, 2013). Research also shows that students with SLD are more likely to act as bully/victims in bullying episodes (Kokkinos & Antoniadou, 2013). Therefore, it is critical to provide SLD students with special care. Since the passage of the Education for All Handicapped Children Act (EAHCA), the first federal special education law in 1975, SLD has been a recognized type of disability for which students can be eligible for special education services. The most recent amendments of IDEA passed in 2004 required children with disabilities including SLD to have the opportunity to receive a free appropriate public education, just like other children.

CASE STUDY

Reason for Referral

Nancy is a 10-year-old child enrolled in fifth grade. She was referred for a speech-language assessment because of her slow progress in gaining more abstract language in English and her difficulties with reading and writing in English.

Client's Background Information

Nancy is 10 years old and lives with her biological parents and her younger brother. They emigrated from China when Nancy was 8 years old. Nancy spoke only Mandarin when she was in China and the dominant language used at home is Mandarin. She began to learn English after moving to the United States. All of Nancy's current schooling is in English. Nancy's parents work at a local computer company, and they speak both Mandarin and English. Both parents are eager to see their children achieve at school. According to them, Nancy's motor, cognitive, and social developments were normal. They indicated that Nancy's academic performance in China was poor, but her parents thought it was because of Nancy's lack of effort. The reports of latest vision and hearing screenings conducted at school were unremarkable.

Nancy was recently diagnosed with SLD by her school psychologist. Currently diagnosis of a student with SLD is open to subjective judgement (Counts, Katsiyannis, & Whitford, 2018) and SLD identification methods are not consistent across states (Maki et al., 2015; Maki & Adams, 2018). Although populations with SLD are heterogeneous (Fletcher et al., 2019), they all exhibit severe deficits in achievement. That is, they demonstrate struggles to achieve a level which is commensurate with their peers (Fletcher et al., 2013). Therefore, the reauthorization of IDEA in 2004 required states to use response to intervention (RtI) as an approach to identifying SLD. RtI is a multi-tiered service delivery model. The first level (Tier One) is for all students to receive instruction. Students' progress reports are reviewed periodically to determine if the students who are falling behind on benchmark skills and if they would qualify for more intense support in Tier Two. If a student still fails to make adequate progress to meet the grade-level expectations (i.e., fail to respond to the interventions provided in Tier Two), the student will be considered for more intensive intervention in Tier Three. Nancy's classroom teachers reported that Nancy had persistent difficulties in reading, writing, and mathematics in spite of intense support from teachers. It was noted that Nancy's reading was slow, effortful, and inaccurate, and she also had difficulty remembering and describing facts/details from a story which was read to her. In writing, Nancy had difficulty spelling, expressing details, using compound and complex sentences, and organizing sentences in longer essays. Her written expression was poor and lacked clarity. Her mathematical reasoning skills were also insufficient. These difficulties impeded her progress through the general education curriculum. According to her test scores in class, Nancy's reading level was two grade levels behind in vocabulary development and three grade levels behind in reading comprehension. Nancy's teachers indicated that Nancy had struggles doing mathematical calculations and applying mathematical concepts to daily tasks.

Nancy was referred to the school SLP because of her slow progress in gaining more abstract language in English and her difficulties with reading and writing in English. Her teachers were concerned that Nancy was not advancing academically at the same/similar rate as her fellow students. She mixed her languages (English and Mandarin) including words, phrases, and sentences (i.e., code-switching). Sometimes, hesitation was observed in Nancy prior to her speaking. Primary concerns centered on Nancy's language level and academic skills (reading and writing).

Assessment Process

Nancy's school SLP decided to conduct a comprehensive assessment of Nancy's language skills using the following test materials.

1. Peabody Picture Vocabulary Test -Fifth Edition (PPVT-5) (Dunn, 2018) PPVT-5 is a norm-referenced test to access receptive vocabulary of a client aging between 2:6-90+. A broad range of receptive vocabulary levels are covered in the test, and 20 categories of content areas (e.g., tools, actions, etc.) and parts of speech (e.g., nouns, verbs, attributes) of various levels of difficulty are evaluated.
2. Expressive Vocabulary Test – Second Edition (EVT-2) (Williams, 2007) The EVT-2 is a norm-referenced test to assess expressive vocabulary and word retrieval for a client whose age is between 2:6-90+.
3. Clinical Evaluation of Language Fundamentals – Fifth Edition (CELF-5) (Wiig, Semel, & Secord, 2013) The CELF-5 is designed to assess language and communication skills in an individual between the ages of 5 and 21 to determine the presence of a language disorder, describe the nature of the language disorder, and/or plan for intervention/treatment.
4. A language sample taken from Nancy's story telling using Myer's (1969) wordless book: Frog, where are you? Nancy's parents indicated that Nancy's languages (English and Mandarin) were at the same/similar level based on their observation. They also pointed out that Nancy was using more and more English at home. When the school SLP asked Nancy the question "Which language is easier for you? English or Mandarin?", Nancy said "Same".

Observations

Nancy was briefly observed in her classroom. It was noted that she was able to follow class routines well. When students were asked questions about a story which had been read to them, Nancy never answered any questions. When students were asked to write down their answers on paper, Nancy's handwriting

Table 1. Test results of Nancy's language skills

Test/Task	Standard Score	Percentile Rank
PPVT-5	85	16
EVT-2	78	7
CELF-5 Core Language Score Receptive Language Index Expressive Language Index Language Content Index Language Structure Index	70 77 71 69 68	2 6 3 2 2

was labored. The SLP asked Nancy's teachers to rate her attention and performance in class. Most of the teachers indicated that Nancy was usually attentive and had good listening skills, but her grades were mostly Cs. During a one-on-one Interaction, Nancy was attentive and cooperative. She was more active and spoke more in individual than in group discussions. It seemed that Nancy liked individual attention. Nancy responded well to verbal praising and stickers.

It was also noted that Nancy did better when pictures were available to pair with questions since she did not have to elaborate on her answers. Hesitations, repetitions, pauses, and code-switching between English and Mandarin were observed when she narrated a story from the wordless book.

Results and Discussion

Test results of Nancy's language assessment are summarized in Table 1.

Test results indicated that Nancy had difficulties with both receptive and expressive vocabulary. The Core Language Score of 70 on CELF-5 placed Nancy's overall performance in the very low range. Specifically, she had difficulties in the following areas:

- **Sentence Comprehension:** Interpreting spoken sentences of increasing length and complexity.
- **Word Structure:** Applying word structure rules (morphology).
- **Word Classes:** Understanding relationships between words based on semantic class features, function, etc.
- **Following Directions:** Interpreting and following spoken directions of increasing length and complexity.
- **Formulated Sentences:** Formulating complete, semantically and grammatically correct sentences.
- **Recalling Sentences:** Repeating sentences without changing meaning and structure.
- **Understanding Spoken Paragraphs:** Answering questions about the content of auditorily presented paragraphs.

However, it should be noted that the results from each test needs to be interpreted more carefully since the English version was standardized on monolingual English-speaking speakers.

LANGUAGE COMPREHENSION/PROCESSING

Nancy was able to comprehend information in conversations and interact with her communicative partners well. However, she had difficulty answering questions about a story/paragraph (CELF-5 Understanding Spoken Paragraphs subtest). Nancy's vocabulary was limited. For example, she missed words such as *wrench* and *refueling* on the PPVT. These words are quite common in textbooks, lecture handouts, exam papers, essays, assignments, etc. Therefore, insufficient knowledge in academic vocabulary has important impact on academic performance. In addition, it was noted that Nancy had difficulty repeating sentences of various lengths and complexities.

Language Expression

Syntax: Nancy used sentences of various types and complexity depending on the topic. She used almost all the major parts of speech in her language expression: nouns, pronouns, adjectives, verbs, adverb, prepositions, conjunction, and interjection words. She also used declaratives, interrogatives, imperatives, and exclamatory sentences. However, grammar and syntax mistakes were observed in Nancy's speech and language. For example, she said "*My best friend Jessica, she is cute. Her mom drived her home yesterday, and she forget her backpack, she cannot do her homework.*" When there were visual cues such as with the use of the wordless book, her grammar and syntax were more correct. It was also noted that her overall ability to expand simple sentences to more complex constructions was restricted.

Semantics: Nancy understood concrete words better than abstract words. She struggled with some concrete words such as *shield* and abstract words such as *freedom*. Concrete words are perceivable and spatially embedded. That is, concrete words identify objects, things, events, etc. that can be observed and measured, and they are intangible in some way. For example, *table, mouse*, etc. are concrete words. Abstract words refer to the terms that are not physically or spatially constrained such as *freedom, affection*, etc. Her restricted vocabulary knowledge negatively affected her receptive and expressive language. She had difficulties with word naming and word description. For example, when she was asked to name *telescope,* she said "*you can see things*." Nancy's descriptions of words were short, and she could not provide enough details. When she was asked to describe *computer*, she only said "*you can work*." Tasks such as antonyms and synonyms were challenging for Nancy too.

Pragmatics: Nancy was pleasant and friendly during the entire session. She was able to carry on conversations. For example, she felt comfortable initiating, maintaining, and changing topics. She was able to make requests, follow directions/commands, attend to tasks, take turns, make eye contact, and respond to greetings. However, it was noticed that her ability to expand on topics was restricted. Although Nancy was able to respond to the SLP's questions and comments, her answers were generally brief. For example, when she was asked why she wanted to be a doctor in the future, she said "to help people," but she could not expand on that. It was noted that Nancy was able to perceive and understand other people's mental states. The ability to attribute mental states to other people to infer their thoughts, feelings, emotions, intentions, and motivation is referred as theory of mind (ToM). This capacity is important not only for language interactions, but also for understanding stories/narratives since ToM is needed to infer story characters' mental states such as emotions (e.g., *"happy", "sad"*), cognition (e.g., *"thinking", "guessing"*), evaluation (e.g., *"good", "bad"*), modality (e.g., *"have to"*, *"should"*), physiology (e.g., *"tired"*, *"thirsty"*), and affective particles (e.g., *"really"*, *"absolutely"*) (Kauschke & Klann-Delius, 1997).

Writing

When Nancy was asked to make up sentences using given words and write them down (the Formulated Sentences subtest of CELF), it was noted that Nancy had difficulty spelling and organizing sentences. Her written expressions were poor and lacked clarity.

Summary of the Test Results

Nancy is a 10-year-old child growing up in a Mandarin-English bilingual environment where Mandarin is the home language and English is the language used in school and the community. Classroom teachers were concerned about her academic progress. The school psychologist recently diagnosed Nancy with SLD because of Nancy's persistent difficulties in reading, writing, and mathematics in spite of teachers' intense support (i.e., nonresponse to intervention). Nancy was usually attentive in class and had good listening skills; however, it was noted that her attention and participation were better during one-on-one interaction.

Grammar and syntax mistakes were observed in Nancy's speech and language; however, the syntactic errors improved when there were visual cues. Nancy had difficulty with vocabulary. Semantic tasks such as word naming, word descriptions, antonyms, and synonyms were challenging for Nancy. It was noted that she had difficulty understanding the concepts that she was reading about and remembering/retelling details from a story. Nancy did better when pictures were available to pair with questions since she did not have to elaborate on her answers. Hesitations, repetitions, pauses, and code-switching between English and Mandarin were observed when she narrated a story from the wordless book.

The challenges noted above prevented Nancy from benefiting from the curriculum. Her academic skills were below the average range of scores in language, reading, writing, and math. Nancy's teachers indicated that such difficulties interfered with her academic achievement.

Questions for the Reader

1. How would you appropriately assess Nancy's language considering her CLD background?
    a. Should Nancy be assessed in only English or both languages (English and Mandarin)?
    b. How to appropriately assess Nancy's language skills?
    c. Are Nancy's code-switching and hesitation prior to speaking signs of disability?
2. How would you appropriately provide intervention services to Nancy considering her CLD background and SLD diagnosis?
    a. Which language would you choose for Nancy's intervention: Her first language (Mandarin) or second (English)?
    b. What accommodations and strategies can be implemented in the intervention process?

Discussion of the Questions for the Reader

1. How would you appropriately assess Nancy's language considering her CLD background?

Think about the language background of Nancy again. She emigrated from China when she was eight and spoke only Mandarin when she was in China and the dominant language used at home is Mandarin. She began to learn English after moving to the United States. Specifically, consider the following questions:

a. Should Nancy be assessed in only English or both languages (English and Mandarin)?

The simultaneous exposure to and use of more than one language does not constitute a high-demanding cognitive task to the CLD individuals if the language learning occurs in a positive environment where the individual has sufficient support for the development of the languages (Langdon, 2008). A bilingual individual may be at a different proficiency levels in each of the languages depending on the person's exposure to the language as well as the support that the person receives. If the mainstream language (English in Nancy's case) happens to be the less familiar language for her, then the diagnosis or placement of Nancy based on this mainstream language assessment is biased against her. This is because a bilingual tends to process information slower with the less proficient language (Ascher, 1990), and a bilingual is more easily disturbed by external environmental conditions of the test, which may pose negative effect on the test score (Ascher, 1990; Figueroa, 1989; Oller, 1997, 2000, 2001). Therefore, it is not sufficient to just assess one language for Nancy since it cannot provide the whole picture or adequate information about her real language proficiency as manifested across the two languages (Langdon, 2018). Instead, both languages should be assessed.

b. How to appropriately assess Nancy's language skills?

Language assessment plays an essential role in screening communication disorders (Damico, 1991; Damico & Damico, 1993; Hegde & Pomaville, 2008; Marquardt, 1999; Owens, Metz & Haas, 2002). Currently, discrete point standardized language tests continue to be widely used with children from CLD backgrounds (Williams & McLeod, 2012). However, a CLD individual like Nancy may perform poorer on such standardized tests (Hoff et al., 2012; De Houwer, Bornstein, & Putnick, 2014). Think about the fact that Nancy emigrated from China two years ago, and she spoke only Mandarin when she was in China. In addition, the dominant language used in her home was Mandarin. Her exposure to English was obviously not enough. If a standardized language test in English is administered to Nancy, two types of test bias might be identified, content bias and linguistic bias (De Lamo White & Jin, 2011). Content bias refers to the influence of Nancy's unfamiliarity with language/culture-bound content of the test, and linguistic bias may arise when an examiner is not familiar with Nancy's culture and/or language. Goh and Ng (2015; also in Goh et al., 2017) indicated that standard language test items may be biased across different levels of bilingual exposure. In Nancy's case, some features or characteristics of one language might be manifested in the other language. That is, her languages (Mandarin and English) influence each other. Traditional discrete point language tests, however, do not measure this influence (Valdes & Figueroa, 1994). These issues may result in the disproportionate representation phenomenon, over-representation of CLD individuals as disordered and under-representation of them as gifted (Yan,

2009, 2013; Yan & Oller, 2007). Therefore, discrete point standardized language tests alone are not the answer to appropriate assessment of Nancy's language skills.

Campbell et al. (1997) proposed the so-called "processing-dependent measures" (PDMs; Dollaghan & Campbell, 1998; Ellis Weismer et al., 2000; Gathercole & Alloway, 2006; Laing & Kamhi, 2003; Reuterskiold-Wagner, Sahlen & Nyman, 2005; Rodekohr & Haynes, 2001) to assess CLD individuals. Campbell and colleagues, and their successors who have used or recommended PDMs, are trying to reduce bias in assessment by eliminating the language factor in PDMs. They described PDMs as depending on psycholinguistic processing instead of knowledge of and experience with a particular language. According to them, PDMs can be used to validly assess individuals like Nancy in a language that she does not know well, or that perhaps she does not know at all. However, Yan and Oller (2007) examined the PDM tasks in detail and indicated that the PDMs do not and cannot escape the need for knowledge and background experience with the language used in the test. Performing the PDM tasks is not possible for individuals who do not have sufficient exposure to the language of the tasks/assessment. Therefore, PDMs are biased against CLD individuals like Nancy and cannot remove the bias that leads to over-representation of language minorities as disordered and their under-representation as gifted (Yan & Oller, 2007).

Obviously, it is not an easy task to appropriately assess Nancy's language. The use of language involves linguistic, social, and cultural domains, and in this vein, assessment of language should also take these issues into consideration. That is, the appropriate assessment of Nancy's language should be dynamic and synergistic, and stress assessing her language performance in rich, naturalistic, and functional communication contexts (Oller, 1979). The procedure is not limited to the collection of the speech and language samples, but is meaning-based and integrative. For example, SLPs can observe and evaluate Nancy's language skills in more natural and realistic environments such as Nancy talking to friends, ordering foods at cafeteria, answering questions in class, etc.

Ethnography can also be used with Nancy. SLPs may take the role as an ethnographer to collect case history information from Nancy, her parents, classroom teachers, school psychologist, etc., and observe the Nancy's language behaviors in both English and Mandarin in multiple settings. In this process, collaborating with interpreters and translators is needed.

One alternative to standardized testing is dynamic assessment. The concept of dynamic assessment was developed by Vygotsky. Vygotsky (1978, 1986) proposed that there was a difference between what a person can do without help and what the person can do with help. That is, there is a gap between a person's actual development level and potential development level, which is called the zone of proximal development (ZPD). ZPD is the area in which a learner cannot complete certain tasks without the scaffolding/teaching from a more capable person. That is, SLPs identify the language skills that Nancy possesses and her learning potential, provide support or teach Nancy new language skills, and then analyse how Nancy responds to scaffolding/teaching in acquiring new language skills.

Re-evaluation functions as a "safety net" for those who are at a high risk for being misdiagnosed or misplaced (Jalomo, 2000). Portfolio assessment is a testing form that contains collection of performances of a student over time, which can function as a follow-up re-evaluation to reduce the bias or errors of language assessment (Cook-Benjamin, 2001; Fouriea & van Niekerk, 2001; Hanson & Gilkerson, 1999; Hoepfl, 1993; Palardy, 1994). SLPs can create a portfolio for Nancy to record the growth/development of her language abilities.

c. Are Nancy's code-switching and hesitation prior to speaking signs of disability?

SLPs should understand the use and interaction between two languages to avoid misdiagnosing a communication disorder. Nancy mixed her languages (Mandarin and English) including words, phrases, and sentences. This phenomenon is called code-switching, which happens when a language user alternates back and forth between various languages (de Jong & Harper, 2011; de Jong et al., 2013). A bilingual individual may mix two languages by inserting a word from one language while communicating with the other (Genesee et al., 2004). This phenomenon is quite common with many bilingual/multilingual individuals (de Jong & Freeman, 2010) and should not be regarded as a sign of a disability. Although hesitation was observed prior to Nancy's speaking, this is a common practice among bilingual children (de Jong, 2011). At school, classroom teachers and/or SLPs should allow time for Nancy to think and decide on the correct words, phrases, and/or sentences to use.

2. How would you appropriately provide intervention services to Nancy considering her CLD background and SLD diagnosis?
   a. *Which language would you choose for Nancy's intervention: Her first (Mandarin) or second language (English)?* When a choice of language is available, the first decision to make while planning intervention for Nancy is to determine which language to use for intervention: Mandarin or English? It has been determined that learning two languages simultaneously does not create additional cognitive load to a child (Kohnert & Bates, 2002; Langdon, 2008). Langdon (2008) indicated that the first language can be selected for intervention in the following situations:
      - The first language is still the student's dominant language.
      - The student acquired his/her background knowledge and experience in the first language.
      - The first language is important for the student to continue communicating with family members who only speak the first language.
      - The first language is the cultural environment in which the student was raised.

Of course, other factors should also be considered such as the availability of SLPs, treatment goals for the student, etc. People who are important to Nancy such as her teachers, school personnel, etc. should be educated to have a positive, respectful, and encouraging attitude toward her use of first language to help the student to sustain the motivation to use that language.

Consider which language should be used with Nancy. Although Nancy still uses Mandarin at home, she speaks more and more English. Both Nancy and her parents rated her English vs. Chinese language level the same/similar. All of Nancy's current schooling is in English and her parents and teachers are eager to see her achieve at school. In addition, one major intervention goal for Nancy is to improve her English language skills and reading and writing abilities. Based on these considerations, English should be used with Nancy for intervention.

b. *What accommodations and strategies can be implemented in the intervention process?* The primary intervention concerns centered on Nancy's language level and academic skills (reading and writing). Therefore, it is critical that the intervention for her should focus on the goals of effective communication and learning. Along this line, the following practices are recommended.

CULTURALLY RESPONSIVE PRACTICES:

With the increasing number of CLD students attending schools in the United States, it is important to provide culturally responsive services to the clients. The United States recognized the need for SLD students from CLD backgrounds to receive language assessment and instruction/intervention (Scott, Hauerwas, & Brown, 2014). However, SLD practices are not uniform across the United States. As discussed previously, RtI is a commonly used approach for identifying SLD. However, there is no consistent nonresponse standard, and accordingly, the identification decisions vary across nonresponse criteria (Barth et al., 2008) and such thresholds may not be stable (Brown Waesche et al., 2011). RtI has not been sufficiently researched with CLD populations (Klinger & Edwards, 2006; Linan-Thompson, Cirino, & Vaughn, 2007), and studies are scant on how RtI would affect SLD identification and assessment (Scott, Hauerwas, & Brown, 2014). In addition, few states have provided regulations on specific practices for the identification of SLD in CLD students (Scott, Hauerwas, & Brown, 2014). Appropriate assessment leads to identification. Further research is needed to refine the assessment and identification of SLD in individuals who come from CLD backgrounds. There is a need for the development of reliable and valid measures for special education service eligibility which are specifically for CLD populations with SLD (Morgan et al., 2015). Currently, there are no nationwide requirements to mandate all teachers and school personnel to receive special training to work with CLD populations (Counts, Katsiyannis, & Whitford, 2018). The increasing diversity of classrooms in the United States, however, makes the integration of culturally responsive practices a necessity instead of just an option (Ford, 2012). For instance, Nancy's parents should advocate for their child, since they know their child best and can help to educate the assessment and/or intervention team about their family's cultural and linguistic beliefs and practices.

Interprofessional Collaboration:

Educators such as teachers and other school personnel are encouraged to work together with the other professionals such as psychologists, SLPs, etc. to provide better assessment and/or intervention services to CLD clients with SLD. When working with Nancy, an English as a Second Language (ELL) teacher can be included in the assessment and/or intervention team (Counts, Katsiyannis, & Whitford, 2018). Team members should understand the complex relationship between acquiring a 2nd language and literacy development in L1 and L2 (Genesee et al., 2005). Nancy's overall performance in English was in the very low range; however, she needs sufficient time to develop her 2nd language (English) proficiency, and 2nd language learners generally need language support for years, not weeks as usually indicated in RtI models (Scott and colleagues, 2014).

Home-school Partnerships:

Research indicates the importance of regular communication between schools and parents (Minke et al., 2014; Pewewardy & Fitzpatrick, 2009). A goal of IDEA is to train students with disabilities and their parents to advocate to obtain the educational support or accommodations they may need (Rossignol & Paasche-Orlow, 2013). Nancy's parents should be encouraged to actively engage in collaborating with schoolteachers and/or SLPs. Opportunities should also be provided for parents to receive education on SLD and CLD.

In addition, the following accommodations and strategies can be implemented in the intervention process to account for the cultural and linguistic diversity of Nancy and her SLD:

- Use authentic and functional communication. For example, instead of asking Nancy to sequence cards, the SLP can involve the student in talking about the steps of an event that she already experienced or will experience.
- Plan intervention activities around a theme or event. For example, instead of asking Nancy to give the past verb forms in isolation, the SLP can have Nancy talk/write about a past event.
- Incorporate Nancy's home/cultural events into intervention activities.
- Create chances for Nancy to generalize the intervention activities to a larger curriculum context.
- Connect the oral and written language components for as much as possible.
- Create an environment in intervention activities to elicit a wider range of responses from Nancy. For example, SLPs can ask Nancy to predict a story orally and/or in written after reading a short paragraph.
- Integrate form (grammar), content (meaning), and use in language activities.
- Make each language strategy specific, clear, and straightforward as much as possible.
- Involve Nancy in small group or one-on-one instruction whenever possible.
- Use visual cues and graphic organizers such as outlines, guided notes, maps.
- Simplify instructions or tasks for the client.
- Repeat instructions or explanations to the client.
- Clarify instructions.
- Provide oral instructions whenever possible since auditory cues are beneficial for the client's understanding.
- Questions or tasks can be read aloud to Nancy whenever possible.
- Build peer tutoring for Nancy. This can help to enhance the client's academic performance and to improve social skills.
- Model tasks to help the client to understand the expected performance.
- Provide extended time for the client to complete her work.
- Frequently check the client's understanding of the topic.
- Provide SLP services in a one-on-one setting, utilizing noise buffers, and highlighting key points.

KEY POINTS

- With the constantly rising multilingualism in the United States, culturally and linguistically diversity is gradually becoming more and more present in the schools throughout the country. Therefore, there is a critical need for resources to support SLPs to work with culturally and linguistically diverse (CLD) clients.
- SLD is a disorder characterized by one or more significant impairments in reading, spelling, writing, or mathematical skills, which are not the direct result of other disorders or inadequate schooling.
- SLPs have to adjust to a variety of populations from culturally and linguistically diverse backgrounds instead of relying on "one-size-fits-all paradigm".
- Discrete point standardized language tests are not the answer in assessing CLD populations.

- The so-called processing-dependent measures (PDMs) do not and cannot escape the need for knowledge and background experience with the language used in the test. Therefore, PDMs are biased against CLD individuals and cannot remove the bias that leads to over-representation of language/dialect minorities as disordered and their under-representation as gifted.
- The appropriate assessment of a CLD individual's speech and language should be pragmatic and dynamic.
- Dynamic assessment is one alternative to standardized testing methods. The concept of dynamic assessment was developed by Vygotsky. A learning component is integrated within the assessment.
- Re-evaluation functions as a "safety net" for those who are at a high risk for being misdiagnosed.
- Portfolio assessment can be used to record the growth/development of an examinee's speech and language abilities.
- Code-switching and hesitation prior to speaking in a second language (observed in Nancy) are not signs of disability.
- When a choice of language is available, and in particular cases (as discussed in the chapter), the first language can be selected for intervention for CLD clients.
- Specific intervention strategies can be incorporated in planning intervention for CLD clients.

REFERENCES

Ali, K., Dahra, D., Coelho, C., Jones, G., & Tredwin, C. (2017). Academic performance of undergraduate dental students with learning disabilities. *British Dental Journal*, *222*(3), 205–208. doi:10.1038j.bdj.2017.125 PMID:28184079

Antoniadou, N., & Kokkinos, C. (2013). A review of research on cyber-bullying in Greece. *International Journal of Adolescence and Youth*, *20*(2), 185–201. doi:10.1080/02673843.2013.778207

Ascher, C. (1990). Assessing bilingual students for placement and instruction. *ERIC/CUE Digest No. 65*.

Backhouse, G., & Morris, K. (2005). *Dyslexia?* London: Hodder Murray.

Banai, K., & Ahissar, M. (2006). Auditory processing deficits in dyslexia: Task or stimulus related? *Cerebral Cortex*, *16*(12), 1718–1728. doi:10.1093/cercor/bhj107 PMID:16407480

Barth, A. E., Stuebing, K. K., Anthony, J. L., Denton, C. A., Mathes, P. G., Fletcher, J. M., & Francis, D. J. (2008). Agreement among response to intervention criteria for identifying responder status. *Learning and Individual Differences*, *18*(3), 296–307. doi:10.1016/j.lindif.2008.04.004 PMID:19081758

Brown Waesche, J. S., Schatschneider, C., Maner, J. K., Ahmed, Y., & Wagner, R. K. (2011). Examining agreement and longitudinal stability among traditional and RTI-based definitions of reading disability using the affected-status agreement statistic. *Journal of Learning Disabilities*, *44*(3), 296–307. doi:10.1177/0022219410392048 PMID:21252372

Campbell, T., Dollaghan, C., Needleman, H., & Janosky, J. (1997). Reducing bias in language assessment: Processing-dependent measures. *Journal of Speech, Language, and Hearing Research: JSLHR*, *40*(3), 519–526. doi:10.1044/jslhr.4003.519 PMID:9210111

Casalis, S., Colé, P., & Sopo, D. (2004). Morphological awareness in developmental dyslexia. *Annals of Dyslexia, 54*(1), 114–138. doi:10.100711881-004-0006-z PMID:15765006

Centeno, J. G. (2015). Assessing services with communicatively impaired bilingual adults in culturally and linguistically diverse neurorehabilitation programs. *Journal of Communication Disorders, 58*, 58–73. doi:10.1016/j.jcomdis.2015.10.005 PMID:26513217

Cook-Benjamin, L. (2001). Portfolio assessment: Benefits, issues of implementation, and reflections on its use. *Assessment Update, 13*(4), 6–7.

Cortiella, C. (2011). *The state of learning disabilities*. New York, NY: National Center for Learning Disabilities.

Counts, J., Katsiyannis, A., & Whitford, D. K. (2018). Culturally and linguistically diverse learners in special education: English Learners. *NASSP Bulletin, 102*(1), 5–21. doi:10.1177/0192636518755945

Damico, J. S. (1991). Descriptive assessment of communicative ability in limited English proficient students. In E. V. Hamayan & J. S. Damico (Eds.), *Limiting bias in the assessment of bilingual students* (pp. 157–217). Austin, TX: PRO-ED.

Damico, J. S., & Damico, S. K. (1993). Clinical forum: Language and social skills in the school-age population. *Language, Speech, and Hearing Services in Schools, 24*, 236–243. doi:10.1044/0161-1461.2404.236

De Houwer, A., Bornstein, M. H., & Putnick, D. L. (2014). A bilingual-monolingual comparison of young children's vocabulary size: Evidence from comprehension and production. *Applied Psycholinguistics, 35*(6), 1189–1211. doi:10.1017/S0142716412000744 PMID:29527076

De Jong, E. J. (2011). *Foundations of multilingualism in education: From principles to practice*. Philadelphia, PA: Caslon Publishing.

De Jong, E. J., & Freeman, R. (2010). Bilingual approaches. In C. Leung & A. Creese (Eds.), *English as an additional language. A reader for teachers working with linguistic minority pupils* (pp. 108–122). UK: Sage publications.

De Jong, E. J., & Harper, C. A. (2011). Accommodating diversity: Pre-service teachers' views on effective practices for English language learners. In T. Lucas (Ed.), *Teacher preparation for linguistically diverse classrooms. A resource for teacher educators*. New York: Routledge.

De Jong, E. J., Harper, C. A., & Coady, M. (2013). Enhanced knowledge and skills for elementary mainstream teachers of English Language Learners. *Theory into Practice, 52*(2), 89–97. doi:10.1080/00405841.2013.770326

De Lamo White, C., & Jin, L. (2011). Evaluation of speech and language assessment approaches with bilingual children. *International Journal of Language & Communication Disorders, 46*(6), 613–627. doi:10.1111/j.1460-6984.2011.00049.x PMID:22026564

Dollaghan, C., & Campbell, T. (1998). Nonword repetition and child language impairment. *Journal of Speech, Language, and Hearing Research: JSLHR, 41*(5), 1136–1146. doi:10.1044/jslhr.4105.1136 PMID:9771635

Dunn, D. M. (2018). Peabody Picture Vocabulary Test – Fifth Edition (PPVT-5). Minneapolis, MN: Pearson Education.

Earland, J., Gilchrist, M., McFarland, L., & Harrison, K. (2011). Dietetics students' perceptions and experiences of interprofessional education. *Journal of Human Nutrition and Dietetics*, *24*(2), 135–143. doi:10.1111/j.1365-277X.2010.01141.x PMID:21332834

Ellis Weismer, S., Tomblin, B., Zhang, X., Buckwalter, P., Chynoweth, J., & Jones, M. (2000). Nonword repetition performance in school-age children with and without language impairment. *Journal of Speech, Language, and Hearing Research: JSLHR*, *43*(4), 865–878. doi:10.1044/jslhr.4304.865 PMID:11386474

Figueroa, R. A. (1989). Psychological testing of linguistic-minority students: Knowledge gaps and regulations. *Exceptional Children*, *56*(2), 145–153. doi:10.1177/001440298905600206 PMID:2792161

Fletcher, J. M., Lyon, G. R., Fuchs, L. S., & Barnes, M. A. (2019). *Learning disabilities: From identification to intervention* (2nd ed.). New York, NY: Guilford Press.

Fletcher, J. M., & Miciak, J. (2017). Comprehensive cognitive assessments are not necessary for the identification and treatment of learning disabilities. *Archives of Clinical Neuropsychology*, *32*, 2–7.

Fletcher, J. M., Stuebing, K. K., Barth, A. E., Denton, C. A., Cirino, P. T., Francis, D. J., & Vaughn, S. (2011). Cognitive correlates of inadequate response to reading intervention. *School Psychology Review*, *40*(1), 3–22. PMID:23125475

Fletcher, J. M., Stuebing, K. K., Morris, R. D., & Lyon, G. R. (2013). Classification and definition of learning disabilities: A hybrid model. In H. L. Swanson, K. R. Harris, & S. Graham (Eds.), *Handbook of learning disabilities*. New York, NY: The Guilford Press.

Ford, D. Y. (2012). Culturally different students in special education: Looking backward to move forward. *Exceptional Children*, *78*(4), 391–405. doi:10.1177/001440291207800401

Fouriea, I., & van Niekerk, D. (2001). Follow-up on the use of portfolio assessment for a module in research information skills: An analysis of its value. *Education for Information*, *19*(2), 107–126. doi:10.3233/EFI-2001-19202

Gathercole, S. E., & Alloway, T. P. (2006). Practitioner review: Short-term and working memory impairments in neurodevelopmental disorders: Diagnosis and remedial support. *Journal of Child Psychology and Psychiatry, and Allied Disciplines*, *47*(1), 4–15. doi:10.1111/j.1469-7610.2005.01446.x PMID:16405635

Geary, D. C., & Hoard, M. K. (2001). Numerical and arithmetical deficits in learning-disabled children: Relation to dyscalculia and dyslexia. *Aphasiology*, *15*(7), 635–647. doi:10.1080/02687040143000113

Genesee, F., Lindholm-Leary, K., Saunders, W., & Christian, D. (2005). English language learn-ers in U.S. schools: An overview of research findings. *Journal of Education for Students Placed at Risk*, *10*(4), 363–385. doi:10.120715327671espr1004_2

Ginieri-Coccossis, M., Rotsika, V., Skevington, S., Papaevangelou, S., Malliori, M., Tomaras, V., & Kokkevi, A. (2013). Quality of life in newly diagnosed children with specific learning disabilities (SpLD) and differences from typically developing children: A study of child and parent reports. *Child: Care, Health and Development*, *39*(4), 581–591. doi:10.1111/j.1365-2214.2012.01369.x PMID:22372869

Goh, S. K. Y., & Ng, C. W. (2015). Hard truths about Chinese language policy and planning in Singapore. *Global Chinese*, *1*, 267–279.

Goh, S. K. Y., Tham, E. K. H., Magiati, I., Sim, L., Sanmugam, S., Aiu, A., ... Rifkin-Graboi, A. (2017). Analysis of item-level bias in the Bayley-III Language Subscales: The validity and utility of standardized language assessment in a multilingual setting. *Journal of Speech, Language, and Hearing Research: JSLHR*, *60*(9), 2663–2671. doi:10.1044/2017_JSLHR-L-16-0196 PMID:28813555

Haft, S., Duong, P. H., Hp, T., Hendren, R., & Hoeft, F. (2018). Anxiety and attentional bias in children with specific learning disorders. *Journal of Abnormal Child Psychology*. Retrieved from https://link.springer.com/article/10.1007/s10802-018-0458-y

Hanson, M. F., & Gilkerson, D. (1999). Portfolio assessment: More than ABCs and 123s. *Early Childhood Education Journal*, *27*(2), 81–86. doi:10.1023/A:1026044126583

Hedge, M. N., & Pomaville, F. (2008). *Assessment of communication disorders in children*. San Diego, CA: Plural Publishing.

Hoepfl, M. (1993). Portfolio assessment. *Technology Teacher*, *53*(2), 28–29.

Hoff, E., Core, C., Place, S., Rumiche, R., Señor, M., & Parra, M. (2012). Dual language exposure and early bilingual development. *Journal of Child Language*, *39*(1), 1–27. doi:10.1017/S0305000910000759 PMID:21418730

Jalomo, R. Jr. (2000). Assessing minority student performance. *New Directions for Community Colleges*, *112*(112), 7–18. doi:10.1002/cc.11201

Kids Count Data Center (KCDC). (2018). *The number of bilingual kids in America continues to rise*. Retrieved from https://datacenter.kidscount.org/updates/show/184-the-number-of-bilingual-kids-in-america-continues-to-rise?utm_source=eblast&utm_medium=email&utm_campaign=KIDS-COUNT

Kids Count Data Center (KCDC). (2019). *Children who speak a language other than English at home in the United States*. Retrieved on Sep 28th, 2019 online from https://datacenter.kidscount.org/data/tables/81-children-who-speak-a-language-other-than-english-at-home#detailed/1/any/false/871,870,573,869,36,868,867,133,38,35/any/396,397

Klingner, J. K., & Edwards, P. A. (2006). Cultural considerations with response to intervention models. *Reading Research Quarterly*, *41*(1), 108–117. doi:10.1598/RRQ.41.1.6

Kohnert, K., & Bates, E. (2002). Balancing bilinguals II: Lexical comprehension and cognitive processing in children learning Spanish and English. *Journal of Speech, Language, and Hearing Research: JSLHR*, *45*(2), 347–359. doi:10.1044/1092-4388(2002/027) PMID:12003516

Laing, S., & Kamhi, A. (2003). Alternative assessment of language and literacy in culturally and linguistically diverse populations. *Language, Speech, and Hearing Services in Schools*, *34*(1), 44–55. doi:10.1044/0161-1461(2003/005) PMID:27764486

Langdon, H. W. (2008). *Assessment and intervention for communication disorders in culturally and linguistically diverse populations*. Clifton, NY: Cengage.

Langdon, H. W. (2015). For parents raising their children bilingually with important messages for those who have children with special needs. *Health Psychology Review*, *3*(2), 1–9.

Levey, S., Cheng, L.L., & Langdon, H.W. (2013). The relationship between ethical principles and clinical practice in working with culturally and linguistically diverse (CLD) populations: A tutorial. *Speech and Hearing Review: A bilingual Annual, 11*, 77-104.

Linan-Thompson, S., Cirino, P. T., & Vaughn, S. (2007). Determining English Language Learners' Response to Intervention: Questions and some answers. *Learning Disability Quarterly*, *30*(3), 185–195. doi:10.2307/30035563

Maki, K. E., & Adams, S. R. (2018). A current landscape of specific learning disability identification: Training, practices, and implications. *Psychology in the Schools*, *56*(1), 18–31. doi:10.1002/pits.22179

Maki, K. E., Floyd, R. G., & Roberson, T. (2015). State learning disability eligibility criteria: A comprehensive review. *School Psychology Quarterly*, *30*(4), 457–469. doi:10.1037pq0000109 PMID:25581001

Marquardt, T. P., & Gillam, R. B. (1999). Assessment in communication disorders: Some observations on current issues. *Language Testing*, *16*(3), 249–269. doi:10.1177/026553229901600302

Migration Policy Institute. (2016). *ELL information center*. Retrieved from http://www.migrationpolicy.org/programs/ell-information-center

Minke, K. M., Sheridan, S. M., Kim, E. M., Ryoo, J. H., & Koziol, N. A. (2014). Congruence in parent-teacher relationships. *The Elementary School Journal*, *114*(4), 527–546. doi:10.1086/675637

Morgan, P. L., Farkas, G., Hillemeier, M. M., Mattison, R., Maczuga, S., Li, H., & Cook, M. (2015). Minorities are disproportionately underrepresented in special education: Longitudinal across five disability conditions. *Educational Researcher*, *44*(5), 278–292. doi:10.3102/0013189X15591157 PMID:27445414

Myer, M. (1969). *Frog, where are you?* New York: Dial Press.

Myers, P., & Hammill, D. (1976). *Methods for learning disorders*. New York, N.Y.: Wiley.

Oller, J. W. Jr. (1979). *Language tests at school*. Longman Group UK Limited.

Oller, J. W. Jr. (1997). Monoglottosis: What's wrong with the idea of the IQ meritocracy and its racy cousins? *Applied Linguistics*, *18*(4), 467–507. doi:10.1093/applin/18.4.467

Oller, J. W. Jr, Kim, K., & Choe, Y. (2000). Testing verbal (language) and non-verbal abilities in language minorities: A socio-educational problem in historical perspective. *Language Testing*, *17*(3), 341–360. doi:10.1177/026553220001700304

Oller, J. W. Jr, Kim, K., Choe, Y., & Jarvis, L. H. (2001). Testing relations between language (verbal) and nonverbal abilities in children and adults acquiring a nonprimary language. *Language Testing*, *18*(1), 33–54. doi:10.1177/026553220101800102

Ooi, C. C.-W., & Wong, A. M.-Y. (2012). Assessing bilingual Chinese – English young children in Malaysia using language sample measures. *International Journal of Speech-Language Pathology*, *14*(6), 499–508. doi:10.3109/17549507.2012.712159 PMID:23039126

Owens, R. E. Jr, Meta, D. E., & Haas, A. (2002). *Communication disorders: A life span perspective*. New York, NY: Pearson Education.

Palardy, J. M. (1994). Theoretical underpinning of portfolio assessment. *Journal of Instructional Psychology*, *21*(1), 90–93.

Pewewardy, C., & Fitzpatrick, M. (2009). Working with American Indian students and families: Disabilities, issues, and interventions. *Intervention in School and Clinic*, *45*(2), 91–98. doi:10.1177/1053451209340223

Reuterskiold-Wagner, C., Sahlen, B., & Nyman, A. (2005). Non-word repetition and non-word discrimination in Swedish preschool children. *Clinical Linguistics & Phonetics*, *19*(8), 681–699. doi:10.1080/02699200400000343 PMID:16147409

Rodekohr, R. K., & Haynes, W. O. (2001). Differentiating dialect from disorder: A comparison of two processing tasks and a standardized language test. *Journal of Communication Disorders*, *34*(3), 255–272. doi:10.1016/S0021-9924(01)00050-8 PMID:11409607

Rossignol, L. N., & Paasche-Orlow, M. K. (2013). Empowering patients who have specific learning disabilities. *Journal of the American Medical Association*, *310*(14), 1445. doi:10.1001/jama.2013.278068 PMID:24052008

Rumbaut, R. G., & Massey, D. S. (2013). Immigration & language diversity in the United States. *Daedalus*, *142*(3), 141–154. doi:10.1162/DAED_a_00224 PMID:25018562

Schultz, E. K., Simpson, C. G., & Lynch, S. A. (2012). Specific learning disability identification: What constitutes a pattern of strengths and weaknesses? *Learning Disabilities*, *18*(2), 87–97.

Scott, A. N., Hauerwas, L. B., & Brown, R. D. (2014). State policy and guidance for identifying learning disabilities in culturally and linguistically diverse students. *Learning Disability Quarterly*, *37*(3), 172–185. doi:10.1177/0731948713507261

Sharfi, K., & Rosenblum, S. (2014). Activity and participation characteristics of adults with learning disabilities - a systematic review. *PLoS One*, *9*(9), e106657. doi:10.1371/journal.pone.0106657 PMID:25184315

Simons, G. F., & Fennig, C. D. (Eds.). (2017), *Ethnologue: Language of the world* (12th ed.). Dallas, TX: SIL International. Retrieved from http://www.ethnologue.com

Uhry, J., & Clark, D. (1995). *Dyslexia: Theory & practice of instruction*. Austin, TX: Pro-ed.

Valdes, G., & Figueroa, R. A. (1994). *Bilingualism and testing: A special case of bias*. Norwood, NJ: Ablex.

Vygotsky, L. S. (1978). *Mind in society: The development of higher psychological processes*. Cambridge, MA: Harvard University Press.

Vygotsky, L. S. (1986). *Thought and language*. Cambridge, MA: The MIT Press.

Wiig, E. H., Semel, E., & Secord, W. A. (2013). Clinical Evaluation of Language Fundamentals –Fifth Edition (CELF-5). Bloomington, MN: NCS Pearson.

Williams, C. J., & McLeod, S. (2012). Speech-language pathologists' assessment and intervention practices with multilingual children. *International Journal of Speech-Language Pathology*, *14*(3), 292–305. doi:10.3109/17549507.2011.636071 PMID:22472031

Williams, K. T. (2007). Expressive Vocabulary Test – Second Edition (EVT-2). Circle Pines, MN: American Guidance Service.

Yan, R. (2009). *Assessing English language proficiency in international aviation: Issues of reliability, validity, and aviation safety*. Saarbrucken, Germany: VDM.

Yan, R. (2013). Assessing the English language proficiency of international aviation staff. In A. J. Kunnan (Ed.), *The companion to language assessment (CLA)* (pp. 484–496). Chichester, UK: Wiley-Blackwell. doi:10.1002/9781118411360.wbcla050

Yan, R., & Oller, J. W. Jr. (2007). Processing-dependent measures as a failed solution to the assessment of individuals from language and dialect minorities. *Communicative Disorders Review*, *1*(3-4), 201–213.

Zirkel, P. A. (2018). The legal meaning of special education eligibility: The latest case law. *Communique*, *46*(7), 14–16.

ADDITIONAL READING

Gort, M., Glenn, W. J., & Settlage, J. (2011). Toward culturally and linguistically responsive teacher education: The impact of a faculty learning community on two teacher educators. In T. Lucas (Ed.), *Teacher preparation for linguistically diverse classrooms. A resource for teacher educators* (pp. 178–194). New York: Routledge.

Kauschke, C., & Klann-Delius, G. (1997). The acquisition of verbal expressions for internal states in German. A descriptive, explorative, longitudinal study. In S. Niemeier & R. Dirven (Eds.), *The language of emotions* (pp. 173–194). Amsterdam: Benjamins. doi:10.1075/z.85.13kau

Kim, K., & Ko, L. (2014). Attitudes toward interprofessional health care teams scale: A confirmatory factor analysis. *Journal of Interprofessional Care*, *28*(2), 149–154. doi:10.3109/13561820.2013.857645 PMID:24329713

Learning Disabilities Association of America. (2018). *New to LD*. Retrieved August 24, 2018, from https://ldaamerica.org/support/new-to-ld/

Robben, S., Perry, M., van Nieuwenhuijzen, L., van Achterberg, T., Rikkert, M. O., Schers, H., ... Melis, R. (2012). Impact of interprofessional education on collaboration: Attitudes, skills, and behavior among primary care professionals. *The Journal of Continuing Education in the Health Professions*, *32*(3), 196–204. doi:10.1002/chp.21145 PMID:23008082

Uro, G., & Barrio, A. (2013). *English Language Learners in America's great city schools: Demographics, achievement, and staffing*. Washington, DC: Council of Great City Schools.

Yan, R. (2009). *Assessing English language proficiency in international aviation: Issues of reliability, validity, and aviation safety*. Saarbrucken, Germany: VDM.

KEY TERMS AND DEFINITIONS

Content Bias: The influence of a CLD student's unfamiliarity with language/culture-bound content of the test.

Disproportionate Representation: Over-representation of CLD individuals as disordered and under-representation of them as gifted.

Dynamic Assessment: One alternative to standardized testing methods. The concept of dynamic assessment was developed by Vygotsky, and a learning component is integrated with the assessment.

Interprofessional Collaboration: Multiple health care workers from different professional backgrounds that work together with patients, families, etc. to deliver the highest quality of care to patients.

Linguistic Bias: The influence caused by an examiner's being unfamiliar with the examinee's culture and/or language.

Portfolio Assessment: A testing format that contains a collection of performances of a student over time.

Specific Learning Disability (SLD): A disorder characterized by one or more significant impairments in reading, spelling, writing, or mathematical skills, which are not the direct result of other disorders or inadequate schooling.

Chapter 8
Working With Deaf and Hard-of-Hearing Children From Linguistically Diverse Backgrounds

Karen Garrido-Nag
Gallaudet University, USA

James McCann
Gallaudet University, USA

EXECUTIVE SUMMARY

An increasing number of deaf and hard-of-hearing (D/HH) children live in homes where languages other than English or American Sign Language (ASL) are used. This chapter reviews issues of culture and linguistic diversity when working with D/HH multilingual learners (DMLs) from identification and early intervention through school entry. The authors will provide two case studies to explore the issues of service delivery to DMLs and their families: 1) Ji-Hun, who appears to use several spoken languages, including Korean, Japanese, and English, and 2) Ana, who is a recent immigrant to the USA and appears to use ASL, spoken Spanish, and spoken English. The discussion of these two case studies will encompass some cultural differences, including 1) openness to engagement with providers, 2) cultural beliefs about hearing loss, 3) community systems and familiar support, 4) perceptions of systems and authorities. The case studies presented are not based on actual clients but are drawn from the clinical experiences of the authors.

INTRODUCTION

According to National Center for Education Statistics (2019), English language learners (ELLs) account for 9.5% of all the students who are enrolled in public schools. The most recent data available from the Gallaudet Research Institute Annual Survey (Gallaudet Research Institute, 2013) indicated that 18.3%

DOI: 10.4018/978-1-7998-2261-5.ch008

of deaf or hard-of-hearing (D/HH) children in public schools were identified as ELLs. Furthermore, 35% of the families in the Gallaudet Research Institute survey reported using a language other than English or American Sign Language (ASL) in the home, suggesting that identification of ELLs for the purposes of the *No Child Left Behind* initiative reporting may underestimate the number of D/HH children in multilingual environments. Even though these statistics indicate a significant proportion of D/HH children are D/HH multilingual learners (DMLs), compared to the hearing multilingual population, very little information is available about how to provide appropriate services that account for their diversity. Furthermore, the literature on service provision to DMLs may be obscured by philosophical issues related to communication modality.

It is well documented that children who are D/HH are at risk for poor language, social-emotional, and academic outcomes (Spencer & Marschark, 2010). The primary risk factor is not the hearing loss itself, but the lack of an accessible language (Knoors & Marschark, 2014; Lederberg, Schick, & Spencer, 2013). Children living in the U.S. who come from households where English is not the primary language face a more challenging task because they may need to negotiate English, ASL, and the spoken and/or signed language(s) which they use in the home. Linguistic and cultural diversity has implications for service delivery from diagnosis through transition to post-secondary settings.

Pediatric hearing loss is estimated to affect 5-15% of the population (Centers for Disease Control & Prevention, 2016). One percent of school-age children with an individualized education program (IEP) receive services based on a code related to hearing loss (American Speech-Language-Hearing Association, 2016; U.S. Department of Education, Office for Special Education, 2019). More than 90% of deaf children are born to hearing parents (Mitchell & Karchmer, 2004), and 35-40% have other conditions/disabilities (Gallaudet Research Institute, 2010; Yoshinaga-Itano, Sedey, Coulter, & Mehl, 1998). Almost 45% of speech-language pathologists (SLPs) who work in a school setting regularly serve children with hearing loss. Early Hearing Detection and Intervention programs have significantly decreased the age at which childhood hearing loss is diagnosed and early intervention services can be initiated (Gaffney, Green, & Gaffney, 2010; Yoshinaga-Itano, 2003). The younger age of diagnosis and subsequent early intervention have shown promising results for developmental outcomes. However, no known studies specifically on outcome measures for DMLs exist.

Upon the diagnosis of hearing loss, families face a decision in determining the communication modality (Table 1) they will use with their children (Decker, Vallotton, & Johnson, 2012). Parents receive and must consider this new information while still processing the emotional response to the diagnosis (Stredler-Brown, 2010). The selection of a communication approach is stressful to families, and they report valuing accurate, impartial, and respectful information (Meadow-Orlans, Sass-Lehrer, & Mertens, 2003). With earlier age of diagnosis, the historical debate of the correct approach is being replaced with the notion of parental informed choice. Informed choice includes the provision of comprehensive, meaningful, relevant, and evidence-based information, so that parents are empowered to make decisions for their children (Moeller, Carr, Seaver, Stredler-Brown, & Holzinger, 2013; Young et al., 2006). For families from developing countries, attitudes and cultural beliefs towards disability play an important role. There may be a delay in acceptance of a disability, and in the case of hearing loss, hearing technology that may draw further attention to the disability (Olusanya, Luxon, & Wirz, 2004). Counseling services for families should consider diverse cultural orientations.

Furthermore, new opportunities to acquire and develop a variety of skills mean that commitment to a single approach is not necessary. Families report a desire for their children to develop skills and flexibility to choose what is best for them in a variety of contexts (Wainscott, Sass-Lehrer, & Croyle,

Table 1. Educational/communication choices in pediatric cases

Communication Modality	Definition and Use in Practice
Total communication	Philosophy of educating children with hearing loss that incorporates all means of communication (i.e., formal signs, natural gestures, fingerspelling, body language, listening, lipreading and speech). While in philosophy total communication supports the use of all the necessary means, in practice it frequently becomes speaking and signing at the same time.
ASL/English bilingual	Philosophy of education supporting development of both ASL and English (written and/or spoken) as separate, but equal languages.
Bimodal-bilingual	Philosophy supporting acquisition of at least one oral language and at least one sign language.
Auditory/oral	Approach that focuses on acquisition of spoken and written language.
Cued speech	Visual mode of communication that uses handshapes and placements in combination with the mouth movements of speech to make the phonemes of a spoken language look different from each other. *It is usually considered an auditory/oral approach, as the goal is to develop the spoken language.*
Listening and spoken language	Approach that uses primarily audition provided by a hearing aid or a cochlear implant (CI) for understanding speech and learning to talk.
Augmentative alternative communication	System of communication that uses supports or alternatives to spoken or signed languages including devices, whether low- or high- technologies, for individuals who have motor, cognitive, and/or social limitations that limit their acquisition of sign/spoken language.

2008, as cited in Sass-Lehrer, 2017). The Joint Committee on Infant Hearing (2007, 2013), the Joint Committee of the American Speech-Language-Hearing Association (2008), the Council on Education of the Deaf, and an international panel of experts in the field (Moeller et al., 2013) advocate for providing families with unbiased, but evaluative information to make an informed choice and then following up with services that support their choice. When there is a language used in the home besides English or ASL, decisions regarding language choice and communication preference are more complex. The choice involves consideration of sign, spoken English, and signed or spoken languages of the home (Leigh & Crowe, 2015). Families must consider the purposes of each of the languages to which the child will be exposed. When a child transitions from home-based to school-based services, the philosophy of the program will drive communication opportunities at school, where the child will spend most of their day. The parents may choose to align their home-based approach with the school's approach, or they may choose to continue with the strategies they have been using at home. For DMLs, the maintenance of spoken or signed language(s) of the home becomes a center issue for decision making. The family may ask professionals for input. Service providers should listen carefully to the family's concerns and goals for home communication. They counsel the family on the benefits of multilingualism, along with realistic expectations given their child's access or lack of access to the languages in their environment. For a child who has limited access to spoken language, it may not be realistic to use the spoken language of the home. Also, without efforts on behalf of the parents to use the child's communication system, there is risk of the child losing his/her bond with the family.

When working with DML children, it is important to have a good profile of all the languages they use. Standardized assessments are a common assessment strategy. While many assess English language skills, they are not normed on a multilingual sample, which makes scores difficult to interpret. A limited number of assessments of Spanish exist. Very few tests have been developed to assess languages other than English and Spanish, including ASL. Translations of tests which are designed to assess English skills may be attempted by SLPs who are bilingual in the target language, or through an interpreter. The challenge with translated tests is cultural bias toward a mainstream American approach to assessment. Furthermore, by translating, items may increase or decrease in complexity and thereby not assess what they are intending. Working with DMLs requires flexibility to use standardized assessments in a meaningful way, so interpretation does not lead to inaccurate conclusions. The use of supplemental and/or alternate strategies should also be considered. These may include parent report/interview, portfolio assessment, observation in natural settings, and dynamic assessment. Dynamic assessment has been shown to differentiate normal hearing ELL children with typically developing language from ELL children with language disorders (Kapantzoglou, Restrepo, & Thompson, 2012; Pena, Gillam, & Bedore, 2014). Dynamic assessment also has utility with the assessment of a child's ASL acquisition (Mann, Pena, & Morgan, 2014), making it a promising approach for DMLs.

While assessment provides practitioners with a child's current language abilities, progress monitoring of growth is important. Little information is available about how to monitor language growth in the early years even for monolingual children (Gillam & Justice, 2010). The most frequently reported language assessment tools used by professionals working with D/HH children compare a child's language development to same age peers at a single moment in time and are not suitable to measuring incremental changes over brief periods (Gillam & Justice, 2010; Luckner & Bowen, 2006). Monitoring a DML's language acquisition requires consideration of the entire language system and the purposes each serves.

The two case studies in the following section have very different backgrounds, but hearing loss is a common factor.

CASE 1

Questions for the Reader

1. When and where is it appropriate to use an interpreter when working with DML families?
2. How valuable are standardized testing materials for DML cases?
3. How should a monolingual therapist work with multilingual families?

Description of the Case

Ji-Hun Kim is a two-year and eight-month-old multilingual (Korean, Japanese, and English) male who attends a preschool early intervention program five days a week. He has congenital severe to profound bilateral sensorineural hearing loss. His case followed the Joint Committee on Infant Hearing's "1-3-6" goals; his loss was detected via universal newborn hearing screening at birth, diagnosed with audiologic measures appropriate for a three-month-old child, fitted with binaural hearing aids soon after, and enrolled in early intervention services by six months of age. Currently, he has binaural amplification, hearing aid on the left ear, and CI on the right ear that was activated at 20 months of age. The family requested a comprehensive evaluation to assess if Ji-Hun could be transitioned to a regular preschool.

Background Information

Ji-Hun is the only child of immigrant parents and lives in the Washington DC metropolitan area. The household is multigenerational, with parents and maternal grandparents. The mother, Mrs. Kim, speaks mostly Korean with some English and the grandparents speak solely Korean. The father, Mr. Kim, speaks Korean, Japanese, and has some conversational skills in English. The family owns several small shops in the area, and all are involved in running their businesses. Both parents are college educated in Korea. Ji-Hun was born in a local hospital which provided newborn hearing screening according to the District of Columbia-Maryland-Virginia law. Upon failing the newborn hearing screening, the family was referred for follow-up at the audiological clinic in the hospital. The clinic is fully equipped for pediatric testing and is closely tied to a local representative for the Infant and Toddler program for families with infants and toddlers who are D/HH.

There were no reports of complications during pregnancy or delivery. Ji-Hun did not pass his newborn otoacoustic emissions hearing screening, when it was first administered. A follow-up screening was done just before being discharged from the hospital. He did not pass the rescreen on both ears, and the nurses made an appointment with the audiological clinic for evaluation. The nurses used a telephone interpreter to explain to the mother and grandparents the results of the screening and subsequent appointment.

The follow-up appointment was scheduled three weeks after Ji-Hun's birth. A severe to profound hearing loss was diagnosed that day, and hearing aid fitting was scheduled at three months of age. During the same meeting, the parents were connected with the local infant-toddler program representative, who then proceeded to make an in-home appointment for an evaluation. At this point, the parents were hesitant to have strangers come to their house, until it was further explained through an interpreter that the team of professionals that would work with them would help assist in the use of the hearing aids and the development of Ji-Hun's listening skills.

Ji-Hun was fitted with binaural hearing aids at four months of age. At this point, a team comprised of an SLP and a teacher of the deaf worked with the family and Ji-Hun in developing his listening and language skills. The team also worked on counseling the parents regarding communication options, educational options for the future, and participation in group settings where the child had access to D/HH peers and adults as language, communication, and cultural models. The family expressed that they wanted a CI for Ji-Hun. It was explained to the family that at Ji-Hun's age hearing aids would provide him access to sounds and language until he could become a candidate for implantation. The family decided they wanted to use sign-supported speech, primarily focusing on language access through auditory means, but using some signs to aid in understanding of key concepts. A Korean-English interpreter was present the first few weeks of the sessions, until Mrs. Kim expressed, through her husband, wanting communication to be done via written English and would no longer need an interpreter. Intervention sessions were conducted in spoken English; coaching was established through written communication. Mr. and Mrs. Kim and Ji-Hun's grandparents continued to communicate with Ji-Hun in Korean and Japanese. Mr. Kim did switch back and forth between Korean and English with some routines in Japanese. At 20 months of age, Ji-Hun's CI was activated on the right ear. All throughout this time, both the SLP and teacher continued to counsel the family on use of signs to support language development. The family was very resistant on the use of sign and expressed that they thought it would stop Ji-Hun from listening. It was explained to the family that the use of two modalities does not hinder the development of one or the other. The visual reinforcement, thru signs, increased Ji-Hun's access to language. The mother and grandmother initially communicated with Ji-Hun only in spoken English, even though they did this with great difficulty. It was emphasized to the family that the use of Korean is natural and would aid in developing Ji-Hun's language skills. Although they were offered a Korean therapist and/or teacher, the family refused. The family established a good connection with the SLP and teacher of the deaf and did not want to introduce changes to the intervention team. At 24 months of age, a reevaluation was conducted at the request of Ji-Hun's parents for consideration of transition to a regular preschool.

Findings of the Evaluation

Ji-Hun's speech and language skills were assessed in Korean, English, and Japanese even though Mr. and Mrs. Kim only wanted the evaluation to be conducted in English. The team had to explain to his parents that Ji-Hun is multilingual, and his language and speech skills would be best measured in all languages that are used at home and in the community. Knowing his strength in one language would help in determining Ji-Hun capacity for progress. Most of the tests used are normed for monolingual speakers of each language and not necessarily for bi/multilingual speakers.

In order to assess Ji-Hun's skills, the following tests were used:

- Rosetti Infant-Toddler Language Scale (English and Korean)
- Goldman-Fristoe Test of Articulation-2 (English)
- Assessment of Phonology and Articulation for Children (Korean)
- The MacArthur-Bates Communicative Development Inventories (English, Korean and Japanese)
- Audiological testing.

Audiology

Electrophysiological testing was conducted at two months for diagnosis and prior to CI implantation that established the diagnosis of bilateral severe to profound sensorineural hearing loss. Behavioral observation audiometry (BOA) was also conducted before and after hearing aid fitting at four months of age. Visual reinforcement audiometry (VRA) was conducted pre- and post-CI fitting at 20 months of age. For the transition evaluation at 24 months, conditioned play audiometry (CPA) was used. During all three testing situations BOA, VRA, and CPA, the parents were able to observe their child, hear the stimuli, and see their child's responses. This establishes for parents a better sense of what their child is hearing and the importance of moving forward with amplification and confirmation of the electrophysiological test results. These three testing conditions also provided information on how a child is able to attend to auditory stimulation and measure the benefits of amplification.

Language

Ji-Hun's communication was assessed using the Rossetti Infant-Toddler Scale (Rosetti, 2006). It is designed to track development in children over the period birth to 36 months. Information is obtained via caregiver report, clinician observation, and clinician elicitation. The scale assesses preverbal and verbal areas of communication and interaction including interaction-attachment, pragmatics, gesture, play, language comprehension, and language expression. Testing was conducted in both Korean (with an interpreter) and in English. Skills in interaction-attachment, pragmatics, gestures, and play were within

Table 2. Aided thresholds for Ji-Hun obtained via BOA at age 4 months of age, VRA at age 20 months and play audiometry at age 24 months

Method	Age	Threshold (dB HL)				
		250 Hz	500 Hz	1000 Hz	2000 Hz	4000 HZ
BOA	4 months	40	50	50	50	60
VRA	20 months	40	40	50	50	50
CPA	24 months	20	20	25	25	25

normal limits in the Rossetti scale. The results of the testing for language comprehension and language expression were as follows:

- **Language Comprehension:** Ji-Hun's language comprehension skills were solid at the 12-15 months' range, with scattered skills in the 15-18 months' range, indicating a 37% delay. Ji-Hun was reported and/or observed to: Look at person saying child's name, perform a routine activity upon verbal request, follow one-step commands during play, respond to "give me" command, identify three body parts, and choose two familiar objects upon request. Ji-Hun benefited when speech was presented with gestures/signs. Ji-Hun appeared to have more scattered skills at 18 months of age, when he was tested in Korean, with his parents reporting that he could understand at least 50 words and complete two requests with one object. Ji-Hun was neither reported nor observed to find familiar objects not in sight, understand meaning of action words, and understand the command "sit down and come here" without gestures. Comprehension was supported with gestures and simple signs.
- **Language Expression:** Ji-Hun's language expression skills in English were solid at the 12-15 months' range, with scattered skills at the 15-18 months' range, indicating a 37% delay. Ji-Hun was reported and/or observed to: Say 15 meaningful words, ask for more, imitate words, and imitate environmental noises. Ji-Hun was neither reported nor observed to use two-word phrases and use new words regularly. Ji-Hun's language expression skills in Korean were higher than his English skills demonstrated by having more of a scatter at the 18-21 months' range. He imitated two-word phrases and had started to use two-word phrases spontaneously. He was also reported to be using sentence-like intonational patterns once in a while.

Phonology

Two tests were used to assess Ji-Hun's articulation and phonology:

1. The Goldman-Fristoe Test of Articulation-2 (Goldman & Fristoe, 2000), which assesses the child's production of English consonant sounds in single words and in sentences. This test was attempted to assess consonants in various word positions. However, testing could not be completed, as Ji-Hun could not name or imitate names of most of the stimulus pictures. Based on progress reports, parental report, and observation of Ji-Hun's one-word productions and vocalizations, Ji-Hun's phonemic repertoire included /p, b, m, k, l, h/ and his vowel repertoire included most vowel sounds when he imitated. However, spontaneous production of vowels tended to be turned into a schwa

Figure 1. Overlap in Korean and English consonants and vowels

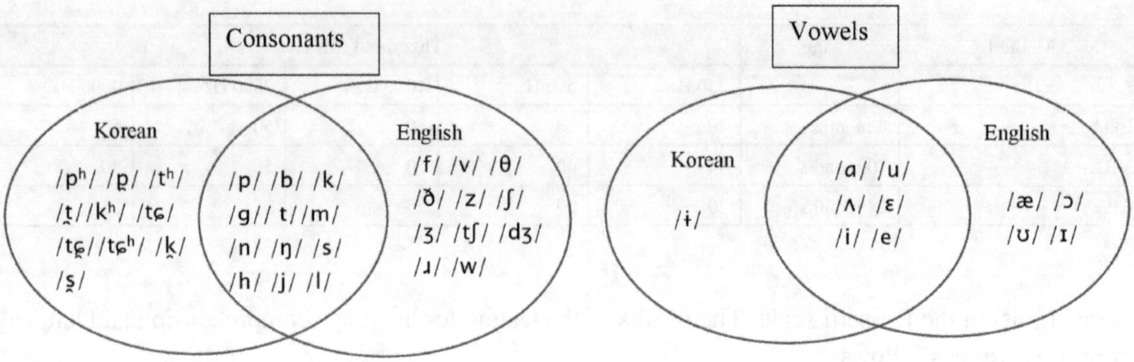

/ə/. His syllable shapes were primarily consonant-vowel (CV) and CVCV. Ji-Hun would also talk, using a wide variety of sounds and intonations. Ji-Hun's speech intelligibility was on average rated at 50%.

2. Assessment of Phonology and Articulation for Children (Kim, Pae, & Bak, 2007), which assesses the child's production of Korean consonant and vowel speech sounds in single words and connected speech, as well as phonological processes. Ji-Hun's phonemic and vowel repertoire mirrored that of his English productions. However, Ji-Hun had longer utterances with some CVC words in Korean aside from CV and CVCV. Ji-Hun's speech intelligibility in Korean was on average rated at 75% by his parents.

Ji-Hun used gestures to communicate including waving, pointing, and leading with his hand, and bodily gestures, such as indicating going to the bathroom and wanting to eat. Figure 1 shows the phonemic overlap between Korean and English.

Vocabulary

The MacArthur-Bates Communicative Development Inventories (Fenson et al., 2007) are parent report instruments which capture important information about children's developing abilities in early language, including vocabulary comprehension, production, gestures, and grammar. The infant form (level I) was used to assess Ji-Hun's vocabulary inventory (Table 3). Ji-Hun performed at less than the 1st percentile for all three languages he uses. However, he performed better in Korean than in English. He had a few words in Japanese that he used but these words were mostly related to specific routines he engaged in with his father.

Recommendations

Based on the results of the assessment and progress with intervention services, the individualized family service plan (IFSP) team recommended that Ji-Hun continue with his individual and group therapy and transition to a D/HH Preschool Program that would focus on language and communication skills devel-

Table 3. Infant form level 1 results for Ji-Hun

	Understands	Understands and Says	Percentile
Korean	50	30	<1th
English	30	15	<1th
Japanese	5	5	<1th

opment along with preacademic skills. The team also recommended a total communication approach to communication, with emphasis on a bilingual/multilingual approach (Korean-English-Sign). Some of the specific recommendations included:

1. Continue to encourage the parents to use gestures and signs when communicating with Ji-Hun. Reintroduce resources for group activities, parental support groups, and community activities.
2. Provide continuous and consistent counselling on the role each language plays (Korean, English, and Sign language) on Ji-Hun's speech and language development, especially since he was newly implanted and changes in his hearing skills would have probably occurred. Counseling should emphasize the importance of access to language.
3. Take a tour of different preschool settings for Ji-Hun. His parents had a strong desire to send Ji-Hun to a regular preschool program and this might not be the best setting for Ji-Hun at his current stage of development.
4. Continuously monitor Ji-Hun's cognitive, preacademic, social-emotional, speech, and language development in all his languages. Bi/multilingual cases are often complex, with multiple factors (i.e., each language, cultural differences, and interaction differences) influencing development. With limited evidence for best practice, assessment tools and treatment approaches, it is crucial that intervention should be based on a thorough assessment via dynamic assessment of Ji-Hun's skills.

Discussion of Questions for the Reader

1. *When and where is it appropriate to use an interpreter when working with DML families?* An interpreter is a person trained to convey spoken or signed communications from one language to another. Interpretation services may be provided in person; by phone; using videoconferencing services; and/or using apps available via electronic devices, such as tablets, computers, and smartphones. Sometimes an interpreter may act as a cultural or linguistic broker. A broker is a person knowledgeable about the child's culture and/or community or communication environment. When working with interpreters, service providers remain responsible for planning the session, selecting culturally relevant materials, and appropriately administering assessment and treatment. The interpreter assists the clinician in gathering the appropriate data and provides language support for services appropriate to the child.

The use of an interpreter is both necessary and required when dealing with multilingual speakers particularly if the service provider does not share all the languages with the child. It is mandated by IDEA that assessment materials and procedures should not be racially and culturally discriminatory and should be provided in the client's native language. It is also the ethical step to follow to avoid incorrectly labeling a child and in determination of eligibility for services.

The service provider is responsible for optimizing the collaboration with the interpreter. Successful interpretation could happen when: (1) selecting an interpreter who could be trained to meet the qualifications, skills and knowledge required for effective interpretation, 2) preparing the interpreter for the assessment or intervention process, and (3) observing verbal and non-verbal cues from both the child and the interpreter to ensure validity of the process.

In the case of Ji-Hun an interpreter was used for multiple instances from his newborn hearing screening at the hospital to his most recent re-evaluation. This guaranteed a valid and reliable assessment result as well as full access to communication during intervention, not only for Ji-Hun but also for his family.

2. *How valuable are standardized testing materials for DML cases?* Standardized test scores or norm-referenced testing, are not valid for an individual who is not included in the normative sample for that assessment. However, these types of assessments could provide descriptive information regarding the child's abilities or limitations in a given language. A test given in English will inform us of the child's ability in English while a test given in Korean will inform us the child's ability in Korean. Standardized assessments that are not normed to multilingual populations are only to be used as informal probes without use of scores. Criterion-referenced assessment tools could be given in a standardized manner and be can used to evaluate a child's strength and weakness. A profile of the child's strength and weaknesses could serve as a guideline for intervention setting or as a starting point for a more naturalistic evaluation such dynamic assessment.

As best as possible, use linguistically and culturally adapted test equivalents in both languages or in multiple languages to compare strengths and weaknesses of the child. Modifications or accommodations to standardized assessments may be needed to gain insight into the child's performance. It is crucial that these modifications or accommodations be reported for proper interpretation of the data. Examples of modifications and accommodations are rewording questions, providing additional cues, using an alternative scoring rubric, and allowing extra time for responses.

As for the case of Ji-Hun, assessment relied heavily on use of criterion-referenced tests that created a profile of his strengths and weaknesses. Standardized measures were used for each language spoken at home, but results were used in a descriptive manner.

3. *How should a monolingual therapist work with multilingual families?* Service provision for children who are multilingual varies depending on the linguistic and cultural profile of the child. Bilingual or multilingual interventionist, who may have the expertise, may not always be available. Service providers should also know their own linguistic and cultural proficiency and determine if they can meet the demands of the child and the family.

When bilingual or multilingual service providers are not available, using an interpreter is the second option. Please see the answer to question #a on how to collaborate with interpreters.

Ethically, service providers are bound to provide linguistically and culturally appropriate services that include assessment, diagnosis, treatment, and discharge. Service provision should always include consideration of how communication disorders might be demonstrated in the child's linguistic and cultural community.

In the case of Ji-Hun, his service providers were both proficient in English and ASL and did not share the dominant language used in the home. Interpreters were used on multiple occasions and even after a Korean speaking SLP and teacher were found, the family decided to stay with their current providers. A communication method that was effective for both the family and service providers was established.

CASE 2

Questions for the Reader

1. How does diagnosis of a significant hearing loss affect speech-language assessment with children from a culturally and linguistically diverse background?
2. How does family language use contribute to language acquisition for DMLs?
3. How do service providers use interprofessional practice in assessment and intervention with DMLs who use sign language?

Background Information

Ana is a four-year, 11-month-old female who is navigating a multilingual environment. She lives with her parents, two older siblings, paternal grandparents, paternal aunt, and one older cousin. Her family uses primarily spoken Spanish at home, although her two older siblings (ages eight and 12) and older cousin (17) speak English to each other. She also attends a D/HH prekindergarten program five days a week for six hours a day. The school uses a total-communication philosophy, which includes spoken English, ASL, and sign-supported speech. Because Ana has made good progress since her initial eligibility and she will be transitioning to Kindergarten, the team recommended having her reevaluation early, at the end of her prekindergarten year. The IEP team recommended an updated speech-language assessment as part of the evaluation process.

Ana immigrated to the U.S. with her family from a rural village in Honduras when she was two years and eight months old. She currently lives in a suburban community in Maryland, outside of Washington DC. She had limited medical care in her country of origin. By the time her family moved to the US, they were becoming increasingly concerned by her lack of spoken language. During her first visit to the pediatrician in the U.S., the parents shared their concerns, but also reported that family members had told them not to worry since many children start to talk late and she was a "very smart child." Their concerns included that Ana did not use any speech to communicate and that she only listened when she was looking at them and when they gestured. The pediatrician referred Ana for an audiological exam.

Ana was seen for an audiological exam at two years and 11 months old. Otoscopy was unremarkable. Immittance testing was consistent with the type and degree of hearing loss. The audiologist used conditioned play audiometry in the sound field to obtain pure tone results. Results indicated a severe at 500Hz and 1000Hz sloping to profound at 2000Hz sensorineural hearing loss in the better ear. Ear specific information was not obtained at this time.

The audiologist counseled the family regarding the hearing loss, its impact on spoken language development, communication modalities, and hearing assistive technology. She also referred the family to the Child Find office of the Local Education Agency. The family indicated they were not opposed to sign language as part of Ana's communication profile, but also wanted her to develop spoken language.

They expressed primary interest in spoken English so she could function in the American educational system and be successful in the US, but also spoken Spanish so she could participate in the family and home community. They expressed concern about sign language preventing her from using any form of spoken language.

Ana was fit with bilateral digital hearing aids obtained from the state hearing aid loan bank. Following a trial period, it was noted that Ana received little benefit from the hearing aids; information about CIs was provided. The family initially expressed hesitation with the CI surgery due to concern about putting their young child through sedation. The educational team counseled the family on realistic expectations for developing spoken language in either English or Spanish given Ana's limited progress in auditory development with the hearing aids. The family ultimately decided to go forward with a unilateral CI on the right ear. Ana's CI was activated when she was three years and eight months old.

Ana was evaluated by the Child Find team at three years old. The Preschool-Language Scales, 5th Edition Spanish (PLS-5 Spanish) (Zimmerman, Steiner, & Pond, 2012) were administered by a bilingual SLP. Due to Ana's significant hearing loss, she did not demonstrate comprehension of any spoken language, nor did she produce any intelligible words. Results from the PLS-5 indicated receptive and expressive language skills that were significantly discrepant from same age peers but provided limited information for treatment planning. Even though choosing the PLS-5 demonstrated sensitivity to language background, it was not sensitive to the needs of a child with severe to profound hearing loss who has not had access to speech or sign. The SLP described gesture and play to inform treatment planning. Ana was observed to follow directions that were gestured when given an object. She pointed to direct the clinician's attention to preferred objects and pointed followed by an "uh-oh" gesture to comment when a toy fell off the table. The family reported that she understood familiar home gestures for "drink" and "garbage." She engaged in joint attention using eye gaze between the clinician and objects and participated in play routines that were initiated by the SLP. She demonstrated relational and symbolic play. Her parents reported that at home she combines actions into entire play scenarios; she loves to feed and dress dolls and put them to bed. While she did not use any spoken language during the evaluation, she did vocalize to get attention from the SLP and her parents. Given her intentional gestures and play skills, the prognosis for language acquisition was reported to be good once language was accessible.

Due to Ana's documented hearing loss, a teacher of the D/HH participated in place of the special education evaluator who typically administers the developmental assessment battery covering cognitive, fine and gross motor, social-emotional, and adaptive domains. Ana demonstrated age-appropriate fine and gross motor skills. Scores on the developmental battery suggested cognitive, social-emotional and adaptive skills that were discrepant from same age peers. Early childhood assessments of cognitive, social-emotional, and adaptive skills often rely on some stimuli that require language for comprehension or expression. For a child with late-identified hearing loss, the severe language delays may confound results from other domains. The teacher of the D/HH completed an items analysis and determined that reporting these scores would be invalid and potentially provide a skewed picture of her skills. Instead, she used qualitative data to indicate that although Ana does not yet demonstrate many skills in the areas of cognitive, social-emotional, and adaptive development due to significant language delays, her development in these domains, considering nonverbal actions and behaviors, is not discrepant from children of her same age. She indicated that the school-based team should monitor her thinking, problem-solving, social, and adaptive skills, but targeting non-linguistic aspects of those domains was not warranted. The focus of Ana's intervention plan should be on development of language which should also allow her to demonstrate improvement in other developmental domains.

Based on the results of the initial evaluation, Ana was determined to be eligible for special education and related services under the IDEA code of deafness. Her IEP was developed and she received special instruction by a teacher of the D/HH, the related service of speech-language therapy, and consultative audiology services. She enrolled in the local three-year total-communication program for D/HH children with speech-language therapy provided six times per month for a duration of 30 minutes each. The school used a total-communication philosophy that included ASL, spoken language, and simultaneous communication.

Findings of the Current Evaluation

At the age of four years and 11 months, Ana was referred to the IEP team for reevaluation. The team recommended a comprehensive speech-language assessment to support IEP decisions for her transition into Kindergarten. An important note is that assessment tools in use were developed for D/HH children from homes that used spoken English and/or ASL, and age criteria were derived from children with that background. Due to Ana's complex communication profile, additional information about her spoken Spanish skills was obtained through parents' report and interaction with a Spanish speaking paraprofessional in the classroom.

The following tools were used:

- Profile of Multiple Language Proficiencies (PMLP)
- Ski-Hi Language Development Scale (Ski-Hi LDS)
- Visual Communication and Sign Language Checklist (VCSL)
- Auditory Skills Checklist (ASC)
- Phonetic/phonemic inventory

An interview with Ana's parents revealed that the family used primarily spoken English with limited sign support when communicating with Ana at home. The parents indicated that their limited English impacts the amount of language they provide when interacting with their daughter. They reported that they depended on the older siblings and cousin to provide spoken language input in English. They worried that speaking to her in Spanish would confuse her and that the school would look down on them for using their limited English skills. They reported that they were not opposed to using sign language in the home, but that financial, time, and transportation issues prevented them from accessing sign language learning opportunities in the community.

Audiology

Ana's most recent audiological evaluation was conducted when she was four years and nine months old. Otoscopy was unremarkable and immittance testing was consistent with her type and degree of hearing loss. Conditioned play audiometry was used to obtain pure tone and speech detection thresholds. Unlike the initial exam, the audiologist obtained ear specific measures. Results indicated a severe at 500 Hz and 1000 Hz sloping to profound at 2000 Hz sensorineural hearing loss in her left ear and a relatively flat profound sensorineural hearing loss in her right ear. Speech detection thresholds were consistent with pure-tone results. Pure tone thresholds were also obtained in the sound field while Ana was wearing her CI. She demonstrated responses at 25 dB HL across the frequencies.

Language

Profile of Multiple Language Proficiencies. The PMLP (Goldstein & Bebko, 2003) provides a global indicator of a child's competencies in spoken English and/or sign communication based on language sampling and observation. Eight levels characterize important milestones/transitions in language development: Prelinguistic, Word Combination, Beginning Sentence, Full Simple Sentence, Compound Sentence, Complex Sentence, Early Fluency, and Full Fluency. Levels are provided for a child's use of English, whether spoken or signed English, and ASL. At Ana's early stage of language development, there is significant overlap between items considered signed English and ASL, therefore, a single sign communication level is provided. Ana is currently functioning at Level-II, Word Combination. She uses one- and two-word sign structures, uses at least 25 recognizable signs, is beginning to use adjectives such as "big" and "happy", and indicates a preference when given a choice. She does not use at least 100 recognizable signs, construct short, and novel language samples, or spontaneously related experiences in simple terms.

Ski-Hi Language Development Scale. The Ski-Hi LDS (Ski-Hi Institute, 2004) is a criterion referenced assessment that was designed for D/HH children who use any communication modality. The child may demonstrate the skills through spoken language or sign. For example, a receptive language item at 8-10 months is "regularly stops activity to 'no' (said or signed)." Ana demonstrated all receptive language skills up to the 22-month level. She was observed or reported to: Love to have simple books read (signed) to her, recognize name for many common objects and pictures of common objects, follow three directions/requests signed about the same object, and understand a couple of descriptive words, such as "dirty" or "wet". She was neither reported nor observed to: Understand many signed sentences which may have more than one idea (e.g., "get the book and we'll read the story"), understand concepts of "here" and "now," or follow four directions/requests about the same object. Ana demonstrated all expressive language skills up to the 22-month level. She was observed or reported to: Have a vocabulary of at least 20-50 words, imitate two- and three-word (sign) sentences, combine words into simple ideas ("mommy come"), and answer many requests with "no" (spoken or signed). She was neither reported nor observed to: Use place terms (signs) such as "here," "over there," sign simple negatives such as "no night-night," or have a vocabulary of 50-100 words (signs).

Visual Communication and Sign Language Checklist. The VCSL (Simms, Baker, & Clark, 2013) is an assessment tool that documents sign language growth and identifies gaps or delays in typical language development. It is intended to assist teachers and early childhood service providers in planning language instruction. The VCSL stimulus items are marked as "not yet emerging," "emerging," "inconsistent use," or "mastered." The SLP completed the VCSL using direct observation and input from the teacher and other service providers. Ana obtained a basal of 20 months. Of the children in the norming group, 75% had mastered the language skills which were represented by the items on the checklist to this point by 20 months. Ana demonstrated scattered skills through 32 months. In the two-three-year age range, she demonstrated mastery of the following skills: Request help when needed, use possessives (e.g., my and your), name at least three colors, count from one to five, and identify/match colors. She demonstrated emerging or inconsistent use of the following skills: Use descriptive classifier (e.g., CL: F "spots"), name objects/animals/people in pictures when asked, and point to noun and verb combinations (e.g., "frog jump"). She did not produce three/four sign utterances, demonstrate a vocabulary range of >150 signs, or use commands with two steps (e.g., "you go to room, bring book.").

Spoken Language

Auditory Skills Checklist. The ASC (Meinzen-Derr, Wiley, Creighton, & Choo, 2007) is an evaluation tool that assesses and tracks a child's auditory skill development. The ASC uses a combination of caregiver report and clinician observation. The hierarchy of auditory skills has four levels (Erber, 1982): Detection, discrimination, identification, and comprehension. Detection is the ability to recognize the presence of a sound. Discrimination is the ability to notice whether two sounds are the same or different. Identification is the ability to label, by pointing or repeating back, the speech stimulus that the person hears. Comprehension refers to the ability to understand the meaning of a spoken message by following directions, answering a question, paraphrasing, or participating in a conversation. Ana's parents and young adult cousin served as informants. Ana has demonstrated all the skills at the detection level. She wears her CI during all waking hours, shows awareness of speakers by looking for a source, and detects the Ling Six Sounds (/ɑ/, /u/, /i/, /m/, /s/, and /ʃ/). At the discrimination level, she discriminates the voice of a speaker from environmental sounds, types of environmental sounds, singing from conversation, and family member voices. She does not discriminate minimal pairs or similar sounding phrases and sentences. At the identification level, she identifies when her name is called. She also identifies the Learning to Listen animal and vehicle sounds from a closed set of three, the Ling Six Sounds, and familiar songs through pointing to object or picture representations. She continues to need support with speech production to identify sounds and syllables through repeating back a stimulus. She demonstrates emerging identification of words that differ by syllable number during structured tasks. She does not yet identify highly contrastive words with the same number of syllables (e.g., "house," "man," "sock"), or minimal pairs with segments that vary by multiple place/manner/voice features (e.g., "fight," "night," "kite") or one place/manner/voice feature (e.g., "key," "pea," "tea") which may be expected due to her delays in overall language skills. She does not demonstrate auditory skills at the comprehension level.

Phonetic and phonemic inventories. Phonetic and phonemic inventories were collected through elicitation of a language sample and observation. Ana demonstrates a limited repertoire of intelligible speech sounds. In English, she produces the word "no", the animal sound "moo," the exclamation "uh-oh," and the following approximations: "Stop," /ɑp/; "yes," /jə/; "my," /mɑ/; "want," /wʌ/; "wait," /we/. She also approximates the animal sound "quack", /wə/. These approximations are intelligible to familiar listeners in context. By parent report, in Spanish, she produces the word "no" and approximations of "más" (more), /mɑ/, and "leche" (milk), /le.ə/. She has not demonstrated use of Spanish approximations at school, even when interacting with the Spanish-speaking paraprofessional. She also produces the following sounds in isolation during structured activities: /ɑ/, /u/, /i/, /m/, /x/ (when attempting to imitate both /s/ and /ʃ/).

- **Phonetic:** /ɑ, u, i, e, ə, o, ʌ, j, p x, m, w, n, d, b/ and "raspberry."
- **Phonemic:** /ɑ, ʌ, i, u, o, e, j, p, m, w, n, l/.

Impressions

Data from the PMLP, Ski-Hi LDS, VCSL, and informal observations are consistent and suggest that Ana's overall language skills are significantly below age expectations. She demonstrates solid skills through 22-months, with scattered skills through 32-months. This is not surprising, given the language deprivation she experienced before her hearing loss was identified. Although Ana demonstrates language skills that are approximately three years below those of her same age peers, she has made significant gains in language acquisition. It is important to note that she only has exposure to sign language during school hours based on the family's report that sign is not used in the home. The trial hearing aid period gave her little benefit in accessing spoken language information, so she has only had consistent access to speech information since activation of her CI. Yet, she has made steady progress in her auditory and spoken language skills in approximately one year's time.

Based on the short duration of access to sign language thus far and her progress up to this point, the prognosis for Ana's sign language development is good given continued enrollment in a supportive school environment that specifically addresses language acquisition. In terms of auditory skill and spoken language development, while Ana has made steady progress, it is unlikely that spoken language will be a primary way by which she receives or expresses curriculum information at this time. Continued spoken language development is warranted, as it may support literacy acquisition as well as improve communication with family and others who do not use sign language.

Ana should be placed in a total-communication or ASL/English bilingual kindergarten classroom with a teacher of the D/HH, with the expectation of meeting the requirements of the general education curriculum provided accommodations for her hearing loss and language delay.

Recommendations

The following measures are recommended to support her continued language development.

Family Counseling

1. Encourage all family members to learn sign language. Provide available free community and online resources. Establish a home-school communication system to provide lists of most important vocabulary from the classroom for home reinforcement. Emphasize that the family should attempt to include any signs they know when interacting with Ana, even if they do not have the sign for each word in their message.
2. Encourage family members to use their most comfortable spoken language when talking to Ana. Counsel the parents on the importance of ongoing language input and that Spanish will not interfere with Ana's English development; the most important point is that they present a language-rich environment.

School-Based Services

1.. Interprofessional collaboration for language learning:
   a. The SLP and teacher of the D/HH will identify language goals based on Ana's current functioning, and the College and Career Readiness for ASL: K-12 Standards (2018).
   b. Language goals for the IEP should address skills that may be less frequently expected to occur naturally in the classroom. For example, asking and answering questions is a common practice in the educational setting and will be targeted even without a direct

IEP goal. A more appropriate goal may be expressing personal and observed events, which is less likely to occur naturally and repeatedly in the classroom and require more direct additional opportunities/support. This skill can then be applied to retelling events from texts presented through sign, an important skill for literacy acquisition.

c. The SLP and teacher of the D/HH will identify opportunities throughout the day to implement language learning instructional strategies that complement content area instruction. For example, during math lessons, the use of sign duplication to express plurals may be modeled. This will not distract from the content lesson but provide additional targeted language modeling of specific ASL structures.
d. The SLP and teacher of the D/HH will establish a shared progress monitoring strategy to evaluate the effectiveness of the interventions and change goals as needed to increase language demands.
e. The SLP and teacher of the D/HH will train support staff to incorporate language strategies throughout the day. Strategies will include modeling, recasting, expansion, and engineering the environment (communication sabotage).
f. The IEP team, including the parents, will collaborate to determine what accommodations and program supports are needed. Examples of program supports may include audiology consult services, monitoring of hearing assistive technology, and visual supports in the classroom.

2. Direct SLP services:
    a. The SLP will provide 60 minutes of direct speech language therapy per week.
    b. Direct therapy services will address the language goals which are identified through collaborative practice and incorporate auditory and spoken language development.
    c. Auditory skills will include analytic and synthetic training using curriculum materials. Although sound-object correspondences such as animal or vehicle sounds were appropriate in the preschool setting, auditory training should incorporate the use of real words or sound-letter associations to be more age- and school-appropriate and align with the content standards.
    d. Spoken language development will connect to auditory training activities to establish the perception production loop. Important considerations will be to expand the repertoire of syllable shapes and increase the variety of features produced. Maximally contrastive targets may support an expanded repertoire.
    e. Direct services will be provided in a small group setting which may include pull-out or collaborative services in the classroom.
3. Additional IEP documentation:
    a. Services for students who are D/HH: The IEP team should document Ana's unique communication needs, and opportunities for direct communication with teachers for direct instruction and peers for socialization.
    b. Services for students who are ELLs: The IEP should document that the language of the home is Spanish. Due to the needs for direct communication, services which are provided by an ESOL teacher may not be supported (unless the ESOL teacher is a fluent signer). However, the teacher of the D/HH may collaborate with the ESOL teacher on second language teaching and learning strategies that may apply to Ana learning English primarily through reading and writing.

Discussion of Questions for the Reader

1. *How does diagnosis of a significant hearing loss affect speech-language assessment with children from a culturally and linguistically diverse background?* As evidenced by Ana's case, when a child presents with a significant hearing loss, it is important to consider their language access prior to assessment to inform interpretation of results. One consideration is quantity and quality of access to sign and spoken language(s). Due to her hearing loss, Ana experienced a period of language deprivation where no formal language was accessible to her. In this case, examination of prelinguistic behaviors is critical. The SLP should consider the child's comprehension and use of gesture, symbolic play, and nonverbal interaction. The assessment of these domains should consider cultural differences that may exist between the norms of the child's home culture and the majority culture. Once formal language is introduced, quantity and quality continue to inform interpretation and recommendations. Many D/HH children have very limited access to sign at home. This limited access may result in slower than expected growth even when prelinguistic skills are strong. For spoken language, the SLP must consider the quantity and quality of sound input. Hearing aids amplify the acoustic signal. Depending on the degree, type, and configuration of the child's hearing loss, speech information through hearing aids may be inaccessible, just audible, or distorted to a degree that the child does not benefit from the hearing aids. Careful monitoring of the child's benefit will inform prognosis and next steps. If a child does not demonstrate benefit from hearing aids, cochlear implants may be considered. Cochlear implants do not amplify sound, but rather provide direct electrical stimulation to the auditory nerve. Cochlear implants are a promising alternative for access to the speech signal that hearing aids may not provide. Even with direct stimulation, the perception of sound is not consistent with typical hearing. A child must learn to listen to and interpret what they hear. A child's progress in auditory skill development is a critical component of the speech-language assessment and will inform goal setting and service provision recommendations. For the multilingual child, it is important to consider their access to both English and their home language(s). Because therapy in the US is provided primarily by monolingual therapists, it is likely that home language stimulation will be provided in less structured environments. Family report of home language behaviors will add information about the child's overall language profile.
2. *How does family language use contribute to language acquisition for DMLs?* Family language use influences a child's language development. For a child who is acquiring sign, family use in the home plays a critical role. Adult sign acquisition is a difficult process, and many D/HH children's families do not acquire sign skills beyond labeling common objects in the child's environment. For a child who has not developed functional spoken language through hearing technology, this means they are vulnerable to having little language access at home. This may impact not only language, but also social-emotional development. For a child who has access to spoken language information through a hearing aid or cochlear implant, families may decide to use only their native language, only English, or a combination of both. Parents who believe that using their native language will negatively impact their child's development of spoken English, such as Ana's, may unintentionally reduce the richness of the language and the interactive environment provided in the home. Furthermore, the number of waking hours the child uses their hearing technology will impact accessibility of spoken language. Some families may perceive a stigma associated with their child's technology use in their community. Others may fear losing the expensive device. Asking families

about language and device use in the home and community and providing culturally sensitive counseling may support the child's language and social-emotional outcomes.

3. *How do service providers use interprofessional practice in assessment and intervention with DMLs who use sign language?* Interprofessional practice involves collaboration between professionals from different disciplines and the family. For a child with hearing loss, this includes the family, the teacher of the D/HH, the SLP, the audiologist, the school psychologist and possibly others. The team should collaborate on assessment strategies, data collection, and interpretation of results. As the case with Ana, a severe language delay may appear to impact other areas of development that rely on language comprehension and expression. Through collaborative efforts, the team identifies developmental strengths, needs, and priorities. The interprofessional team identifies instructional and therapeutic strategies and makes service provision recommendations. Collaboration helps to ensure all areas of needs are addressed in an effective and efficient manner. Engaging the family in the decision-making process by considering their concerns, priorities, preferences, and cultural and linguistic differences is an important component. This may occur during formal meetings, but to consider the family as part of the interprofessional team, communication between the team and family should be ongoing.

KEY POINTS

DMLs are an increasing proportion of SLPs' caseloads. Expertise in only working with D/HH or hearing bi/multilingual learners does not capture the unique needs with which multilingual learners with significant hearing loss present. When assessing DMLs, it is critical to consider all languages equally and counsel families on the role of each language. The lack of available standardized assessments for this population means that scores may not provide an accurate picture of strengths and weakness, and that clinical judgment and dynamic assessment are needed. Working with DMLs requires cultural sensitivity of all the involved cultures, as well as the changes that occur with cultural adaptation. The family may even use the professionals working with them as a guide in this process. Interprofessional practice is crucial to make sure all involved professionals are working towards the same goals and provide support to each other in what may be a complex case.

REFERENCES

American Speech-Language-Hearing Association. (2008). *Service provision to children who are deaf and hard of hearing, birth to 36 months*. Joint Committee of the American Speech-Language-Hearing Association and Council on Education of the Deaf. Retrieved from http//www.asha.org/policy/ps2013-0339

American Speech-Language-Hearing Association. (2016). *2016 Schools Survey report: SLP workforce/work conditions*. Retrieved from https://www.asha.org/uploadedFiles/2018-Schools-Survey-Workforce-Report.pdf

Cannon, J. E., Guardino, C., & Gallimore, E. (2016). A new kind of heterogeneity: What we can learn from d/Deaf and hard of hearing multilingual learners. *American Annals of the Deaf, 161*(1), 8–16. doi:10.1353/aad.2016.0015 PMID:27156914

Centers for Disease Control & Prevention. (2016). *Summary of 2016 national CDC EHDI data*. Retrieved from https://www.cdc.gov/ncbddd/hearingloss/2016-data/01-2016-HSFS-Data-Summary-h.pdf

Decker, K. B., Vallotton, C. D., & Johnson, H. A. (2012). Parents' communication decision for children with hearing loss: Sources of information and influence. *American Annals of the Deaf*, *157*(4), 326–339. doi:10.1353/aad.2012.1631 PMID:23259352

Erber, N. (1982). *Auditory training*. Washington, DC: Alexander Graham Bell Association for the Deaf.

Fenson, L., Marchman, V. A., Thal, D. J., Dale, P. S., Reznick, J. S., & Bates, E. (2007). *MacArthur-Bates Communicative Development Inventories: User's guide and technical manual* (2nd ed.). Baltimore, MD: Brookes.

Gaffney, M., Green, D. R., & Gaffney, C. (2010). Newborn hearing screening and follow-up: Are children receiving recommended services? *Public Health Reports*, *125*(2), 199–207. doi:10.1177/003335491012500208 PMID:20297746

Gallaudet Research Institute. (2010). *Annual survey of deaf and hard of hearing children & youth*. Retrieved from https://www.gallaudet.edu/research-support-and-international-affairs/research-support/research-resources/demographics

Gallaudet Research Institute. (2013). *Regional and National Summary Report of Data from the 2011-12 Annual survey of deaf and hard of hearing children and youth*. Washington, DC: GRI, Gallaudet University.

Gallaudet University Laurent Clerc National Deaf Education Center and California School for the Deaf-Riverside. (2018). *The College and Career Readiness for ASL: K-12 Standards*. Washington, DC: Clerc Center, Gallaudet University.

Gillam, S., & Justice, L. (2010). Progress monitoring tools for SLPs in response to intervention (RTI): Primary grades. *The ASHA Leader*, *9*(21).

Goldman, R., & Fristoe, M. (2000). *Goldman-Fristoe Test of Articulation-2*. Circle Pines, MN: American Guidance Service, Inc.

Goldstein, G., & Bebko, J. M. (2003). The profile of multiple language proficiencies: A measure for evaluation language samples of deaf children. *Journal of Deaf Studies and Deaf Education*, *4*(8), 452–463. doi:10.1093/deafed/eng027 PMID:15448075

Joint Committee on Infant Hearing. (2007). Year 2007 position statement: Principles and guidelines for early hearing detection and intervention programs. *American Academy of Pediatrics*, *120*(4), 898–921. PMID:17908777

Joint Committee on Infant Hearing. (2013). Supplement to the JCIH 2007 position statement: Principles and guidelines for intervention after confirmation that a child is deaf or hard of hearing. *American Academy of Pediatrics*, *131*, 1324–1349. PMID:23530178

Kapantzoglou, M., Restrepo, M. A., & Thompson, M. S. (2012). Dynamic assessment of word learning skills: Identifying language impairment in bilingual children. *Language, Speech, and Hearing Services in Schools*, *43*(1), 81–96. doi:10.1044/0161-1461(2011/10-0095) PMID:22052970

Kim, M., Pae, S., & Bak, C. (2007). *Assessment of phonology and articulation for children (APAC)*. Inchon, South Korea: Human Brain Research and Consulting Company.

Knoors, H., & Marschark, M. (2014). *Teaching deaf learners; psychological and developmental foundations*. New York, NY: Oxford University Press. doi:10.1093/acprof:oso/9780199792023.001.0001

Lederberg, A. R., Schick, B., & Spencer, P. E. (2013). Language and literacy development of deaf and hard-of-hearing children: Successes and challenges. *Developmental Psychology*, *49*(1), 15–30. doi:10.1037/a0029558 PMID:22845829

Leigh, G., & Crowe, K. (2015). Responding to cultural and linguistic diversity among deaf and hard-of-hearing learnings. In H. Knoors & M. Marschark (Eds.), *Educating deaf learners: Creating a global evidence base* (pp. 68–91). New York, NY: Oxford University Press. doi:10.1093/acprof:oso/9780190215194.003.0004

Luckner, J. L., & Bowen, S. (2006). Assessment practices of professionals serving students who are deaf or hard of hearing: An initial investigation. *American Annals of the Deaf*, *151*(4), 410–417. doi:10.1353/aad.2006.0046 PMID:17225635

Mann, W., Pena, E. D., & Morgan, G. (2014). Exploring the use of dynamic language assessment with deaf children, who use American Sign Language: Two case studies. *Journal of Communication Disorders*, *52*, 16–30. doi:10.1016/j.jcomdis.2014.05.002 PMID:24908340

McFarland, J. (2016, February 18). *Diversity in home languages: Examining English learners in public schools.* Retrieved from https://nces.ed.gov/blogs/nces/post/diversity-in-home-languages-examining-english-learners-in-u-s-public-schools

Meadow-Orlans, K. P., Sass-Lehrer, M., & Mertens, D. M. (2003). *Parents and their deaf children: The early years*. Washington, DC: Gallaudet University Press.

Meinzen-Derr, J., Wiley, S., Creighton, J., & Choo, D. (2007). Auditory skills checklist: Clinical tool for monitoring functional auditory skill development in young children with cochlear implants. *The Annals of Otology, Rhinology, and Laryngology*, *116*(11), 812–818. doi:10.1177/000348940711601104 PMID:18074665

Mitchell, R. E., & Karchmer, M. A. (2004). Chasing the mythical ten percent: Parental hearing status of deaf and hard of hearing students in the United States. *Sign Language Studies*, *4*(2), 138–163. doi:10.1353ls.2004.0005

Moeller, M. P., Carr, G., Seaver, L., Stredler-Brown, A., & Holzinger, D. (2013). Best practices in family-centered early intervention for children who are deaf or hard of hearing: An international consensus statement. *Journal of Deaf Studies and Deaf Education*, *18*(4), 429–445. doi:10.1093/deafed/ent034 PMID:24030911

National Center for Education Statistics. (2018). *Table 204.30. Children 3-21 years old served under Individuals with Disabilities Education Act, Part B, by type of disability: Selected years, 1976-77 through 2011-12*. Retrieved from https://nces.ed.gov/programs/digest/d13/tables/dt13_204.30.asp

National Center for Education Statistics. (2019, May). *English language learners in public schools.* Retrieved from https://nces.ed.gov/programs/coe/indicator_cgf.asp

Ogura, T., Watamaki, T., & Inaba, T. (2016). *The Japanese MacArthur-Bates Communicative Development Inventories*. Kyoto: Nakanishiya Co.

Olusanya, B. O., Luxon, L. M., & Wirz, S. L. (2004). Benefits and challenges of newborn hearing screening for developing countries. *International Journal of Pediatric Otorhinolaryngology*, *68*(3), 287–305. doi:10.1016/j.ijporl.2003.10.015 PMID:15129939

Pae, S., & Kwak, K. C. (2011). *Korean MacArthur-Bates Communicative Development Inventories (K M-B CDI)*. Seoul: Mindpress.

Pena, E. D., Gillam, R. B., & Bedore, L. M. (2014). Dynamic assessment of narrative ability in English accurately identifies language impairments in English language learners. *Journal of Speech, Language, and Hearing Research: JSLHR*, *57*(6), 2208–2220. doi:10.1044/2014_JSLHR-L-13-0151 PMID:25075793

Rossetti, L. (2006). *The Rossetti infant toddler language scale*. East Moline, IL: Linguisystems.

Sass-Lehrer, M. (2017). Early intervention for children birth-3: Families, communities, & communication. In L. R. Schmeltz (Ed.), *The NCHAM e-book: A resource guide for early hearing detection and intervention* (pp. 17-1–17-16). Logan, UT: National Center for Hearing Assessment and Management.

Simms, L., Baker, S., & Clark, M. D. (2013). The standardized visual communication and sign language checklist for signing children. *Sign Language Studies*, *14*(1), 101–124. doi:10.1353ls.2013.0029

Ski-Hi Institute. (2004). *Ski-hi language development scale* (2nd ed.). North Logan, UT: Hope, Inc.

Spencer, P. E., & Marschark, M. (2010). *Evidence-based practice in educating deaf and hard-of hearing students*. New York, NY: Oxford University Press.

Stredler-Brown, A. (2010). Communication choices and outcomes during the early years: An assessment and evidence-based approach. In M. Marschark & P. E. Spencer (Eds.), *The Oxford handbook of deaf studies, language, and education* (Vol. 2, pp. 291–315). New York, NY: Oxford University Press.

U.S. Department of Education, Office of Special Education. (2019). Children and youth with disabilities. In National Center for Education Statistics. *The Condition of Education.* Retrieved from https://nces.ed.gov/programs/coe/pdf/coe_cgg.pdf

Yoshinaga-Itano, C. (2003). From screening to early identification and intervention: Discovering predictors to successful outcomes for children with significant hearing losses. *Journal of Deaf Studies and Deaf Education*, *8*(1), 11–30. doi:10.1093/deafed/8.1.11 PMID:15448044

Yoshinaga-Itano, C., Sedey, A. L., Coulter, D. K., & Mehl, A. L. (1998). Language of early- and later-identified children with hearing loss. *Pediatrics*, *102*(5), 1161–1171. doi:10.1542/peds.102.5.1161 PMID:9794949

Young, A., Carr, G., Hunt, R., McCracken, W., Skipp, A., & Tattersall, H. (2006). Informed choice and deaf children: Underpinning concepts and enduring challenges. *Journal of Deaf Studies and Deaf Education*, *11*(3), 322–336. doi:10.1093/deafed/enj041 PMID:16717258

Zimmerman, I. L., Steiner, V. G., & Pond, R. E. (2012). Preschool Language Scales (5th ed.). Bloomington, MN: Pearson. (in Spanish)

KEY TERMS AND DEFINITIONS

American Sign Language (ASL): Visual-spatial language used by the Deaf community in the US and Canada. ASL if a natural language with a lexicon, grammar, and discourse pattern that is distinct from other world sign languages and spoken English.

Cochlear Implant: Hearing technology that converts the acoustic signal into an electrical signal and directly stimulates the auditory nerve.

Deaf or Hard-of-Hearing Multilingual Learner (DML): D/HH children from families where languages other than or in addition to English and/or ASL are used in the home.

Dynamic Assessment: Language assessment strategy that identifies the skills a child possesses as well as their learning potential. The procedure emphasizes the learning process and accounts for examiner effort in diagnosis.

Early Hearing Detection and Intervention (EHDI): Practice of screening every newborn for hearing loss prior to hospital discharge, diagnosing hearing loss before three months old, and initiating early intervention by six months old.

Fingerspelling: The use of a manual alphabet to represent the letters of a writing system.

Hearing Aid: Hearing technology that amplifies the acoustic signal. Conventional hearing aids (air conduction) deliver the sound into the ear canal. Bone conduction hearing aids deliver the sound to the inner ear via bone vibration.

Individualized Education Plan (IEP): The IEP is a written statement of the educational program designed to meet a child's individual needs. Every child who receives special education services must have an IEP.

Individualized Family Service Plan (IFSP): The IFSP is a written treatment plan that maps out the EI services your child will receive, as well as how and when these services will be administered. It details your child's current levels of functioning, specific needs and goals for treatment.

Chapter 9
Sickle Cell Disease and Hidden Hearing Loss

Diane Scott
https://orcid.org/0000-0002-7472-7208
North Carolina Central University, USA

EXECUTIVE SUMMARY

Sickle cell disease (SCD) is an autosomal recessively inherited group of red blood cell disorders. It is more commonly found in African Americans and Hispanics in the United States. The sickle-shaped cells characteristic of the disease cause physiological problems, including hemolytic anemia and vaso-occlusion. Research has linked hearing loss to sickle cell disease. Studies have shown that children and adults with sickle cell disease may have higher rates of sensorineural and central auditory hearing impairment. This case study examines hidden hearing loss in an African American boy with SCD who presents with normal hearing thresholds. It also discusses the role of audiologists in the care of individuals with sickle cell disease and hearing loss.

INTRODUCTION

Sickle Cell Disease

Sickle cell disease (SCD) is a group of autosomal recessively inherited red blood cell disorders. Red blood cells contain a protein called hemoglobin (Hb). Hemoglobin gives blood its characteristic red color, and its job is to transport and release oxygen throughout the body. People who have sickle cell disease have abnormal hemoglobin in their red blood cells. The abnormal hemoglobin, known as hemoglobin S (HbS), causes sickle cell disease.

Red blood cells that contain normal hemoglobin are disc-shaped and flexible so that they can move easily through large and small blood vessels of the body to deliver oxygen. Since red blood cells are soft and pliable, they can squeeze through blood vessels that are narrower than themselves. This flexibility (pliability) occurs because the normal hemoglobin remains dissolved in the presence of low levels of oxygen. Sickle hemoglobin is not like normal hemoglobin. Problems occur when oxygen levels in the

DOI: 10.4018/978-1-7998-2261-5.ch009

Figure 1. Normal and sickled red blood cells (U.S. National Library of Medicine)

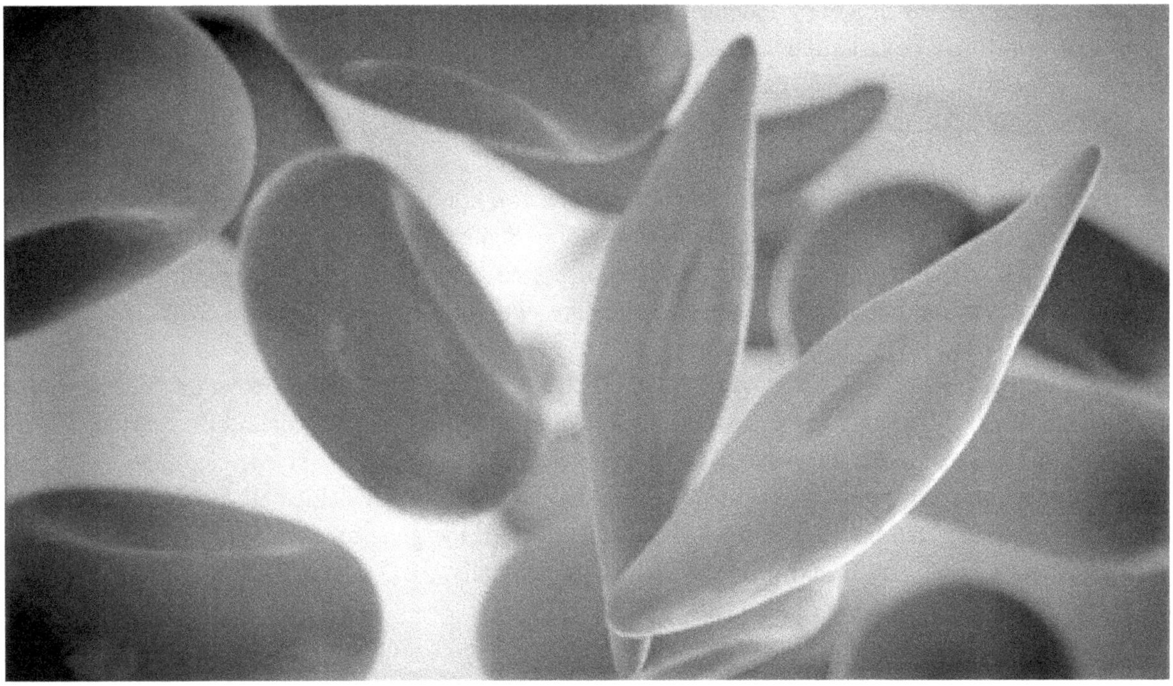

blood are lower, which happens once the hemoglobin has delivered oxygen to cells in the body's tissues. With less oxygen present, the abnormal hemoglobin can cause rigid, nonliquid protein strands to form within the red blood cell. These rigid strands can then change the shape of the cell, producing the sickled red blood cell that gives the disease its name.

Because sickle-shaped cells are not flexible, they can stick to vessel walls, causing a blockage that slows or stops the flow of blood, referred to as vaso-occlusion. When this happens, oxygen cannot reach nearby tissues. The lack of oxygen in tissues can cause attacks of sudden severe pain, otherwise known as pain crises. Pain crises can occur without warning, and individuals who have them often need to go to the hospital for effective treatment.

Given that sickle cells cannot change shape easily, they tend to burst apart. Normal red blood cells live about 90 to 120 days in the body, but sickle cells last only 10 to 20 days. The body is always making new red blood cells to replace the old cells. In the case of sickle cell disease, the body may have trouble keeping up with replacing the old red blood cells given how quickly the old cells are being destroyed. Under these circumstances, the number of red blood cells circulating in the body is usually lower than normal. This condition is called hemolytic anemia, which can lead to fatigue and jaundice (National Heart, Lung, and Blood Institute, 2019).

Over time, SCD can lead to major complications such as infections, delayed growth, and more pain crises. Most children who have sickle cell disease are pain-free between crises, but adolescents and adults may also suffer with chronic, ongoing pain. Over a lifetime, SCD can harm an individual's spleen, brain, eyes, lungs, liver, heart, kidneys, penis, joints, bones, or skin (National Heart, Lung, and Brian Institute, 2019).

SCD is a term used to refer to sickle cell anemia and sickle cell variants, which are combinations of the sickle cell gene (HbS) and another gene responsible for hemoglobin production. Other types of abnormal genes may be inherited with HbS. People who have SCD inherit two abnormal hemoglobin genes, one from each parent. The various types of sickle cell disease include the following: hemoglobin SS, hemoglobin Sβ0 thalassemia, hemoglobin Sβ+ thalassemia, hemoglobin SC, hemoglobin SD, and hemoglobin SE.

In all types of sickle cell disease, at least one of the two abnormal genes causes a person's body to make hemoglobin S. When a person has two hemoglobin S genes (hemoglobin SS), the disease is called sickle cell anemia. This is the most common and often most severe type of sickle cell disease. Hemoglobin SC disease and hemoglobin Sβ thalassemia are two other common types of SCD. Hemoglobin SD and hemoglobin SE are much less common.

Sickle cell disease occurs in approximately 100,000 Americans, though the exact number of people living with SCD in the United States is unknown (Centers for Disease Control and Prevention (CDC), 2019). In the United States, most people who have sickle cell disease are of African ancestry. While approximately one in every 365 African American babies is born with sickle cell disease, roughly one in 13 African American babies is born with sickle cell trait, the gene for hemoglobin S (CDC, 2019; National Heart, Lung, and Blood Institute, 2019). Additionally, SCD occurs in approximately one out of every 16,300 Hispanic American births (CDC, 2019).

While SCD is among the most common hemoglobinopathies globally affecting millions of people throughout the world, it is particularly common among those whose ancestors came from sub-Saharan Africa, Spanish-speaking regions in the Western Hemisphere (South America, the Caribbean, and Central America), Saudi Arabia, India, and Mediterranean countries such as Turkey, Greece, and Italy. Sickle cell disease occurs more often among people from these parts of the world because malaria is or was common. It is believed that people who carry the sickle cell trait are less likely to have severe forms of malaria. The mechanism by which people carrying the gene for sickle cell disease are protected from malaria has been identified. The sickle cell gene does not protect against infection by the malaria parasite, as was previously thought. Instead, it prevents the disease from taking hold after a person has been infected (de Lange, 2011).

In the United States universal newborn screening programs for sickle cell disease (which also identify sickle cell trait) exist in all 50 states and the District of Columbia and in Puerto Rico and the U.S. Virgin Islands. Universal newborn screening is one factor that has led to the dramatically improved survival rates of young children with SCD over the past several decades. Sickle cell-related death among African American children younger than 4 years of age fell by 42% from 1999 through 2002. This drop coincided with the introduction of vaccinations against *Haemophilus influenzae* type b and *Streptococcus pneumoniae*, the use of prophylactic penicillin, and universal newborn screening (Quinn, Rogers, McCavit, & Buchanan, 2010; Yanni, Grosse, Yang, & Olney, 2009). Compared to the rate for the period 1983 through 1986, the SCD mortality rate for the period 1999 through 2002 decreased by:

- 68% at ages 0 through 3 years;
- 39% at ages 4 through 9 years; and
- 24% at ages 10 through 14 years (Yanni et al., 2009).

Quinn et al. (2010) studied the Dallas Newborn Cohort (DNC) to estimate contemporary 18-year survival for newborns with SCD and document changes in the causes and ages of death over time. Of the 940 children followed, most children with sickle cell anemia (93.9%) and nearly all children with milder forms of SCD (98.4%) now live to become adults. The incidence of death and the pattern of mortality changed over the duration of the cohort. Sepsis, which can be a consequence of infections, was no longer the leading cause of death. All the recent deaths in the cohort occurred in patients 18 years or older, most shortly after the transition to adult care. As adults, individuals with SCD no longer received the same level of medical care they did as children. SCD is not just a disease of childhood; it is a lifelong, chronic medical condition.

An additional factor in improving the survival rate of individuals with SCD is hydroxyurea. Hydroxyurea is an oral medicine that has been shown to reduce or prevent several sickle cell disease complications. This medicine increases the amount of fetal hemoglobin (hemoglobin F) in the blood. Increased hemoglobin F provides some protection against the effects of hemoglobin S (CDC, 2019). The Food and Drug Administration has also approved a new medicine to reduce the number of sickle cell crises in adults and children older than age five; it is called Endari (AKA L-glutamine oral powder) (CDC, 2019). Another treatment, which can actually cure SCD, is a stem cell transplant (also called a bone marrow transplant). This procedure infuses healthy cells, called stem cells, into the body to replace damaged or diseased bone marrow (bone marrow is the center of the bone where red blood cells are made) (CDC, 2019).

The early life of a child with SCD may look like this. At birth 50-95 percent of the child's hemoglobin is fetal hemoglobin (HbF). After birth the percentage drops off at a rate of 3 to 4 percent each week, changing to HbA, HbS, or another hemoglobin. Thus, by 4 to 5 months of age, red blood cells in children with SCD are capable of sickling. Once the red blood cells in children with SCD are capable of sickling, SCD can then begin to affect bodily functions. During early infancy, the child is usually without symptoms. Infections can start after 2-3 months, but many children remain symptom-free for a year or more. In the absence of prophylactic antibiotics or vaccines, children often die of infections between the ages of 1 and 3 years. In early childhood, hand-foot syndrome (blocked blood flow in the bones of the hands and feet causing local swelling accompanied by pain and fever) is often the first presenting problem.

In summary, SCD is a genetically determined disorder of the red blood cells. The gene for sickle cell disease, HbS, has survived in the gene pool because it provides protection for individuals who may be exposed to malaria. The gene prevents malaria from taking hold after a person has been infected. Though, at the same time, the individuals with SCD experience significant morbidity and mortality. The sickle-shaped red blood cells associated with SCD have pathophysiologic disadvantages, including hemolytic anemia and vaso-occlusion. Normal red blood cells live about 90 to 120 days, but sickle cells last only 10 to 20 days because sickle cells cannot change shape easily. Consequently, they tend to burst apart. The body replaces old red blood cells with new red blood cells on a regular basis. In the case of sickle cell disease, the body may have trouble keeping up with replacing the old red blood cells given how quickly the cells are being destroyed. Under these circumstances, the number of red blood cells is usually lower than normal. This condition is called hemolytic anemia. In addition, sickle-shaped cells are not flexible and can stick to vessel walls, causing a blockage that slows or stops the flow of blood, vaso-occlusion. The sequelae (after affects) of hemolytic anemia and vaso-occlusion include local hypoxia, more sickling, and spread of the occlusion to adjacent tissue. This, in turn, can lead to pain crises and possible organ malfunctions in individuals with SCD.

SCD and Hearing Loss

Considering the nature of SCD, the potential for damage to the auditory system is not unexpected. The auditory system is just as susceptible to the effects of SCD as the rest of the body. Histopathological changes have been observed in the temporal bone and organ of Corti in individuals with SCD. A study conducted approximately 50 years ago was the first to report inner ear abnormalities including a clumped mass of sickle-shaped red blood cells in the organ of Corti of a child with SCD and hearing loss (Morganstein & Manace, 1969). The findings are consistent with hypoxia (a chronic deficiency in oxygen) and with the nature of the microvasculature of the cochlea. The organ of Corti is sensitive to hypoxia and infarction due to the sizeable metabolic requirements necessary to maintain the ionic balance of endolymph within the inner ear (Miller & Dengerink, 1988).

The most accepted theories in the development of sensorineural hearing loss (SNHL) in SCD involve clumped sickle-shaped blood cells that lead to decreased blood flow in the cochlear venous system, which in turn leads to a chronic deficiency in oxygen in the organ of Corti and death of the outer hair cells (Serjeant, Norman, & Todd, 1975). Studies have reported that the vascular endothelium influences the formation of cell clusters that interact with vessel walls, culminating in vaso-occlusive processes. Reduced flow-mediated vasodilatation is considered an early marker of vascular alterations in patients with SCD (Belhassen et al., 2001). The relationship between endothelial dysfunction (ED) and SNHL is documented in sudden SNHL and idiopathic SNHL, supporting the presence of vascular damage (Berjis, Moeinimehr, & Nasiri, 2016; Casale et al., 2016). This also may be a mechanism for the development of hearing impairment in individuals with SCD.

Adults and children with SCD may present with higher rates of peripheral and central auditory impairment compared to adults and children with normal hemoglobin. The prevalence of sensorineural hearing loss among individuals with SCD is higher than in the general population; however, the estimated prevalence has a wide range. For example, Crawford et al. (1991) and Gould et al. (1991) studied the prevalence of hearing impairments in adults with sickle cell disease. Of the 75 subjects with audiological test results, 31 subjects (41%) were identified with sensorineural hearing loss. The percentage of adults with hearing loss varied by type of sickle cell disease. For adults with hemoglobin SS, 18 out of 50 (36%) adults had sensorineural hearing loss, no adults with hemoglobin Sβ0 thalassemia had hearing loss, 4 out of 8 (50%) adults with hemoglobin Sβ+ thalassemia had hearing loss, and 9 out of 13 (69%) of adults with hemoglobin SC had hearing loss.

Compared to adults with SCD, children with SCD appear to have a lower prevalence of sensorineural hearing loss. Studies examining the prevalence of hearing impairment in pediatric patients have been conducted for decades. Friedman, Luban, Herer, and Williams (1980) examined 43 children ages 7 to 18 years, all of whom had sickle cell anemia (HbSS). Five of the 43 (12%) children were identified with sensorineural hearing loss. In addition, three of the five children with SNHL had a history of cerebrovascular accidents (CVAs) of varying severity. In a study from 1999, McDonald, Bauer, Cox, and McMahon examined 84 children who all had sickle cell anemia (HbSS). The mean age of the children was 7.8 years. Three or 3.5% of the children had sensorineural hearing loss, while 19 or 22.6% of the children had conductive hearing loss.

More recently, Farrell, Landry, Yee, Leu, and Goudy (2019) conducted a retrospective review of a database of patients with SCD followed at a pediatric tertiary referral center from 2010 through 2016. Out of 2600 patients with SCD 181 met the study criteria of having a SCD diagnosis of any type and results from audiological testing. Of the 181 patients, 153 were HbSS, 19 HbSC, and 9 HbSβ thalassemia. Ninety-six percent had passed a newborn hearing screen. The mean age for their first audiograms was 8.9 ± 5.2 (range of 0 to 19.6 years). Patients were referred for audiological testing due to 1) hearing concern (48 or 26.5%), 2) history of cerebrovascular accident (5 or 2.8%), 3) history of ototoxic medication (105 or 58.0%), 4) history of recurrent ear infections (9 or 5.0%), or 5) to establish a hearing baseline (14 or 7.7%). Twelve patients (6.6%) had SNHL. Ten of the twelve patients had HbSS (sickle cell anemia) and two had HbSC. Three patients had documented cerebrovascular disease prior to the first audiogram. Patients had both unilateral and bilateral hearing losses and the hearing losses ranged from normal to profound (> 80 dB HL). In addition, seven of the nine patients tested had absent distortion product otoacoustic emissions (DPOAEs).

The results of this study would suggest that hearing loss may be acquired later in life given the number of children with SCD who passed the newborn hearing screen (Farrell et al., 2019). In addition, for the children born with HbS in this study, the left ear thresholds were consistently poorer than the right ear thresholds across all frequencies. The majority of patients were referred for audiological testing to monitor their hearing secondary to receiving ototoxic medication rather than for damage caused by SCD. This suggests that the relationship between SCD and hearing impairment is complex.

Other studies support the findings of the Farrell et al. (2019) study in that (apparently) normal hearing children with SCD can present with subclinical cochlear damage in the form of abnormal otoacoustic emissions compared to age- and sex-matched children with normal hearing (Downs, Stuart, & Holbert, 2000; Stuart, Jones, & Walker, 2006; Stuart & Preast, 2012; Walker, Stuart, & Green, 2004). Normal hearing children with SCD have also demonstrated abnormal acoustic reflexes and auditory brainstem responses (Rissatto-Lago et al., 2019).

Stuart and Smith (2019) examined a large medical and research database from the Children's Hospital of Philadelphia to investigate the emergence and prevalence of hearing loss in children with HbSS. Normal hearing was defined as hearing thresholds ≤ 15 dB HL for pure tone air conduction testing and £ 20 dB HL for sound-field testing. Hearing loss was defined as any pure tone threshold at any frequency above 15 dB HL or minimal response level above 20 dB HL for sound-field testing. Degree and type of hearing loss were also determined.

One hundred and twenty-eight children with HbSS and at least one audiogram were identified. The prevalence of hearing loss in the children with SCD ranged from 34 to 51% depending on the definition of hearing loss used. When defining hearing loss as the presence of one elevated hearing threshold, the prevalence was 51%. When using the three frequency average of the thresholds at 500, 1000, and 2000 Hz, prevalence rates were lower at 34%. These prevalence rates for hearing loss are higher than those usually reported for children in North America (Feder, Michaud, McNamee, Fitzpatrick, Ramage-Morin, & Beauregard, 2017; Su & Chan, 2017).

In the light of recent research, healthcare professionals need to be aware of the relationship between SCD and hearing loss. Research indicates that SCD can affect the auditory system, specifically the blood vessels within the cochlea and other larger vessels within the central auditory system. Children with SCD may present with higher rates of peripheral and central auditory impairment compared to children with normal hemoglobin. Children with HbSS, as compared to other types of SCD, are more likely to exhibit a hearing loss.

CASE STUDY

Background Information/Clinical History

Brian was a 12-year-old African American male. He was the youngest of three children who lived with both of his parents and his two siblings, one brother (15 years old) and one sister (17 years old). His mother, who was 39 years old, was a school librarian, while his father, who was 42 years old, was a police officer. Brian had sickle cell anemia (HbSS) of mild to moderate severity. His siblings had normal hemoglobin. The parents were not screened for the sickle cell gene until the birth of their second son. Brian passed his newborn hearing screening.

Brian attended daycare and public schools and was absent from time to time when he was having a crisis. He had been hospitalized four times due to SCD. He had his first bout of otitis media at 10 months of age and had two more over several years. Brian was vaccinated to protect against invasive pneumococcal disease and given prophylactic penicillin until he was 5 years old. While he was small for his age, which is not uncommon for children with SCD, his developmental milestones were within normal limits. The audiologist noted that Brian's family seemed to be handling his chronic health problems fairly well. The family was self-educated about SCD. Brian's physician became aware of the possible effects of SCD on the auditory system, so Brian had been referred for annual hearing evaluations since about he was about 6 years of age.

Brian was doing well in school with no major concerns about his school progress. Brian had no family history of hearing loss, had not had a bout of otitis media since he was about 5 years of age, and had not been exposed to ototoxic medications. He had no comorbidities, such as genetic syndromes, obesity, diabetes mellitus, stroke, hypercholesterolemia, neurological disease, or lung disease. His annual audiological testing had always revealed normal otoscopic results, pure tone thresholds within normal limits, and Type A tympanograms (i.e., normal middle ear pressure and compliance). He came to the speech and hearing clinic for his annual hearing evaluation.

Clinical Evaluations

The otoscopic examination revealed clear ear canals along with a clear visualization of the tympanic membrane. Immittance testing revealed normal middle ear pressure and compliance bilaterally, basically Type A tympanograms. Brian's acoustic reflexes had not been assessed regularly. Acoustic reflex testing revealed elevated contralateral acoustic reflex thresholds for both ears.

Pure tone testing revealed that Brian had air conduction thresholds $\leq$ 15 dB HL from 250 through 8000 Hz. Bone conduction thresholds were within 10 dB HL of air conduction thresholds. Speech reception thresholds (SRTs) agreed with the pure tone averages. Speech recognition (discrimination) testing was also conducted utilizing NU-6 word lists. Brian's scores were 92% and 96% for the right and left ears respectively.

The results of the evaluation indicated hearing within normal limits across the frequency range of 250 through 8000 Hz. SRTs agreed with pure tone thresholds. Speech recognition scores fell within normal limits; they were excellent in quiet. Otoscopic and tympanometric results all were within normal limits with the exception of contralateral acoustic reflex thresholds, which were elevated.

Questions for the Reader

1. Are there any red flags that should be noted given Brian's audiological test results?
2. Why would an audiologist be concerned about the presence of certain comorbidities, such as obesity, diabetes, and stroke in a pediatric patient?

Discussion of the Questions for the Reader

1. **Are there any red flags that should be noted given Brian's audiological test results?** The fact that Brian has elevated contralateral acoustic reflexes in the presence of normal pure tone thresholds is of concern. Elevated contralateral acoustic reflexes can be due either a peripheral or central auditory system problem. Abnormalities in the acoustic reflex can be linked to cochlear impairment including SNHL. However, elevated acoustic reflex thresholds without SNHL can indicate alterations in brainstem structures (Borg, 1973). There might be transmission problems from the superior olivary complex to the facial nerve, which innervates and activates the stapedius muscle.

Rissatto-Lago et al. (2019) have indicated that there is a gap in the research about the effects of SCD on the central auditory system (CAS). They stated that an investigation into the functional integrity of the CAS may assist in diagnosing deficits in the auditory system due to SCD vasculopathy that do not manifest themselves as decreases in auditory (hearing) thresholds. The researchers designed a study to investigate subclinical damage or hidden hearing loss and its association with clinical variables in a pediatric population with SCD.

Study participants included 37 patients (20 males and 17 females) with sickle cell anemia (HBSS) ages 6-18 years and 44 healthy controls (27 males and 17 females) ages 6-18 years. None of the participants had any associated comorbidities such as genetic syndromes, obesity, and diabetes. Patients with a history of otologic injuries, chronic otitis media, exposure to ototoxic medications, and family history of hearing loss were also excluded from the study. All of the subjects had hearing thresholds with normal limits ($\leq$ 20 dB HL) for frequencies 250 through 8000 Hz as well as normal otoscopic and tympanometric findings (Type A tympanograms and contralateral acoustic reflex threshold in at least one of the analyzed frequencies). Participants' auditory systems were evaluated using pure tone audiometry, tympanometry, acoustic reflexes, otoacoustic emissions, and auditory brainstem responses (ABR).

Results indicated no significant differences between the two subject groups in pure tone thresholds, tympanometric results and distortion product otoacoustic emissions; however, there were differences in acoustic reflex thresholds. The participants with HbSS had a higher percentage of elevated and absent contralateral acoustic reflexes. There was also a significant difference in ABR values between the two subject groups. For the participants with HbSS, the mean latencies of waves III and V and the mean interpeak latencies I-III and I-V were significantly longer when compared to the healthy controls. While the latency differences were statistically different, they were actually within normal limits clinically. The differences may signal some alterations in the central auditory system that could manifest themselves more visibly (clinically) as individuals with SCD age or as the SCD worsens (Rissatto-Lago et al., 2019). The researchers concluded that damage in the auditory system in patients with HbSS can be present in the retrocochlear structures of the auditory system leading to functional deficits without deterioration of hearing thresholds (Rissatto-Lago et al., 2019).

2. **Why would an audiologist be concerned about the presence of certain comorbidities, such as obesity, diabetes, and stroke in a pediatric patient?** The presence of comorbidities can be contributing factors to the presence of any hearing impairment. Obesity is a leading cause of diabetes (Bancks et al., 2017). Moreover, diabetes is more common in African Americans (American Diabetes Association, 2018). Added to that is the fact that hearing impairment has a higher prevalence in individuals with diabetes (Bainbridge, Hoffman, & Cowie, 2008). Neurologic complications are a major cause of morbidity and mortality in sickle cell disease (SCD). One of the leading causes of pediatric strokes is SCD. In children with sickle cell anemia, routine use of transcranial Doppler screening, coupled with regular blood transfusion therapy, has decreased the prevalence of overt stroke from ~11% to 1% (CDC, 2019). Neurologic complications can lead to sensorineural or central auditory hearing impairment.

TREATMENT OPTIONS

Given Brian's elevated contralateral acoustic reflex thresholds, the audiologist recommended that Brian undergo additional testing in the form of distortion product otoacoustic emissions (DPOEs) and auditory brainstem responses (ABRs). DPOAEs are responses generated when the cochlea is stimulated simultaneously by two pure tone frequencies whose ratio is between 1.1 to 1.3. The prevalence of DPOAEs is 100% in normal adult ears. Responses from the left and right ears are often correlated (that is, they are very similar). Auditory brainstem response (ABR) audiometry is a neurologic test of auditory brainstem function in response to auditory stimuli. The ABR test is frequently employed to estimate hearing sensitivity and assess the integrity of the ascending auditory system. It is an evoked potential generated by a brief click or tone pip (tone burst) transmitted from an insert earphone or headphone. The elicited waveform response is measured by surface electrodes typically placed at the vertex of the scalp and the ear lobes.

Outcomes

Brian underwent additional hearing testing using DPOAEs and ABR. There were no significant differences in his distortion product otoacoustic emissions compared to norms. Normal DPOAEs indicate normal functioning within the cochlea. ABR test results indicated that the mean latencies of waves III and V and the mean interpeak latencies I-III and I-V were significantly longer when compared to norms. These differences were not clinically significant. The differences may signal some alterations in the central auditory system that could manifest themselves more visibly (clinically) over the course of time.

Additional Questions for the Reader

1. How should the DPOAEs and ABR test results be interpreted in terms of Brian's current hearing status and his SCD?
2. What concerns about Brian's health may arise as he ages?
3. What recommendations have been formulated for the general care of individuals with SCD?

Discussion of the Questions for the Reader

1. **How should the DPOAEs and ABR test results be interpreted in terms of Brian's current hearing status and his SCD?** Brian's ABR test results indicate prolonged latencies. These results may portend future hearing problems. Prolonged latencies indicate slower transmission of neural signals to the brainstem. A study examining hearing loss in children with SCD reported that one patient with a prolonged III-V interpeak latency in one ear later sustained a unilateral SNHL in the same ear and an infarct of the middle cerebral artery (Koussi et al., 2001).

In a study conducted in 2006, DPOAEs were examined in 15 normal-hearing African American children between the ages of 6 and 14 years with hemoglobin SS and who were on a regimen of hydroxyurea, a drug that reduces inflammatory processes and symptoms of SCD, as well as a matched group of 15 African American children with hemoglobin SS not on hydroxyurea and 15 African American children with normal hemoglobin. DPOAEs were evoked by 13 primary tone pairs with f_2 frequencies ranging from 1000 to 4500 Hz. Increased DPOAE amplitudes, believed to be a precursor of eventual hearing loss, were evident in children with SCD who were not receiving hydroxyurea. Those taking hydroxyurea had DPOAE amplitudes similar to normal controls. These findings suggest that hydroxyurea, in addition to reducing symptoms of SCD, may play a role in inhibiting or preventing cochlear pathology and hearing loss in individuals with SCD. Brian's DPOAE test results indicate normal cochlear function. The case history form did not note if Brian had taken hydroxyurea.

It was recommended that Brian continue having annual hearing evaluations, which should include the basic test battery along with acoustic reflex testing, DPOAE testing, and ABR testing.

2. **What concerns about Brian's health may arise as he ages?** The transition of young adults with SCD from pediatric to adult medical care is a critical priority, given medical advances that have transformed SCD into a lifelong chronic condition, rather than a disease of childhood (Kayle, Docherty, Sloane, Tanabe, Maslow, Pan, & Shah, 2019). A longitudinal analysis of medical records was conducted to describe the clinical course among adolescents and young adults (ages 12–27 years) with SCD during transition to adult care (Kayle et al., 2019). Measures included sociodemographic, complications, SCD severity, and comorbidities. Overall, 339 adolescents and young adults (97% African American, 56% male, and 69% hemoglobin SS) had 10,848 clinic, 3840 hospital, and 3152 emergency department visits. Complications included vaso-occlusive crises (80%) and acute chest syndrome (41%). Comorbidities included depression (19%) and anxiety (14%).
3. **What recommendations have been formulated for the general care of individuals with SCD?** Recently published guidelines provide recommendations for health maintenance, acute care, and monitoring of therapy in persons with SCD. The recommendations include the following. Children with sickle cell anemia should receive prophylactic penicillin from birth through at least five years of age, and all persons with SCD require vaccination to prevent invasive pneumococcal disease. Annual screening with transcranial Doppler ultrasonography is recommended for all children with sickle cell disease beginning at two years of age and continuing through adolescence to evaluate the risk of stroke and to initiate transfusion therapy in those at high risk. Vaso-occlusive crises require immediate and adequate pain management appropriate to the level of patient-reported pain. There is strong evidence to support the promotion and use of hydroxyurea therapy in patients nine months

and older who have sickle cell anemia because its use can decrease the frequency of vaso-occlusive crises and acute chest syndrome with limited adverse effects (Yawn & John-Sowah, 2015).

KEY POINTS

- Sickle cell disease (SCD) is a group of genetically inherited red blood cell disorders. Red blood cells contain a protein called hemoglobin. Hemoglobin gives blood its characteristic red color, and its job is to transport oxygen throughout the body. Individuals who have SCD have abnormal hemoglobin in their red blood cells. The abnormal hemoglobin, known as hemoglobin S, causes sickle cell disease.
- SCD causes normal disc-shaped red blood cells to become sickle-shaped when oxygen levels in the blood are lower. Sickle-shaped cells can stick to blood vessel walls, thus causing a blockage that slows or stops the flow of blood, called a vaso-occlusion. In addition, sickle-shaped cells do not live as long in the body as normal red blood cells. The body may have difficulty keeping up with replacing worn out red blood cells with new ones. Under these circumstances, the number of red blood cells is usually lower than normal. This condition is called hemolytic anemia.
- Over time, SCD can lead to major complications such as infections, delayed growth, and pain crises. Over a lifetime, SCD can harm an individual's spleen, brain, eyes, lungs, liver, heart, kidneys, penis, joints, bones, or skin (National Heart, Lung, and Brian Institute, 2019).
- The auditory system is susceptible to the effects of SCD. Histopathological changes have been observed in the temporal bone and the organ of Corti in individuals with SCD. Sensorineural hearing loss in SCD is theorized to develop from sickle-shaped red blood cells clumping and decreasing blood flow to the cochlear venous system leading to hypoxia in the organ of Corti.
- Adults and children with SCD may present with higher rates of peripheral and central auditory impairment compared to adults and children with normal hemoglobin.
- Studies have found evidence that normal hearing children with SCD may present with subclinical cochlear damage in the form of abnormal otoacoustic emissions. Retrocochlear structures may also be damaged without deterioration of peripheral hearing thresholds.
- Research suggests that it may be beneficial to complete baseline audiological testing as the starting point for monitoring for possible hearing loss in children with SCD. This should be followed by annual audiological testing to check for any changes within the auditory system. Audiologists should serve as advocates for early and ongoing hearing assessments of children with SCD (Stuart, 2019).

Audiometric evaluations should be part of the ongoing assessment of children with SCD, so that hearing loss can be diagnosed and treated as early as possible to minimize any impacts on language, speech, cognition, and academic performance.

REFERENCES

American Diabetes Association. (2018, March 22). *Statistics about diabetes*. Retrieved from http://www.diabetes.org/diabetes-basics/statistics/

Bainbridge, K. E., Hoffman, H. J., & Cowie, C. C. (2011). Risk factors for hearing impairment among U.S. adults with diabetes: National Health and Nutrition Examination Survey 1999-2004. *Diabetes Care*, *34*(7), 1540–1545. doi:10.2337/dc10-2161 PMID:21593298

Bancks, M. P., Kershaw, K., Carson, A. P., Gordon-Larsen, P., Schreiner, P. J., & Carnethon, M. R. (2017, December). Association of modifiable risk factors in young adulthood with racial disparity in incident Type 2 during middle adulthood. *Journal of the American Medical Association*, *318*(24), 2457–2465. doi:10.1001/jama.2017.19546 PMID:29279935

Belhassen, L., Pelle, G., Sediame, S., Bachir, D., Carville, C., Bucherer, C., ... Adnot, S. (2001). Endothelial dysfunction in patients with sickle cell disease is related to selective impairment of shear stress-mediated vasodilation. *Blood*, *97*(6), 1584–1589. doi:10.1182/blood.V97.6.1584 PMID:11238095

Berjis, N., Moeinimehr, M., & Nasiri, S. (2016). Endothelial dysfunction in patients with sudden sensorineural hearing loss. *Advanced Biomedical Research*, *5*, 1–4. PMID:26955626

Borg, E. (1973). On the neuronal organization of the acoustic middle ear reflex. A physiological and anatomical study. *Brain Research*, *49*(1), 101–123. doi:10.1016/0006-8993(73)90404-6 PMID:4349006

Casale, M., Mangiacapra, F., Bressi, E., Pace, A., Sabatino, L., Moffa, A., ... Salvinelli, F. (2016). Idiopathic sensorineural hearing loss is associated with endothelial dysfunction. *International Journal of Cardiology Heart & Vasculature*, *12*, 32–33. doi:10.1016/j.ijcha.2016.05.001 PMID:28616539

Centers for Disease Control and Prevention. (2019, June 12). *Complications and treatments of sickle cell disease*. Retrieved from https://www.cdc.gov/ncbddd/sicklecell/treatments.html

Crawford, M. R., Gould, H. J., Smith, W. R., Beckford, N., Gibson, W. R., & Bobo, L. (1991). Prevalence of hearing loss in adults with sickle cell disease. *Ear and Hearing*, *12*(5), 349–351. doi:10.1097/00003446-199110000-00007 PMID:1783238

de Lange, C. (2011, May 5). How sickle-cell carriers fend off malaria. *New Scientist*. Retrieved from https://www.newscientist.com/article/dn20450-how-sickle-cell-carriers-fend-off-malaria/#ixzz68ag80o2F

Downs, C. R., Stuart, A., & Holbert, D. (2000). Distortion product otoacoustic emissions in normal-hearing African-American children with homozygous sickle cell disease. *Journal of Communication Disorders*, *33*(2), 111–129. doi:10.1016/S0021-9924(99)00027-1 PMID:10834829

Farrell, A. N., Landry, A. M., Yee, M. E., Leu, R. M., & Goudy, S. L. (2019). Sensorineural hearing loss in children with sickle cell disease. *International Journal of Pediatric Otorhinolaryngology*, *118*, 110114. doi:10.1016/j.ijporl.2018.12.002 PMID:30599285

Feder, K. P., Michaud, M., McNamee, J., Fitzpatrick, E., Ramage-Morin, P., & Beauregard, Y. (2017). Prevalence of hearing loss among a representative sample of Canadian children and adolescents, 3 to 19 years of age. *Ear and Hearing*, *38*(1), 7–20. doi:10.1097/AUD.0000000000000345 PMID:27556530

Friedman, E. M., Luban, N. L. C., Herer, G. R., & Williams, I. (1980). Sickle cell anemia and hearing. *The Annals of Otology, Rhinology, and Laryngology*, *89*(4), 342–349. doi:10.1177/000348948008900409 PMID:7416684

Gould, H. J., Crawford, M. R., Smith, W. R., Beckford, N., Gibson, W. R., Pettie, L., & Bobo, L. (1991). Hearing disorders in sickle cell disease: Cochlear and retrocochlear findings. *Ear and Hearing*, *12*(5), 352–354. doi:10.1097/00003446-199110000-00008 PMID:1783239

Kayle, M., Docherty, S. L., Sloane, R., Tanabe, P., Maslow, G., Pan, W., & Shah, W. N. (2019). Transition to adult care in sickle cell disease: A longitudinal study of clinical characteristics and disease severity. *Pediatric Blood & Cancer*, *66*(1), e27463. doi:10.1002/pbc.27463 PMID:30251318

Koussi, A., Zafeiriou, D. I., Kontzoglou, G., Tsatra, I., Noussios, G., & Athanassiou, M. (2001). Hearing loss in children with sickle cell disease. *Acta Oto-Rhino-Laryngologica Belgica*, *55*, 235–239. PMID:11685961

MacDonald, C. B., Bauer, P. W., Cox, L. C., & McMahon, L. (1999). Otologic findings in pediatric cohort with sickle cell disease. *International Journal of Pediatric Otorhinolaryngology*, *47*(1), 23–28. doi:10.1016/S0165-5876(98)90152-5 PMID:10206391

Miller, J. M., & Dengerink, H. (1988, November-December). Control of inner ear blood flow. *American Journal of Otolaryngology*, *9*(6), 302–316. doi:10.1016/S0196-0709(88)80038-3 PMID:3067593

Morganstein, K. M., & Manace, E. D. (1969). Temporal bone histopathology in sickle cell disease. *Laryngoscope*, *79*(12), 2172–2180. doi:10.1288/00005537-196912000-00013 PMID:5362685

National Heart, Lung, and Blood Institute. (2019). *Sickle cell disease*. Retrieved from https://www.nhlbi.nih.gov/health-topics/sickle-cell-disease

Quaranta, N., De Ceglie, V., & D'Elia, A. (2016). Endothelial dysfunction in idiopathic sudden sensorineural hearing loss: A review. *Audiology Research*, *6*(1), 17–21. doi:10.4081/audiores.2016.151 PMID:27588164

Quinn, C. T., Rogers, Z. R., McCavit, T. L., & Buchanan, G. R. (2010). Improved survival of children and adolescents with sickle cell disease. *Blood*, *115*(17), 3447–3452. doi:10.1182/blood-2009-07-233700 PMID:20194891

Serjeant, G. R., Norman, W., & Todd, G. B. (1975). The internal auditory canal and sensorineural hearing loss in homozygous sickle cell disease. *The Journal of Laryngology and Otology*, *89*(4), 453–455. doi:10.1017/S0022215100080580 PMID:1127338

Stuart, A. (2019). Hearing loss in children with homozygous sickle cell disease. *The Hearing Journal*, *72*(7), 16 & 18-19.

Stuart, A., Jones, S. M., & Walker, L. J. (2006). Insights into elevated distortion product otoacoustic emissions in sickle cell disease: Comparisons of hydroxyurea-treated and non-treated young children. *Hearing Research*, *212*(1-2), 83–89. doi:10.1016/j.heares.2005.10.014 PMID:16364581

Stuart, A., & Preast, J. L. (2012). Contralateral suppression of transient evoked otoacoustic emissions in children with sickle cell disease. *Ear and Hearing*, *33*(3), 421–429. doi:10.1097/AUD.0b013e31823effd9 PMID:22246207

Su, B. M., & Chan, D. K. (2017). Prevalence of hearing loss in US children and adolescents: Findings from NHANES 1988-2010. *JAMA Otolaryngology-Head & Neck Surgery*, *143*(9), 920–927. doi:10.1001/jamaoto.2017.0953 PMID:28750123

U.S. National Library of Medicine. (2019, Dec 10). *Your guide to understanding genetic conditions: Sickled cells.* National Library of Medicine (US). Genetics Home Reference. Retrieved from https://ghr.nlm.nih.gov/gallery?start=60

Walker, L. J., Stuart, A., & Green, W. B. (2004). Outer and middle ear status and distortion product otoacoustic emissions in children with sickle cell disease. *American Journal of Audiology*, *13*(2), 164–172. doi:10.1044/1059-0889(2004/021) PMID:15903142

Yanni, E., Grosse, S. D., Yang, Q., & Olney, R. S. (2009). Trends in pediatric sickle cell disease-related mortality in the United States, 1983-2002. *The Journal of Pediatrics*, *154*(4), 541–545. doi:10.1016/j.jpeds.2008.09.052 PMID:19028391

Yawn, B. P., & John-Sowah, J. (2015, December 15). Management of sickle cell disease: Recommendations from the 2014 Expert Panel Report. *American Family Physician*, *92*(12), 1069–1076. PMID:26760593

ADDITIONAL READING

Adams, R. J., McKie, V. J., Hsu, L., ... Waclawiw, M. (1998). Prevention of first stroke by transfusion in children with sickle cell anemia and abnormal results on transcranial Doppler. *The New England Journal of Medicine*, *339*, 5–11. doi:10.1056/NEJM199807023390102 PMID:9647873

Hoppe, C., Klitz, W., Cheng, S., Apple, R., Steiner, L., Robles, L., ... Styles, L. (2004). Gene interactions and stroke risk in children with sickle cell anemia. *Blood*, *103*(6), 2391–2396. doi:10.1182/blood-2003-09-3015 PMID:14615367

Kavanaugh, P. L., Wang, C. J., Therrell, B. L., Sprinz, P. G., & Bauchner, H. (2008). Communication of positive newborn screening results for sickle cell disease and sickle cell trait: Variation across states. *American Journal of Medical Genetics. Part C, Seminars in Medical Genetics*, *148*(1), 15–22. doi:10.1002/ajmg.c.30160 PMID:18200513

Piltcher, O., Cigana, L., Friedriech, J., Quintanilha Ribeiro, F. A., & Selaimen da Costa, S. (2000). Sensorineural hearing loss among sickle cell disease patients from southern Brazil. *American Journal of Otolaryngology*, *21*(2), 75–79. doi:10.1016/S0196-0709(00)85001-2 PMID:10758990

Schatz, J., McClellan, C. B., Puffer, E. S., Johnson, K., & Roberts, C. W. (2008). Neurodevelopmental screening in toddlers and early preschoolers with sickle cell disease. *Journal of Child Neurology*, *23*(1), 44–50. doi:10.1177/0883073807307982 PMID:18160556

Schatz, J., & Roberts, C. W. (2007). Neurobehavioral impact of sickle cell disease in early childhood. *Journal of the International Neuropsychological Society*, *13*(6), 933–943. doi:10.1017/S1355617707071196 PMID:17942011

Scott, D.M. (2005, Nov 29). Hearing research: Children from culturally and linguistically diverse populations. *The ASHA Leader*, p. 4, 22-23.

KEY TERMS AND DEFINITIONS

Acoustic Reflexes: The acoustic reflex is an involuntary muscle contraction that occurs in the middle ear in response to high intensity sounds. When presented with a high intensity sound, the stapedius and tensor tympani muscles contract. The stapedius stiffens the ossicular chain by pulling the stapes (stirrup) of the middle ear away from the oval window of the cochlea, while the tensor tympani muscle stiffens the ossicular chain by pulling the malleus (hammer) in toward the middle ear. The reflex decreases the transmission of acoustic (mechanical) energy to the cochlea.

Auditory Brainstem Response (ABR): Auditory brainstem response (ABR) audiometry is a neurologic test of auditory brainstem function in response to auditory (click) stimuli. The ABR test provides information on how the inner ear, the cochlea, and the brain pathways for hearing are working.

Hemoglobin: Hemoglobin is a protein found in red blood cells. It gives blood its red color, and its job is to transport and release oxygen throughout the body.

Hydroxyurea: Hydroxyurea, a myelosuppressive agent, is the only effective drug proven to reduce the frequency of painful episodes in sickle cell disease. It raises the level of fetal hemoglobin (HbF). It usually decreases the rate of painful episodes by 50%. It was first tested in SCD in 1984. It was developed as an anticancer drug and has been used to treat myeloproliferative syndromes such as leukemia, melanoma, and ovarian cancer (CDC, 2019).

Otoacoustic Emissions (OAEs): Otoacoustic emissions are sounds given off by the inner ear when responding to a sound. There are hair cells in the inner ear that respond to sound by vibrating. The vibration produces a very quiet sound that echoes back into the middle ear. This sound is the OAE that is measured.

Prophylactic Penicillin or Antibiotics: Children who have sickle cell disease and are under the age of five years are at increased risk of life-threatening pneumococcal infection due to absent or non-functional spleens and a decreased immune response. To prevent pneumococcal infection, the American Academy of Pediatrics recommends the use of penicillin prophylaxis in children with SCD under the age of five and in older children who have had a previous severe pneumococcal infection or have functional/surgical asplenia (asplenia is the absence of spleen and/or its functions).

Sickle Cell Disease: Sickle cell disease is a group of autosomal recessively inherited red blood cell disorders. Red blood cells contain hemoglobin. People who have SCD have an abnormal protein in their red blood cells. The protein is called hemoglobin.

Vaso-Occlusion: Vaso-occlusion relates to, results from, or is caused by the blockage of a blood vessel.

Vaso-Occlusive Crisis: A vaso-occlusive crisis occurs when microcirculation of blood vessels is obstructed by sickled red blood cells, causing ischemic injury to the organ supplied and resultant pain.

Section 2

Adult Populations

Chapter 10
Factors Influencing Aphasia Assessment for Bilingual Adults

Leslie W. Johnson
https://orcid.org/0000-0002-6651-4763
North Carolina Central University, USA

EXECUTIVE SUMMARY

This chapter provides a brief overview of stroke, aphasia, and aphasia assessment. Additionally, it considers various issues associated with the standardized assessment of aphasia, including problems related to cultural and linguistic biases. The chapter also includes information on working with people who are bilingual, as well as working with interpreters. A hypothetical case study is presented as a teaching avenue to discuss these topics in greater length. This section contains details regarding how both cultural and linguistic barriers associated with the assessment of the patient's aphasia may have influenced the intervention provided by the speech-language pathologist (SLP). Medical terminology and procedures related to stroke intervention are also discussed as it relates to the SLP's plan of care.

INTRODUCTION

Overview of Stroke and Aphasia

Stroke is the fifth leading cause of death in the United States (Nichols, 2019). A stroke, also known as a cerebrovascular accident (CVA), occurs when there is a change in blood flow to the brain or the area surrounding the brain, which causes injury to the brain's cells. A stroke can happen to anyone at anytime, though there are certain risk factors, such as history of heart disease, high blood pressure, poor diet, age, genetics, and race, that may predispose one person over another to be at an increased risk for stroke (American Stroke Association, 2019).

Brain cells have a dedicated function within the brain that in turn correspond to a specific ability; therefore, how each person is affected by stroke is different, based on where the stroke occurred within the brain, and how much of the brain was damaged. According to the American Stroke Association (2019), some people recover completely from a stroke, but more than two-thirds of survivors will have

DOI: 10.4018/978-1-7998-2261-5.ch010

some type of permanent disability as a result of their stroke. Impairments after stroke can be related to visual disturbances, motor movement of one or more extremities, slurred speech, numbness of one or more parts of the body, balance or coordination issues, or numerous other difficulties (Tatemichi, Desmond, Stern, Paik, Sano, & Bagiella, 1994).

Changes related to a person's language abilities are referred to as aphasia. Aphasia is an acquired disorder due to an injury to the brain and is commonly secondary to stroke (National Institute on Deafness and Other Communication Disorders, 2019). Aphasia can affect any component of language: spoken language expression, auditory language comprehension, reading comprehension, or written expression. It can range in severity from mild to severe. In the most severe cases of aphasia, communication exchanges between the patient and the listener may be almost impossible. Multiple domains of language are typically affected by aphasia, such as naming objects, formulating grammatical sentences, understanding complex directions, or reading paragraphs. Aphasia can be extremely frustrating for some patients as they may know exactly what they want to say, but cannot get the words out to say it. Other patients with aphasia may believe they are speaking perfectly clear and appropriately to their communication partner, when in reality the words coming out of their mouths are merely jargon with no meaningful communicative intent. A person with aphasia often has relatively intact nonlinguistic cognitive skills, though cognitive deficits may co-occur with aphasia (American Speech-Language-Hearing Association [ASHA], 2015).

Aphasia in Culturally and Linguistically Diverse (CLD) Populations

Aphasia intervention within CLD populations is a topic that has gained increased awareness in the field of speech-language pathology over the last several decades (Goral & Conner, 2013; Paniagua & Yamada, 2013; Penn & Armstrong, 2017; Roger, Code, & Sheard, 2000). This is especially important as SLPs are starting to see an increase in the number of patients on their caseload from diverse backgrounds, while also reporting increasing numbers of bilingual speakers (ASHA, 2014). This may be due to a steady increase in the numbers of older minority individuals (Ortman, Velkoff, & Hogan, 2014) or a high incidence of stroke reported in older members of minority groups (Payne, 2014). Cultural and linguistic factors impacting aphasia may include such things as verbal and gestural communication, use of eye contact, number of languages spoken, the patient's level of acculturation or acclimation to a more mainstream culture, and/or paralinguistic aspects of expressive language (ASHA, 2004).

Aphasia in people who speak more than one language involves multiple factors to consider. Grosjean (1994) defined bilingualism as the use of at least two languages in one's daily life. Considerations for bilingual speakers also depend on when and how each language was learned, how frequently each language is used, and how proficient the speaker is for each language (Hallowell, 2017). Multiple studies have demonstrated how people who are bilingual process language in both similar and different ways than people who are monolingual (Fabbro, 2001; Hernandez, Dapretto, Mazziotta, & Bookheimer, 2001; Lorenzen & Murray, 2008). Understanding that the neural pathways for language processing may be different in bilingual speakers is important for any clinician working with someone who has aphasia as this can impact how aphasia presents itself clinically. Language impairment can present differently in bilingual speakers compared to monolingual speakers. For example, in parallel impairment, the most common type of aphasia impairment noted in bilingual speakers (Hallowell, 2017), both languages are impaired in the same manner and to the same degree. There are other types of impairment in bilingual aphasia, such as differential impairment with one language more severely impaired than the other.

Working with interpreters is another common occurrence for SLPs working with CLD populations. ASHA has noted that most certified SLPs feel they have average preparation to address cultural and linguistic influences noted on their caseloads, and tend to rely on interpreters or cultural brokers, such as family members, when working with CLD populations (ASHA, 2013). The use of interpreters within CLD populations can help ensure patient safety, accuracy of service delivery, and improve the efficiency of care for patients. Interpreter services have also been noted to increase patient satisfaction scores, reduce the number of hospital readmissions, demonstrate a dedication to quality care, and improve patient compliance with discharge instructions (Gerrish, 2013). Interpreter services can be provided in person, over the telephone, or via video telepractice, depending on the resources available to the particular healthcare setting.

Aphasia Assessment

SLPs play an essential role in the screening, assessment, diagnosis, and treatment of persons with aphasia. According to ASHA (2015), SLPs are central in providing not only clinical (diagnostic and therapeutic) services for people with aphasia, but also serve as advocates for prevention and education related to aphasia, as well as researchers of aphasia.

A SLP conducts a comprehensive aphasia assessment to determine severity and subtype of aphasia, while also evaluating the impact of the communication impairment on the person's quality of life, including how these functional impairments impact the person's social roles related to the family and community. Aphasia assessment can be performed in both nonstandardized and standardized manners, with each having positive and negative implications based on the specific patient, clinician, and testing environment (Hallowell, 2017). Nonstandardized assessments are typically dynamic and allow for the modification of the test stimuli and variation of acceptable responses. On the other hand, standardized aphasia assessments require all clinicians to administer and all test takers to answer the test items the same way so that the administration and scoring is consistent. This allows the clinician to compare the relative performance of an individual or groups of individuals to their particular patient. Standardized aphasia assessments are evaluation tools with established statistical reliability and validity, but when used alone may not be sufficient enough to determine the extent of a patient's communication disorder (Salter, 2005). Still, standardized tests can provide valuable descriptive information about the patient's abilities and impairments, and can be used to track patterns of recovery, stabilization, or decline. When coupled with nonstandardized assessments and/or discourse analysis, the SLP may be able to achieve a more complete representation of the patient's true communication abilities across varied genres.

Factors Impacting Aphasia Assessment

Aphasia assessment can be impacted by many different confounding factors which may lead to invalid results of the assessment. Skilled clinicians are able to recognize some of the more overt aspects and modify their assessment and intervention plan accordingly. These overt aspects are typically related to the patient's environment and can be modified by reducing noise, improving lighting, or having the patient wear their glasses or hearing aids if needed. However, some of these factors are not as explicit, nor as easily modifiable. These factors may be related to concomitant medical diagnoses, such as hemiparesis, concurrent motor speech disorder, such as dysarthria or apraxia of speech, or the presence of a cognitive impairment. Accommodations and modifications may be necessary to address many of these factors and may help the clinician gain useful information in the assessment of a patient's aphasia; however, these changes may invalidate scores obtained from standardized tests (Turkstra, Coelho & Ylvisaker, 2005).

Other less modifiable factors influencing aphasia assessment may be associated with the patient's cultural background, and ultimately the clinician's ability to provide clinically competent care. These factors may be related to internally driven patient factors, such as patient motivation, their engagement with the assessment process, or their beliefs related to illness and healing. Or they may be linked to the patient's social support system (family members and/or other caregivers) who may either help or hinder a patient's ability to participate appropriately in assessment (Smith, Bottemiller, Flemming, Cutrer, & Strand, 2013). Family dynamics vary from one culture to the next and understanding the roles (i.e., decision maker, caregiver, historian, etc.) of each member within the family unit is vital. Considering how the patient's culture influences healthcare beliefs and family dynamics are both ways to incorporate cultural competence into aphasia assessment. Finally, the interpersonal dynamics between the clinician and the patient being assessed are also important factors during the assessment process and likely influenced by the SLP's cultural competence. This relationship may be influenced by the patient's culture, the clinician's culture, the patient's caregivers, the use of an interpreter, and/or overt or covert stereotypes on behalf of both the clinician and patient (Hallowell, 2017).

In addition to these factors, there are several cultural and linguistic biases in the assessment of aphasia of which clinicians should be responsive. Until recently, many academic and clinical training programs had included minimal education related to building culturally and linguistically contextualized curriculums (Horton-Ikard, Munoz, Thomas, & Keller-Bell, 2009). Increasingly, training programs are appreciating cultural factors that might impact how students learn, how students interact with their patients and clients from CLD backgrounds, and how students can become more informed about cultural and professional competencies related to working with people from diverse backgrounds (Paniagua & Yamada, 2013). Deficiencies in both educational and professional training have been linked to a critical shortage of trained faculty and trained clinicians serving diverse individuals (Horton-Ikard et al., 2009). Centeno (2015) surveyed SLPs working with diverse populations and found that 66.4% reported minimal to moderate preparation for working with neurologically impaired bilingual adults. Improved training related to providing culturally competent care may help to foster sustainable growth and understanding of the diverse populations SLPs are increasingly seeing on their caseloads. Interestingly, despite a gap in professional preparation, it appears SLP are making appropriate decisions for the clinical services they provide to people from culturally and linguistically diverse backgrounds (Centeno, 2015).

Another cultural and linguistic concern related to aphasia assessment is that many aphasiologists in the United States are generally from the more dominant cultural and linguistic discourses (Karanth, 2000; Payne, 2014). There are CLD researchers actively engaged in building the aphasia literature related to diverse populations (Centeno, 2015; Daugherty, Puente, Fasfous, Hidalgo-Ruzzante, & Perez-Garcia, 2017; Penn & Armstong, 2017); however, in general the field of aphasiology lacks sufficient personnel from many global regions (Hallowell, 2017). Therefore, much of the research that has been conducted on aphasia, both related to aphasia assessment and intervention, has been conducted by aphasiologists usually from Western backgrounds on participants from similar backgrounds (Goral & Conner, 2013; Hallowell, 2017; Roger & Code, 2011). Generalization of the findings of many research studies related to aphasia may not be applicable to CLD populations if they were not indeed the population studied (Goral & Conner, 2013). Moreover, administering an assessment tool standardized in English by translating it into another language may invalidate the standardized score of the assessment (Daugherty et al., 2017; Roger & Code, 2011; Turkstra et al., 2005). Finally, although there are some standardized aphasia assessments available in languages other than English and some English originating tests have been translated into other languages (see Ivanova & Hallowell, 2013 for review), there remain relatively few options available for non-English-speaking clinicians in the standardized assessment of aphasia (Paniague & Yamada, 2013).

Because much of the research related to aphasia is conducted on English-speaking populations, the peer-reviewed, evidenced based articles that many clinicians use to guide their practices are found in predominately English written journals (Hallowell, 2017). Therefore, there is an extreme language bias noted in our scholarly journals with over 85% of aphasia research studies based on observations of English-speaking people (Beveridge & Bak, 2011). There appears to be a continued need for aphasiologists who are proficient in English, and who are bilingual/multilingual, to collaborate with people from across the globe to enhance the research literature of people from diverse backgrounds (Isaac, 2002). This is especially important as there is a rapidly expanding aging population, specifically in the relatively under-resourced areas of the world (Orttman et al., 2014).

In addition to language biases, several researchers have presented evidence that neuropsychological examinations, including cognitive linguistic assessments used by SLPs, present with cultural biases too, which may ultimately lead to issues with diagnostic assessment (Daugherty et al., 2017; Fasfous, Hidalgo-Russante, Vilar-López, Catena-Martinez, & Pérez-Garcia, 2013; Norman et al., 2011; Puente, Perez-Garcia, Lopez, Hidalgo-Ruzzante, & Fasfous, 2013). Daugherty et al. (2017) reports that much of the research studying the diagnostic effects of standardized neuropsychological tests on individuals of different cultures has been limited to the U.S. Many of these study only a few minority groups, most often composed of African Americans living in the U.S., and compare them to North American, Anglo-Saxon standards (Norman et al., 2011; Proctor & Zhang, 2008). Daugherty and colleagues (2017) concluded that most studies that aim to evaluate cultural differences in diagnostic standards are merely evaluating ethnic-minority differences, rather than true cultural issues.

Serving adults with aphasia is a complex process, and for those patients from CLD backgrounds, assessment requires the integration of linguistic, cultural, theoretical, and clinical competence to determine if communication is impacted by a disorder (due to neurological damage), or a difference (due to person's unique cultural and/or linguistic background) (Centeno, 2015). Much has been studied related to aphasia in bilingual speakers (ASHA, 2014; Grosjean, 1994; Lorenzen & Murray, 2008; Paradis & Libben, 2014), as this group can demonstrate unique characteristics and heterogeneity, which may challenge clinicians when providing both diagnostic and therapeutic services. Still, minimal has been studied related to specific cultural beliefs and values that may impact communication abilities (Centeno & Ansaldo, 2013). Puente et al. (2013) reported that false positives are likely to occur when neuropsychological tests from one culture group are applied to individuals from another. Daugherty and colleagues (2017) add that diagnostic inaccuracies such as this can augment measurement errors, and subsequent misdiagnoses. Another cultural bias within many aphasia assessment tools can be noted related to presented stimuli used to elicit a response (Battle & Anderson, 1998). For example, the visualization of a swastika to elicit an emotional response, the identification of famous faces, or the use of gestures to supplement verbal communication are all highly culturally dependent testing stimuli.

As appropriate and available, the clinician should select both culturally and linguistically appropriate measures to evaluate their patient; however, many of the current standardized aphasia assessment tools have both cultural and linguistic biases. The ability to appropriately intervene and ultimately help people with aphasia is directly connected to a reflective understanding of various biases associated with the assessment process. Consideration of these issues can help the clinician evaluate the complex nature of each patient's assets and challenges, while remaining sensitive to their real-life needs, including their cultural and language needs.

CASE STUDY PRESENTATION

Medical Evaluation

Karl is a 68-year-old male who speaks only German. Karl moved to the U.S. from Germany to live with his daughter, Gaby, and her family. He has been living in the U.S. for just over one year. Currently, he does not have much interaction with other Americans because of his language barrier and therefore has minimal social interaction outside of Gaby, her husband, and their two children, who are all bilingual in both German and English.

Gaby brought Karl to the hospital after she found him at home sitting slumped to one side in his recliner, talking gibberish, and seemingly not understanding the questions she was asking him. In the emergency department, the neurologists were concerned that Karl had a stroke and started a workup to determine a more definitive diagnosis. They sent him immediately for neuroimaging, using a head computed tomography (CT) to evaluate for any changes within his brain. His head CT showed no acute intracranial abnormalities. The neurologist completed a thorough neurological examination which can aid in determining the precise location of the problem within the nervous system (Oommen, 2017). Karl's neurological examination confirmed right hemiplegia, decreased motor and sensory function of cranial nerves V, VII, IX, and XII, aphasia, and dysarthria. The neurologists also completed the National Institutes of Health Stroke Scale (NIHSS) (Goldstein, Bertels, & Davis, 1989). Karl had an NIHSS score of 16, mainly gaining points in the areas of language, dysarthria, and motor/sensory abilities. The neurology team used Gaby as an interpreter for their completion of the neurological examination and the NIHSS. Despite a negative head CT, the neurology team felt strongly that Karl indeed had had a stroke and believed it was likely ischemic in nature. After considering the results of Karl's neurological examination, as well as his NIHSS score, the neurology team felt confident in their diagnosis of a left middle cerebral artery (MCA) CVA.

The neurology team spoke with Gaby about Karl's condition. She had last spoken to him the night before and felt at that time he was acting "normal". Gaby found Karl the next afternoon around 4:00pm when she returned home from work. She mused that at some point during the day, Karl must have made his way to his recliner, which is where he was found. Consequently, no one could confirm when Karl's symptoms began. Because of this, the neurology team ruled out tissue plasminogen activator (tPA) as a CVA intervention option for Karl. tPA is a protein that can be given intravenously to patients who are candidates to potentially breakdown the blood clot causing their stroke and theoretically restore blood flow to that area of the brain.

Karl was admitted to the intensive care unit (ICU) because of the severity of his stroke. As part of their admitting orders, the neurologist ordered Karl to be kept NPO (nothing by mouth), and also initiated consults to physical therapy (PT), occupational therapy (OT), and speech therapy (ST). Specifically, the SLP was tasked to evaluate and treat Karl's dysphagia, dysarthria, and aphasia.

SLP Evaluation

Karl remained NPO overnight and a nasogastric tube (NGT) was placed through Karl's nasal passages, down his pharynx and esophagus, and into his stomach so that his nurse could give him various medications and give him nutrition via liquid tube feeds. Gaby remained at Karl's bedside to help with her father as needed. She also continued to serve as the primary interpreter to convey information to Karl. When the SLP arrived the next morning, she too used Gaby as an interpreter. The SLP completed the clinical swallow evaluation noting continued weakness, decreased range of motion, and decreased sensation on Karl's right side, intermittent wet vocal quality, and inconsistent signs and symptoms of aspiration. Therefore, the SLP recommended continued NPO except ice chips and water after oral care, and a Modified Barium Swallow Study (MBSS) to further evaluate Karl's dysphagia.

The SLP then shifted her assessment to focus on Karl's communication abilities. Up to this point, the SLP had felt comfortable using Gaby as an interpreter for her session with Karl. She paused and considered using the hospital's interpreter service moving forward with her assessment. The SLP knew that the only interpreters the hospital had on site were Spanish -speaking interpreters, so she would have to use the hospital's contracted interpreter telephone service to find a German interpreter. Considering it important to accurately assess Karl's communication abilities in his native language, the SLP explained to Karl and Gaby that she wanted to continue her assessment using an interpreter and excused herself from Karl's room. She returned shortly with a specialized telephone system the hospital used for interpreter services for many different languages. This telephone system consisted of two handheld telephone receivers, one for the SLP and the other for the patient. A three-way conference call connected the clinician, patient, and interpreter, which took several minutes to set up properly. The SLP briefed the interpreter on Karl's medical status and the reason why the SLP was working with Karl. Gaby helped position Karl in the bed so he could hold the telephone receiver with his left hand and listen to the conversation. Eventually, both the SLP and Karl were ready to proceed.

The SLP decided to use informal assessments to evaluate Karl's aphasia and dysarthria. Karl was able to follow 2/5 one-step commands and 0/5 2-step commands. Karl answered 3/10 simple Yes/No questions accurately and demonstrated the function of 4 common objects (a toothbrush, telephone, remote control, and spoon). Regarding Karl's expressive language abilities, the SLP noted poor naming, 1-2 word responses with picture description testing, 2/6 word level repetitions, and 1-2 word responses to open-ended Wh-questions. Given Karl's increased difficulties with these expressive tasks, the SLP redirected her assessment to more automatic tasks in an attempt to increase Karl's stimuability and perhaps accuracy. Karl completed 2/5 fill in the blank tasks correctly, used 2 appropriate greetings, and demonstrated 3 appropriate hand gestures in conversation (thumbs up, wave, and shoulder shrug). Frequently, the interpreter would pause in an attempt to determine the most appropriate translation of Karl's expressive language. The interpreter reported Karl's words were slurred and difficult to understand. Sometimes he would not make any sense with the word(s) he said, sometimes he repeated words he had already said, and sometimes (as the SLP could witness herself) he did not respond at all to the task. The SLP presumed some of these difficulties were due to Karl's receptive language impairment, but realized Karl had significant expressive difficulties as well. Karl was unable to complete certain tasks to evaluate for dysarthria, such as diadochokinetic rates, but the interpreter consistently reported that Karl had decreased speech intelligibility. Karl was able to demonstrate 1/5 oral movements and 2/5 limb movements on command and the SLP suspected some level of apraxia, though she realized this task could have also been influenced by Karl's poor receptive language.

The SLP concluded her session with Karl and the interpreter by giving some brief statements related to Karl's current language function, anticipated prognosis and need for continued ST follow up, and the role of the SLP moving forward. Gaby asked if there was anything, she could be doing to help her father's language abilities improve and the SLP suggested singing with him; asking him simple, Yes/No questions; and encouraging the use of gestures to supplement his verbal communication. The SLP left the session feeling she did not get an accurate picture of Karl's communication abilities and perhaps she should have actually used Gaby as an interpreter for the language assessment. As the SLP began to complete her documentation for Karl's session, she felt overwhelmed with the extent of Karl's communication and motor speech impairments, and questioned how she could best serve him given the language barrier between the two.

Questions for the Reader

1. Why was Karl's stroke not identified on his head CT?
2. Was it appropriate for the medical practitioners to use Gaby as an interpreter?
3. Why is Karl's NIHSS score of 16 important to know?
4. What made Karl an inappropriate candidate for tPA?
5. What clinical indicators did the neurologists use to diagnose Karl with a left MCA CVA?
6. Why was the SLP hesitant to use Karl's daughter as an interpreter for the communication portion of her evaluation?
7. When working with an interpreter, what are some important things for a SLP to consider?
8. Why did the SLP use informal assessment measures during her initial evaluation of Karl's language abilities?
9. What specific components of Karl's communication may the SLP have had difficulty assessing using an interpreter?
10. Given the clinical information presented, what type of aphasia does Karl most likely have?
11. What are the next steps for the SLP regarding Karl's aphasia and ST intervention?

Discussion of Questions to the Reader

1. *Why was Karl's stroke not identified on his head CT?* A head CT is typically the first neuroimaging test performed upon arrival to the hospital to evaluate for acute neurological changes. It is fast, relatively low-priced, widely available, and highly accurate in the detection of skull fractures and intracranial hemorrhage (Le & Gean, 2009). It provides excellent information related to injuries that may be imperative in decisions of how to initially approach intervention (i.e., need for neurosurgery, or determining candidacy for tPA). However, early in the disease process of ischemic strokes particularly, the head CT may not readily detect this type of stroke (Filho, 2018). Therefore, it is not uncommon to have a negative head CT, as Karl did, and still have had a neurological change, such as a stroke.
2. *Was it appropriate for the medical practitioners to use Gaby as an interpreter?* In periods of neurological change and suspected stroke, time is of the utmost concern because time equals brain, essentially meaning the longer it takes to initiate intervention after stroke onset, the more likely it is that permanent brain damage will occur. A German language interpreter was likely not on site at this facility and the medical practitioners would undoubtedly have to go through the process of

accessing an interpreter via a telephone conferencing service. This process may be time consuming and in an emergency situation such as Karl's would not have been the most advantageous use of the healthcare workers' time. Therefore, the healthcare providers chose to use Gaby as an interpreter to save time, in turn potentially decreasing the lasting effects of Karl's stroke. There are concerns for using a family member as an interpreter which are discussed in one of the subsequent questions to the reader.

3. *Why is Karl's NIHSS score of 16 important to know*? The NIHSS was developed to help physicians objectively rate stroke severity. It is composed of 11 items, each of which assesses a specific ability related to neurological function. Increased scores have been shown to correlate with the size of the stroke infarction on both head CT and MRI evaluation (Glymour, Berkman, Ertel, Fay, Glass, & Furie, 2007). The NIHSS has been shown to be a predictor of both short term and long term outcome for patients with stroke. When assessed within the first 48 hours following the onset of stroke symptoms, NIHSS scores have been shown to correlate with clinical outcomes at the 3-month and 1-year mark (Muir, Weir, Murray, Povey, & Lees, 1996; Yoo, Kim, Kwon, Yun, Koh, & Kang, 2008). Patients with a NIHSS score of 4 or less have generally favorable clinical outcomes and have a high likelihood of regaining functional independence regardless of treatment modality (De Haan, Horn, Limburg, van der Meulen, & Bossuyt, 1993).

A score of 16 places Karl within the moderate to severe stroke severity range. Looking back to what areas of the assessment the patient scored points in can be a useful tool for SLPs to guide their evaluation and intervention of dysphagia, communication, and motor speech disorders. In Karl's situation, careful review of his NIHSS confirmed difficulties with his level of consciousness, facial motor movement, and sensory loss impairment. This should indicate to the SLP that Karl was likely going to have swallowing difficulties. Likewise, the noted cranial nerve impairments should also indicate an increased chance of dysarthria. Furthermore, a high score in the language and following commands items should indicate to the SLP aphasia is a chief symptom of Karl's neurological changes. The initial NIHSS score of 16 indicates moderate to severe stroke severity, but it may also have prognostic value too. Higher initial NIHSS scores often are correlated with poorer overall outcome (Weimar, Konig, Kraywinkel, Ziegler, & Diener, 2004). The SLP may want to consider this when formulating prognostic statements or therapy goals.

4. *What made Karl an inappropriate candidate for tPA?* Current inclusion criterion for tPA administration are 18 years or older, clinical diagnosis of an ischemic stroke which causes a neurological deficit, and time of tPA administration is less than three hours after initial symptom onset (Demaerschalk et al., 2016). Because the physicians could not pinpoint exactly when Karl's symptoms began, they had to assume it was greater than three hours before, which precluded Karl from receiving tPA.
5. *What clinical indicators did the neurologists use to diagnose Karl with a left MCA CVA?* Karl's substantial right hemiplegia and significant difficulties with communication likely aided the neurology team in isolating Karl's stroke to the left MCA. Given his right sided weakness, it can be presumed that Karl's stroke occurred within the left hemisphere as the left side of the brain controls motor movement and sensation of the right side of the body. Moreover, given his communication difficulties, Karl likely had damage to the left hemisphere where the majority of people have the language center of their brain located. As the left MCA supplies blood to much of the frontal and temporal lobes involving portions of the brain essential in language, the neurologists isolated the ischemia there.

6. *Why was the SLP hesitant to use Karl's daughter as an interpreter for the communication portion of her evaluation?* For swallowing evaluations, many clinical signs and symptoms of aspiration can be easily distinguished by simple observation of the patient. In this instance, an interpreter's main role is to explain to the patient what the SLP is going to do and why they are doing it. However, for communication evaluations, the interpreter has a much larger role as they are providing vital information to the SLP regarding the patient's language and speech abilities. The SLP may have been hesitant to use a family member as an interpreter because she may have felt she would not have gotten an accurate representation of Karl's communication abilities. In these instance, there is much more room for the interpreter to provide cues, or additional help, to the patient; to gloss over perceived difficulties; or to minimize the extent of the patient's deficits. A family member may be more likely to fall victim to these concerns, rather than a trained and qualified professional interpreter. Similarly, a family member may be less likely to disclose the extent or severity of a medical diagnosis, or the extent to which recovery can be anticipated, fearing hurting their loved one's feelings or in an attempt to keep their loved one's optimism high. Additionally, many family members may not be well versed in medical terminology and may not know how specific medical terms translate between the two languages (Hallowell, 2017).
7. *When working with an interpreter, what are some important things for the SLP to consider?* It is important that the interpreter with whom the SLP is working has both oral and written fluency in the language used by the patient. Interpreters should hold themselves to a high standard of ethics; and therefore, honest and direct interpretation, as well as maintaining confidentiality, are both critical aspects of this profession. The SLP should train the interpreter in any necessary testing rules and procedures, providing written directions as applicable. The SLP should also review any professional terminology that may be used during the session. It is also important for the SLP to establish the roles of both the interpreter and the clinician and discuss the purpose and goals of the session prior to working together. A short debriefing session after working with the patient may be helpful for the interpreter and the SLP so that both professionals can appropriately and accurately reflect the session in their respective documentation.
8. *Why did the SLP use informal assessment measures during her initial evaluation of Karl's language abilities?* From reading Karl's chart, the SLP likely noted Karl had significant aphasia, thereby assuming he would not be able to complete many of the formalized tasks on more standardized aphasia assessments. Secondly, Karl remained in the ICU, so his medical status was still likely very tenuous. Completing a formalized assessment may not have been a good use of the SLP's or Karl's time if it was likely that Karl's medical status could improve (by spontaneous recovery), or decline (due to extension of his stroke) at any given point. Lastly, given the language barrier, the SLP may have wanted to establish Karl's premorbid use of language through patient/family self-report and initiate a screen of Karl's current abilities to get a better sense of how to direct formalized testing. For example, if the family had reported Karl was bilingual in German and English, the SLP's aphasia assessment may have taken a different route completely.
9. *What specific components of Karl's communication may the SLP have had difficulty assessing using an interpreter?* The SLP may have found it difficult to assess Karl's language abilities due to the nature of the interaction, the decreased ability to quickly change the assessment tasks or stimuli, and/or the inability to accurately detail some aspects of Karl's communication abilities. For example, when working with an interpreter, especially when it is not in person, it can be difficult for many clinicians to establish a good rapport with their patient. Establishing a good patient rapport is key

in any clinician-patient interaction as it helps patients open up about their difficulties, be more vulnerable with their attempts at tasks that may be difficult, and improves patient buy-in to the intervention process (Gerrish, Chau, Sobowale, & Birks, 2004). From the clinician's standpoint, a good patient rapport can improve the clinician's helping behaviors and lead to increased time spent with the patient. Using an interpreter may have negative impacts on building a relationship between some clinicians and their patients.

Another reason why the SLP may have found the assessment difficult may be due to the time constraints of allowing for interpretation of each phrase or sentence uttered. A key benefit of performing informal assessments is that they are dynamic, and the clinician is quickly able to change the targeted stimuli, or provide cues or feedback to determine what level of assistance the patient may need to facilitate accuracy. By using an interpreter, the SLP may have found it difficult to utilize this aspect of informal assessment. Most importantly, the SLP likely missed several important aspects of Karl's language abilities that even a professional interpreter may not have fully been aware of or able to grasp. After all, interpreters are trained to interpret one language to another, and do not understand the many nuances associated with disordered language, such as those present in aphasia. For example, the interpreter often mentioned that Karl was saying words that did not sound like real words. They may have been neologistic paraphasias, which is when the patient uses a nonsense, or made up word, rather than the intended word. Had the SLP been able to hear these types of errors repeatedly, she may have had a better sense of the extent of Karl's aphasia and what may be the best way to treat it. Similarly, the interpreter reported that Karl had very slurred speech, which was difficult to understand, which indicated to the SLP Karl had dysarthria in addition to his aphasia. Had the SLP and Karl spoken the same language, the SLP may have been able to better classify Karl's dysarthria into a specific subtype, which likely would have helped in intervention planning.

10. *Given the clinical information presented, what type of aphasia does Karl most likely have?* Karl most likely has global aphasia. Global aphasia is characterized by poor auditory comprehension, poor repetition, and nonfluent expressive language. Global aphasia is the most severe form of the nonfluent aphasias.
11. *What are the next steps for the SLP regarding Karl's aphasia and ST intervention?* Based on the SLP's assessment of Karl's aphasia, the SLP will likely develop an intervention plan targeting Karl's ability to appropriately convey his wants and needs. Karl's comprehension and expression of language are both severely impacted. The SLP will work to improve both of these abilities. Related to comprehension, Karl needs an accurate Yes/No response so that he can tell his caregivers and medical personnel what he needs. From an expressive language standpoint, the SLP will work on improving Karl's fluency. She may do this through automatic language tasks, such as singing or the use of greetings, or perhaps supplementing Karl's verbal output with the use of alternative and augmentative communication or gestures.

Treatment considerations

Karl continued to be monitored in the ICU for the next three days. The neurology team determined Karl's stroke had been caused by atherosclerosis and carotid artery disease, both contributing to a build-up of plaque within Karl's carotid neck arteries, a major supply of blood flow to the brain. Five days after

Karl's initial symptoms started, he continued to have dense right sided hemiparesis and global aphasia, though both he and his family thought these were improving. The neurology team repeated Karl's head CT one week into his hospitalization. The repeat head CT confirmed the suspected clinical diagnosis of left MCA CVA, with findings indicating a large, left frontotemporal infarct.

The SLP continued to work with Karl while he was in the ICU and after he transferred to the hospital's floor unit. Karl's MBSS showed inconsistent silent aspiration of thin and thick liquids, as well as purees. The SLP recommended continued NPO except ice chips and water after oral care, with a repeat MBSS in the next 7-10 days. Until Karl was able to initiate food and liquid by mouth, he would have to continue tube feedings via his NGT, or a more permanent means of nutrition should this impairment extend for a longer period.

Karl continued to present with significant global aphasia. Both the SLP and Karl found the telephone interpreter system cumbersome to use and as a family member was almost always at Karl's bedside, family became the primary source for interpretation between the SLP and Karl. The SLP formulated an intervention plan targeting establishing an accurate Yes/No response for Karl, implementing gestures to supplement verbalizations, and extending Karl's fluency to 2-4 words per utterance. The SLP planned to work with Karl 2-3 times a week while he remained hospitalized. Improvements in therapy were first noted related to Karl's comprehension. Karl's accuracy for responding to Yes/No questions improved when his communication partner provided Karl with a visual representation of a Yes or No response. Gaby and the other family members continued to sing with Karl to access expressive language. This practice began to carryover in other automatic utterance tasks during Karl's ST sessions, such as with greetings and fill in the blank tasks. Karl's naming abilities remained poor, though he was stimuable to select the correct response when given a choice of 2 options. Repetition remained difficult for Karl, even at the word and 2-3 word phrase level, and the SLP continued to note groping movements for some words, which appeared congruent with apraxia of speech.

Two weeks after his stroke, Karl's physicians asked the rehabilitation team to re-assess Karl's abilities related to each discipline (OT, PT, and ST) to aid in determining if Karl was an appropriate candidate for acute inpatient rehabilitation (AIR). The AIR setting provides intense therapy at least three hours a day to prepare patients for discharge back home and into their communities. This level of acute rehabilitation has been repeatedly shown to increase both short term and long term outcomes after stroke, and other acute neurological events (DaVanzo et al., 2014). Given his clinical improvements, the SLP decided to complete Karl's re-assessment using a formal, standardized aphasia test, using Gaby as the interpreter.

The SLP completed the Western Aphasia Battery (Kertesz, 1982). She provided Gaby with a copy of the testing manual so that she could be prepared to help translate the test. As they progressed through the test, Gaby did not know the literal translation for some of the testing stimuli, so the SLP told Gaby to use a word or phrase that most closely resembled the targeted word or phrase. Again, similar to his previous assessment, Karl's slurred speech made it difficult to understand many of the words he was attempting to say. Other times Gaby was not sure what he said was even a German word, and occasionally he repeated words he had already said. Comparable to his previous assessment, intermittently Karl would not even respond to certain tasks. The SLP attempted to make it through as much of the standardized assessment as she could, but felt limited by both the extent of Karl's aphasia and the ongoing language barrier.

Outcomes

Karl was accepted into AIR and transferred there to complete his intense post-stroke therapy. This occurred approximately three weeks after the onset of his stroke. At his time of discharge from the acute care setting, the SLP did not feel Karl could safely intake anything by mouth other than ice chips and water. The medical team placed a percutaneous endoscopic gastrostomy (PEG) tube into Karl's stomach to provide a means of giving Karl nutrition and hydration. The SLP anticipated a good long-term return to safe intake of food and liquid by mouth for Karl, but suspected his dysphagia would persist for the next several weeks.

At his time of discharge from the acute care setting, Karl continued to present with global aphasia, though it had improved slightly since his initial assessment. The SLP anticipated Karl's communication abilities to continue to improve, though knew he had a difficult road to recovery ahead of him. Not only was he limited by the severity of his stroke, the likelihood of Karl having a language barrier between him and the therapists involved in his treatment would likely be high. Still, he had several positive prognostic indicators, namely his family support and his continued motivation to participate in therapy. The SLP anticipated Karl would need continued ST follow up for many months, likely years to come, first in the AIR setting, then the home health or outpatient setting.

Working with Karl had changed the SLP. The SLP had previously worked with other patients who did not speak English, and some who were bilingual in English and another language, but the case with Karl seemed different. Perhaps it was due to the intricacies of aphasia and the inability of the SLP to ever fully grasp what was going on with Karl's communication without hearing and recognizing the changes for herself. She believed she was losing a great deal of information related to Karl's language and dysarthria abilities through the use of interpreters, no matter if the interpreter was a true medical interpreter (who specialized in the interpreting of medically related situations), or a family interpreter (who knew the patient better and was more vested in the situation). Perhaps the SLP's discontent was related to feelings of inadequacy in serving her patient to the best of her abilities because of the culture and linguistic barriers. Either way, the SLP used this experience to modify her practice when working with patients from different cultural and linguistic backgrounds to ultimately enhance the assessment and treatment services she provides. She continually interweaved cultural competence into all aspects of intervention for all patients on her caseload.

Additional Questions for the Reader

1. Why do SLPs need to know about specific diagnoses, assessments, or typical medical interventions related to the care of patients with stroke?
2. Why is it not standard practice to simply translate an English, standardized aphasia test to use with a patient/client who speaks a language other than English?
3. What are some examples of either overt or covert biases that may have influenced the assessment of Karl's aphasia?
4. What other cultural biases may be noted in Karl's case study?

5. What do you think Karl's overall prognosis is regarding his communication abilities?
6. Karl was not bilingual, but if he had been, what are some considerations related to bilingual aphasia that may be important for the SLP to consider?
7. What other resources related to intervention, support, or community resources are available to Karl and his family?

Discussion of Additional Questions for the Reader

1. *Why do SLPs need to know about specific diagnosis, assessments, or typical medical interventions related to the care of patients with stroke?* SLPs should know about these things as they can often dictate treatment and prognosis. For example, Karl's initial NIHSS provided the SLP with vital information related to the severity of Karl's stroke and his anticipated prognosis. Additionally, Karl had an ischemic stroke. Ischemic strokes are medically managed very differently than hemorrhagic ones, which can impact how and when the SLP may be able to initiate services. Additionally, research has demonstrated that people who have an ischemic stroke have increased disabilities after stroke and poorer long-term outcomes compared to people who have had a hemorrhagic stroke (Varona, Bermejo, Guerra, & Molina, 2004).
2. *Why is it not standard practice to simply translate an English, standardized aphasia test to use with a patient/client who speaks a language other than English?* It is important to realize that because of the wide range of variability from one language to another related to language vocabulary, morphology, and syntactic structure, the idea of simply translating a standardized aphasia test to another language is not a viable option, though it remains common practice (Isaac, 2002; Roger et al., 2000). Roger and Code (2011) reported significant content validity problems when conducting aphasia assessments using English language testing instruments with items interpreted by a trained interpreter. Aphasiologists have largely focused on linguistic differences in diverse populations, such as test translation or the ramifications of working with an interpreter, with less attention being paid to the impact of the broader concept of culture and how that impacts aphasia intervention (Peen & Armstrong, 2017). Perhaps straight translation of a test from one language to another targets the language barrier, though the patient's cultural differences remain unaddressed. In instances such as this, it may be appropriate to use informal assessments to assess aphasia. Some informal strategies listed by SLPs when working with CLD populations include gathering information on pre-morbid language use via conversation using an interpreter, using standardized tests to assess English proficiency in patients who are bilingual, and collecting a discourse sample (Centeno, 2015).
3. *What are some examples of either overt or covert biases that may have influenced the assessment of Karl's aphasia?* Perhaps the biggest overt bias associated with the assessment of Karl's aphasia was the notable language barrier. Although the assessment was completed with an interpreter, there remains aspects of Karl's communication abilities that appeared to be lost in translation. Another overt bias is the limited understanding of how Karl's German culture may impact how Karl performed on the assessment. Because of the linguistic and cultural differences, Karl more than likely did not fit in with the group the assessment tool was normed on, thus potentially invalidating the results of standardized assessment. Covert biases may be related to certain stereotypes the SLP may have related to CLD individuals, or may pertain to the SLP's experience with working with patients with such severe aphasia.

4. *What other cultural biases may be noted in Karl's case study?* Cultural biases may be related to family structure and general healthcare considerations in Karl's case study. It may have been helpful for the SLP to know how families are typically structured within the German culture and who makes key decisions, how these decisions are made, and what role each family member may play. Karl moved from Germany to live with Gaby and her family, but it may be helpful to have more information on the culture's beliefs related to family support for care of adults with disabilities, or considerations of alternative living arrangements if needed. The cultural beliefs related to certain aspects of healthcare, such as access to care, utilization of healthcare, and traditional healing beliefs may have influenced both Karl and Gaby when signs of Karl's stroke were originally noted. Cultural beliefs related to cause of illness, the aging process, and disability may have influenced how Karl interacted with his medical team and how motivated he was to follow through with their recommendations. If the medical team had weighed Karl's cultural preferences more, it may have impacted the team's intervention plan to send Karl to AIR, or the SLP's intervention plan related to specific goals targeted in therapy.
5. *What do you think Karl's overall prognosis is regarding his communication abilities?* Karl likely has an overall fair prognosis regarding his communication abilities. He does have several positive prognostic indicators, including his relative age, strong social support, within the window of continued spontaneous recovery, and motivation to improve. Still, he remains limited by several substantial negative prognostic indicators, including severity and location of his stroke; severity of global aphasia, other concurrent deficits of dysarthria, apraxia, and dysphagia; and relatively minimal progress to date. The most predictive indicator of long-term recovery related to language ability is initial aphasia severity, along with lesion site and size (Plowman, Hentz & Ellis, 2012).
6. *Karl was not bilingual, but if he had been, what are some considerations related to bilingual aphasia that may be important for the SLP to consider?* Bilingualism is often rated on a continuum of language abilities, as proficiency across any of the languages used may fluctuate over time, across social environments, with various conversation partners, or with topics of conversation (Grosjean, 1994). For any SLP working with a patient who is bilingual, there are several aspects of the patient's language abilities that should be considered. First, learning how and at what age the person acquired each language is essential. Some examples of this may include simultaneous bilingualism, sequential bilingualism, dual language learner, or English as a second language learner. Second, it is important for the SLP to learn how frequently each language is used by the patient, in what contexts, and the patient's proficiency of each language. Third, SLPs should be cognizant of the types of impairments typically noted in bilingual aphasia, such as parallel impairment (both languages are impacted similarly), differential impairment (one language is impacted differently than the other), or selective impairment (various aspects of one or more language may be impacted to a different degree) (Hallowell, 2017). There are standardized aphasia assessments for bilingual speakers, the Bilingual Aphasia Test (Paradis & Libben, 1987) and Bilingual English Spanish Assessment (Peña, Gutiérrez-Clellen, Iglesias, Goldstein, & Bedore, 2018) are two notable ones. Additionally, in providing services to bilingual patients, the SLP should consider how the communication disorder may be manifested, identified, or described in the patient's cultural and linguistic community (Lorenzen & Murray, 2008). This information is vital in the SLP's assessment, diagnosis, and intervention plan for the patient. SLPs should be prepared to address the unique needs of their bilingual patients and are ethically obligated to provide culturally and linguistically appropriate services to their patients.

7. *What other resources related to intervention, support, or community resources are available to Karl and his family?* There are a variety of post-stroke resources available to Karl and his family. The American Stroke Association has an enormous amount of information on its website related to life after stroke, help and support after stroke, and ways to get involved to advocate for stroke related issues. This organization can also help find nearby support groups for both Karl and his family. The National Aphasia Association is an organization dedicated to advocating for persons with aphasia and their families. It can be helpful in providing a community of individuals and caregivers all living with aphasia, or being impacted by aphasia, in various ways. Some communities have smaller non-profit organizations dedicated to providing ongoing rehabilitation services to people with aphasia in an outpatient based model. These organizations may be helpful in providing additional services after the person has reached the annual therapy cap allotted by insurance companies. Examples of groups focused on global and multicultural engagement in aphasiology are Aphasia United (www.aphasiaunited.org), The National Aphasia Association (NAA) Multicultural Task Force (MTF) (www.aphasia.org), and Association Internationale d'Aphasie (AIA) (www.aphasia-international.com).

KEY POINTS

Stroke occurs when there is a change in blood flow to the brain or the area surrounding the brain and can be classified as ischemic or hemorrhagic. Stroke is the leading cause of aphasia, which refers to any impairment across the various domains of language, namely expressive language, comprehension of language, written language, and reading comprehension. Understanding how aphasia presents within CLD populations is key for any clinician working in this area. Inherent in the standardized assessment of aphasia remains confounding factors that may impact how a person performs on standardized aphasia assessment, many are related to both cultural and linguistic biases.

Karl's case study presentation demonstrates how important medical information can be used by the SLP in the assessment and intervention of aphasia. It incorporates both medical and SLP interventions to demonstrate how these two fields work closely together for added benefit to the patients they serve. Importantly, it also reviews how one SLP attempted to modify and accommodate her aphasia assessment based on a linguistic barrier. It details how the language barrier affected both the informal and formal assessments, and reviews important aspects for SLPs to consider when working with interpreters or attempting to evaluate aphasia in a language other than English.

REFERENCES

American Speech-Hearing-Language Association. (2013). *ASHA SLP health care survey*. Retrieved from https://www.asha.org/Research/memberdata/Healthcare-Survey/

American Speech-Hearing-Language Association. (2014). *Demographic profile of ASHA members providing bilingual services*. Retrieved from https://www.asha.org/uploadedFiles/Demographic-Profile-Bilingual-Spanish-Service-Members.pdf

American Speech-Hearing-Language Association. (2015). *Person centered focus on function: Aphasia*. Retrieved from https://www.asha.org/uploadedFiles/ICF-Aphasia.pdf

American Speech-Language-Hearing Association. (2004). *Knowledge and skills needed by speech-language pathologists and audiologists to provide culturally and linguistically appropriate services*. Retrieved from http://www.asha.org/docs/html/KS2004-00215.html

American Stroke Association. (2019). *Stroke risk factors*. Retrieved from https://www.stroke.org/en/about-stroke/stroke-risk-factors

Battle, D., & Anderson, N. (1998). Culturally diverse families and the development of language. In D. E. Battle (Ed.), *Communication disorders in multicultural populations* (pp. 213–245). Boston: Butterworth-Heinemann.

Beveridge, M. E., & Bak, T. H. (2011). The languages of aphasia research: Bias and diversity. *Aphasiology*, *25*(12), 1451–1468. doi:10.1080/02687038.2011.624165

Centeno, J. G. (2015). Assessing services with communicatively impaired bilingual adults in culturally and linguistically diverse neurorehabilitation programs. *Journal of Communication Disorders*, *58*, 58–73. doi:10.1016/j.jcomdis.2015.10.005 PMID:26513217

Centeno, J. G., & Ansaldo, A. (2013). Aphasia in multilingual populations. In I. Papathanasious, P. Coppens, & C. Potagas (Eds.), *Aphasia and related neurogenic communication disorders* (pp. 275–294). Boston: Jones and Bartlett.

Daugherty, J. C., Puente, A. E., Fasfous, A. F., Hidalgo-Ruzzante, N., & Pérez-Garcia, M. (2017). Diagnostic mistakes of culturally diverse individuals when using North American neuropsychological tests. *Applied Neuropsychology. Adult*, *24*(1), 16–22. doi:10.1080/23279095.2015.1036992 PMID:27485042

DaVanzo, J. E., Dobson, A., El-Gamil, A., Li, J. W., & Manolov, N. (2014). *Assessment of patient outcomes of rehabilitative care provided in inpatient rehabilitation facilities and after discharge*. Presentation to ARA Research Institute. Retrieved from https://amrpa.org/Portals/0/ARA%20Research%20Institute%20Final%20Dobson%20Da Vanzo%20Senate%20Briefing%207%2010%2014.pdf

De Haan, R., Horn, J., Limburg, M., van der Meulen, J., & Bossuyt, P. (1993). A comparison of 5 stroke scales with measures of disability, handicap, and quality-of-life. *Stroke*, *24*(8), 1178–1181. doi:10.1161/01.STR.24.8.1178 PMID:8342193

Demaerschalk, B. M., Kleindorfer, D. O., Adeoye, O. M., Demchuk, A. M., Fugate, J. E., Grotta, J. C., ... Smith, E. E. (2016). Scientific rationale for the inclusion and exclusion criteria for intravenous alteplase in acute ischemic stroke: A statement for healthcare professionals from the American Heart Association/American Stroke Association. *Stroke*, *47*(2), 581–641. doi:10.1161/STR.0000000000000086 PMID:26696642

Fabbro, F. (2001). The bilingual brain: Bilingual aphasia. *Brain and Language*, *79*(2), 201–210. doi:10.1006/brln.2001.2480 PMID:11712844

Fasfous, A. F., Hidalgo-Russante, N., Vilar-López, R., Catena-Martinez, A., & Pérez-Garcia, M. (2013). Cultural differences in neuropsychological abilities related to perform intelligence tasks. *Archives of Clinical Neuropsychology*, *28*(8), 784–790. doi:10.1093/arclin/act074 PMID:24055883

Filho, J. O. (2018). Neuroimaging of acute ischemic stroke. *UpToDate*. Retrieved from https://www.uptodate.com/contents/neuroimaging-of-acute-ischemic-stroke

Gerrish, K., Chau, R., Sobowale, A., & Birks, E. (2004). Bridging the language barrier: The use of interpreters in primary care nursing. *Health & Social Care in the Community*, *12*(5), 407–413. doi:10.1111/j.1365-2524.2004.00510.x PMID:15373819

Glymour, M., Berkman, L., Ertel, K., Fay, M., Glass, T., & Furie, K. (2007). Lesion characteristics, NIH Stroke Scale, and functional recovery after stroke. *American Journal of Physical Medicine & Rehabilitation*, *86*(9), 725–733. doi:10.1097/PHM.0b013e31813e0a32 PMID:17709996

Goldstein, L. B., Bertels, C., & Davis, J. N. (1989). Interrater Reliability of the NIH Stroke Scale. *Archives of Neurology*, *46*(6), 660–662. doi:10.1001/archneur.1989.00520420080026 PMID:2730378

Goral, M., & Conner, P. S. (2013). Language disorders in multilingual and multicultural populations. *Annual Review of Applied Linguistics*, *33*, 128–161. doi:10.1017/S026719051300010X PMID:26257455

Grosjean, F. (1994). Individual bilingualism. In *The Encyclopedia of Language and Linguistics*. Oxford, UK: Pergamon Press.

Hallowell, B. (2017). *Aphasia and other acquired neurogenic language disorders: A guide for clinical excellence*. San Diego, CA: Plural Publishing.

Hernandez, A. E., Dapretto, M., Mazziotta, J., & Bookheimer, S. (2001). Language switching and language representation in Spanish-English bilinguals: An fMRI study. *Neuroimaging*, *14*(2), 510–520. doi:10.1006/nimg.2001.0810 PMID:11467923

Horton-Ikard, R., Munoz, M. L., Thomas-Tate, S., & Keller-Bell, Y. (2009). Establishing a pedagogical framework for the multicultural course in communication sciences and disorders. *American Journal of Speech-Language Pathology*, *18*(2), 192–206. doi:10.1044/1058-0360(2008/07-0086) PMID:19106206

Isaac, K. (2002). *Speech pathology and cultural and linguistic diversity*. London: Whurr.

Ivanova, M. V., & Hallowell, B. (2013). A tutorial on aphasia test development in any langauage: Key substantive and psychometric considerations. *Aphasiology*, *27*(8), 891–920. doi:10.1080/02687038.2013.805728 PMID:23976813

Karanth, P. (2000). Multilingual/multiliterate/multicultural studies of aphasia – the Rosetta Stone of neurolinguistics in the new millennium. *Brain and Language, 71*(1), 113-115.

Le, T. H., & Gean, A. D. (2009). Neuroimaging of traumatic brain injury. *The Mount Sinai Journal of Medicine, New York, 76*(2), 145–162. doi:10.1002/msj.20102 PMID:19306377

Lorenzen, B., & Murray, L. (2008). Bilingual aphasia: A theoretical and clinical review. *American Journal of Speech-Language Pathology, 17*(3), 299–317. doi:10.1044/1058-0360(2008/026) PMID:18663112

Muir, K. W., Weir, C. J., Murray, G. D., Povey, C., & Lees, K. R. (1996). Comparison of neurological scales and scoring systems for acute stroke prognosis. *Stroke, 27*(10), 1817–1820. doi:10.1161/01.STR.27.10.1817 PMID:8841337

National Institute on Deafness and Other Communication Disorders. (2019). *Aphasia*. Retrieved from https://www.nidcd.nih.gov/health/aphasia

Nichols, H. (2019, July 4). *The top 10 leading causes of death in the United States*. Retrieved from https://www.medicalnewstoday.com/articles/282929.php

Norman, M. A., Moore, D. J., Taylor, M., Franklin Jr, D., Cysique, L., & Ake, C. (2011). Demographically corrected norms for African Americans and Caucasians on the Hopkins Verbal Learning Test–Revised, brief visuospatial memory test–revised, stroop color and word test, and Wisconsin card sorting test 64-card version. *Journal of Clinical and Experimental Neuropsychology, 33*(7), 793-804.

Oommen, K. J. (2004). *Neurological history and physical examination*. Retrieved from https://emedicine.medscape.com/article/1147993-overview

Orttman, J. M., Velkoff, V. A., & Howard, H. (2014). An Aging Nation: The Older Population in the United States Population Estimates and Projections Current Population Reports. *United States Census Bureau*. Retrieved from https://www.census.gov/prod/2014pubs/p25-1140.pdf

Paniagua, F. A., & Yamada, A. M. (Eds.). (2013). *Handbook of multicultural mental health: Assessment and treatment of diverse populations*. Cambridge, UK: Academic Press.

Paradis, M., & Libben, G. (2014). *The assessment of bilingual aphasia*. New York: Psychology Press. doi:10.4324/9781315802138

Payne, J. C. (2014). *Adult neurogenic language disorders: Assessment and treatment. A comprehensive ethnobiological approach*. San Diego, CA: Plural Publishing.

Peña, E. D., Gutiérrez-Clellen, V. F., Iglesias, A., Goldstein, B., & Bedore, L. M. (2018). *Bilingual English Spanish Assessment (BESA)*. Baltimore, MD: Brookes.

Penn, C., & Armstrong, E. (2017). Intercultural aphasia: New models of understanding for Indigenous populations. *Aphasiology, 31*(5), 563–594.

Plowman, E., Hentz, B., & Ellis, C. (2012). Post-stroke aphasia prognosis: A review of patient related and stroke-related factors. *Journal of Evaluating Clinical Practices, 18*(3), 689–694. doi:10.1111/j.1365-2753.2011.01650.x PMID:21395923

Proctor, A., Yairi, E., Duff, M. C., & Zhang, J. (2008). Prevalence of stuttering in African American preschoolers. *Journal of Speech, Language, and Hearing Research: JSLHR*, *51*(6), 1465–1479. doi:10.1044/1092-4388(2008/07-0057) PMID:18664698

Puente, A. E., Perez-Garcia, M., Lopez, R. V., Hidalgo-Ruzzante, N. A., & Fasfous, A. F. (2013). Neuropsychological assessment of culturally and educationally dissimilar individuals. In *Handbook of Multicultural Mental Health* (pp. 225–241). Cambridge, UK: Academic Press. doi:10.1016/B978-0-12-394420-7.00012-6

Roger, P., & Code, C. (2011). Lost in translation? Issues of content validity in interpreter mediated aphasia assessments. *International Journal of Speech-Language Pathology*, *13*(1), 61–73. doi:10.3109/17549507.2011.549241 PMID:21329412

Roger, P., Code, C., & Sheard, C. (2000). Assessment and management of aphasia in a linguistically diverse society. *Asia Pacific Journal of Speech, Language and Hearing*, *5*(1), 21–34. doi:10.1179/136132800807547573

Salter, K., Jutai, J., Foley, N., Hellings, C., & Teasell, R. (2006). Identification of aphasia post stroke: A review of screening assessment tools. *Brain Injury: [BI]*, *20*(6), 559–568. doi:10.1080/02699050600744087 PMID:16754281

Smith, J. H., Bottemiller, K. L., Flemming, K. D., Cutrer, F. M., & Strand, E. A. (2013). Inability to self-report pain after a stroke: A population-based study. *Pain*, *154*(8), 1281–1286. doi:10.1016/j.pain.2013.04.006 PMID:23725781

Tatemichi, T. K., Desmond, D. W., Stern, Y., Paik, M., Sano, M., & Bagiella, E. (1994). Cognitive impairment after stroke: Frequency, patterns, and relationship to functional abilities. *Journal of Neurology, Neurosurgery, and Psychiatry*, *57*(2), 202–207. doi:10.1136/jnnp.57.2.202 PMID:8126506

Turkstra, L. S., Coelho, C., & Ylvisaker, M. (2005). The use of standardized tests for individuals with cognitive-communication disorders. *Seminars in Speech and Language*, *26*(4), 215–222. doi:10.1055-2005-922101 PMID:16278794

Varona, J. F., Bermejo, F., Guerra, J. M., & Molina, J. A. (2004). Long-term prognosis of ischemic stroke in young adults. *Journal of Neurology*, *251*(12), 1507–1514. doi:10.100700415-004-0583-0 PMID:15645352

Wardlaw, J. M., & Mielke, O. (2005). Early signs of brain infarction at CT: Observer reliability and outcome after thrombolytic treatment – systematic review. *Radiology*, *235*(2), 444–453. doi:10.1148/radiol.2352040262 PMID:15858087

Weimar, C., Konig, I., Kraywinkel, K., Ziegler, A., & Diener, H. (2004). Age and national institutes of health stroke scale score within 6 hours after onset are accurate predictors of outcome after cerebral ischemia - Development and external validation of prognostic models. *Stroke*, *35*(1), 158–162. doi:10.1161/01.STR.0000106761.94985.8B PMID:14684776

Yoo, S. H., Kim, J. S., Kwon, S. U., Yun, S. C., Koh, J. Y., & Kang, D. W. (2008). Undernutrition as a predictor of poor clinical outcomes in acute ischemic stroke patients. *Archives of Neurology*, *65*(1), 39–43. doi:10.1001/archneurol.2007.12 PMID:18195138

ADDITIONAL READING

American Academy of CME. (1999). *NIH Stroke Scale – Know stroke*. Retrieved from https://www.stroke.nih.gov/documents/NIH_Stroke_Scale_508C.pdf

American Speech-Hearing-Language Association. (2004). *Classification of aphasia*. Retrieved from https://www.asha.org/uploadedFiles/ASHA/Practice_Portal/Clinical_Topics/Aphasia/Common-Classifications-of-Aphasia.pdf

Birenbaum, D., Bancroft, L. W., & Felsberg, G. J. (2011). Imaging in acute stroke. *The Western Journal of Emergency Medicine*, *12*(1), 67–76. PMID:21694755

Roger, P., & Code, C. (2011). Lost in translation? Issues of content validity in interpreter mediated aphasia assessments. *International Journal of Speech-Language Pathology*, *13*(1), 61–73. doi:10.3109/17549507.2011.549241 PMID:21329412

KEY TERMS AND DEFINITIONS

Communication: Communication is the exchange of information, or the act of conveying meaning.

Computed Tomography: CT, refers to a computerized x-ray imaging procedure in which a narrow beam of x-rays is aimed at a patient and quickly rotated around the body, producing signals that are processed by the machine's computer to generate cross-sectional images of the body.

Hemiparesis: Hemiparesis is the weakness of one entire side of the body. It can be caused by a variety of medical conditions affecting the central nervous system, such as a stroke. Oftentimes, people who have aphasia may also have a hemiparesis, depending on the location and severity of their injury.

Neurological Examination: A neurological examination assesses sensory and motor responses, as well as reflexes, cranial nerves, and mental status to determine whether neurological dysfunction exists. More specifically, it evaluates muscle strength and range of motion, muscle tone and bulk, muscular coordination, sensory function, balance, and gait.

Nonfluent Aphasia: Nonfluent aphasia is expressive language output that is severely reduced and limited to short utterances, generally less than five words per breath group. Examples of nonfluent aphasia subtypes are Global Aphasia, Mixed Nonfluent Aphasia, Transcortical Motor Aphasia, and Broca's Aphasia.

Tissue Plasminogen Activator (tPA): tPA is a naturally occurring protein found on endothelial cells, the cells that line blood vessels. It activates the conversion of plasminogen to plasmin, an enzyme responsible for the breakdown of clots. tPA works by preventing the enlargement of blood clots that obstruct the flow of blood in the brain.

Verbal Communication: Verbal communication can include aspects related to both linguistic and paralinguistic skills. Linguistics aspects targeted by the SLP may be related to expressive and receptive language abilities. Paralinguistic aspects targeted by the SLP may be related to pragmatics, the use of prosody in conversation, and appropriate use of body language or facial expressions.

Chapter 11
Dysphagia Management in Culturally-Linguistically Diverse Populations

Kellyn Dailey Hall
North Carolina Central University, USA

EXECUTIVE SUMMARY

Culturally competent management of adults with swallowing disorders involves more than simply including ethnically appropriate foods in dysphagia therapy. It requires an understanding of the client's health beliefs, challenges, and unique cultural perspective regarding all aspects of food to ensure unbiased and culturally appropriate services are provided. This chapter begins with an overview of dysphagia management followed by a closer look at cultural beliefs regarding food and ethical conflicts that may arise. The strategies for shared decision-making presented help create a culturally sensitive dynamic between the clinician and the patient/family that positively influence therapy outcomes. The chapter concludes with a case study that highlights the importance of ethnographic interviewing needed to establish understanding and trust between the clinician and an elderly Mexican woman and her family. The strategies and techniques presented here can be applied across all cultures to achieve successful management of dysphagia.

INTRODUCTION

The collective practices, rituals, and traditions surrounding food make it clear that eating is deeply rooted in culture. Eating food is much more than the physiologic process of breaking down a bolus that can be safely and efficiently swallowed so that nutrients can be consumed. It is an essential aspect of human social life. When swallowing is impaired, the health, psychosocial well-being, and quality of life (QOL) of an individual is threatened (Kenny, 2015). Approximately one in 25 adults are diagnosed with dysphagia each year (Bhattacharyya, 2014). Although the prevalence of dysphagia in adult populations is not fully known and often underestimated (ASHA, n.d.), even less is known about the prevalence of dysphagia across racial/ethnic groups. In one of the few studies, González-Fernández, Kuhlemeirer, and Palmer

DOI: 10.4018/978-1-7998-2261-5.ch011

(2008) reported that the incidence of poststroke dysphagia was higher in minority groups, particularly Asians, as compared to Caucasians. Similarly, Brussel and González-Fernández (2011) found evidence of increased odds for dysphagia in racial/ethnic minority groups following stroke. Given the presence of racial disparities in general health care (Feldman, McDonald, Eimicke, & Teresi (2019), and the link between dysphagia and common stroke (Bhattacharyya, 2014), it is likely that dysphagia is impacted by such disparities as well.

Hispanics, particularly Mexican Americans, have a higher risk of stroke than non-Hispanics (Lisbeth et al., 2014). According to the U.S. Census Bureau (2016), the terms *Hispanic or Latino* refer to a person of Cuban, Mexican, Puerto Rican, South or Central American, or other Spanish culture or origin regardless of race. Hispanics represent that largest minority group in the U.S. Considering that all minority groups are rapidly growing in the U.S. (U.S. Census Bureau, 2016), SLPs can expect to see growing numbers of culturally-linguistically diverse patients (CLD) with dysphagia on their caseloads and the likelihood that they will be Hispanic is high.

The SLP treating patients with dysphagia from CLD groups must have a firm understanding of the role that culture plays in dysphagia management. This chapter presents an overview of food and culture. Next, strategies and suggestions to promote cultural competence are presented. This chapter focuses on the Hispanic culture and strategies to achieve culturally competent care. However, these strategies can be adapted for use with any patient, regardless of cultural background, and are the first steps toward cultural competence. It is important to realize though, that cultural competence is not limited to text-book knowledge of the customs, beliefs, language, and food preferences of culturally and linguistically diverse groups. Rather, cultural competence encompasses a much broader ability to evaluate one's own culture, including one's inherent biases and values, to better engage with persons from any culture, including one's own (Riquelme & Rosa, 2013).

Food and Culture

The simple act of choosing and eating food has meaning that extends beyond personal choice or survival; it is a socio-cultural road map of one's identity. Food provides an essential connection with others. It is the center piece of family gatherings, religious practices, and social occasions (Padilla, Palmer, & Rodriguez, 2019). In short, safe and efficient swallowing skills are necessary not only for meeting nutritional needs, but for maintaining overall QOL that is so deeply rooted in cultural norms (Maloney & Walsh, 2019).

Culture plays an important role in shaping a patient's beliefs regarding food and health which in turn may impact dysphagia management (Davis-McFarland, 2008). All aspects of cultural food rules (what, where, when, and how) are important variables to consider. For example, beef, pork, horse, dog, guinea pig, and insects all good sources of protein. However, what is considered appropriate, or even a delicacy in one culture, might be inedible or even forbidden in another. There are clear and definite sociocultural rules that influence all aspects of the food experience. This is why it is important that the SLP prepare for working with a CLD patient by reviewing the food preferences of their culture. For example, an internet search for 'cultural foods of Mexico' across multiple sites shows that the staples in a traditional Mexican diet include beans, corn, chilis, rice, chicken, pork, and beef. These are just general guidelines and do not necessarily apply to all Mexican Americans. However, gathering this kind of general background knowledge may prove useful in preparing the SLP to work with a patient who recently immigrated from Mexico.

Religion also influences food choices, for example, the kosher diets of Jews and vegetarian diets of Buddhists. Then again it would be an overgeneralization to characterize a cultural group or individuals by what they eat. For example, all vegetarians are not followers of Buddhism. It is important, though, to be aware of potential influences of religion on food choice.

Where and when food is eaten are also factors to consider. In some households, food is eaten only at the kitchen or dining room table, never in bed or while sitting on the floor. Conversely, sitting on the floor for meals is an ancient culture of many Asian countries. Again, to conclude that this is a cultural norm is unwise. Rather, it is important to be aware that there are rules for eating that are unique to each person and subsequently to each person with dysphagia. Consider two dysphagia patients receiving pureed diets. They may have similar symptoms and severities, but very different attitudes towards eating. One may value food for nutrition, the other may place greater value on the social experience surrounding food. Both will experience the diet change differently. Also, consider the patient, confined to a hospital bed who previously had eaten meals only at the kitchen table. If they now receive dysphagia therapy at mealtimes in bed, they may perceive their swallowing disorder as much worse (Kenny, 2015). Furthermore, most patients with dysphagia will likely have strong attitudes toward food preferences and rituals. If altered, these factors may exacerbate emotional stress that is already occurring in conjunction with their acute or chronic illness (Kenny, 2015).

Time of day when food is eaten is another aspect of food culture. For example, Muslims fast during Ramadan, eating only before sunrise and after sunset. More commonly seen are the individual and household rules/preferences for when meals are eaten. These can range from no restrictions (e.g., eating when hungry) to specific mealtimes (e.g., dinner at 6:00 pm every day). For patients who now must eat dinner at a specified time tied to the hospital or skilled nursing facility (SNF) dining schedule, eating may become more challenging and less enjoyable.

Finally, cultural etiquette dictates how food is eaten. For example, in Western cultures, forks are used for salads and fingers/hands for sandwiches and not the other way around. In other cultures, eating food with the fingers/hands is the proper etiquette. Eating only with the right hand, using three fingers, or licking fingers can be regarded as either polite or impolite depending on the cultural context. The same applies to "slurping" and belching during meals (Polan, 2009).

In summary, it is important to gain a thorough understanding of each patient's eating habits and food preferences so that therapy can be planned appropriately. This is true for patients of any culture, but especially true for the CLD population. Food is not just a preference; it is a way to preserve cultural identity. Be aware, though, that CLD patients may have experienced a level of cultural adaptation (i.e., assimilation) to food through repeated exposure to the mainstream culture. They may maintain certain food rituals and preferences from the original culture but adopt new practices and food preferences from the mainstream culture (Padilla et al. 2019). Thus, each person must be viewed individually, and their own idiosyncratic food rules must be determined.

Cultural Values and Ethical Conflicts

Ultimately, the primary goal of swallowing therapy is to support positive health outcomes. To do this, SLP's must balance their duty of care to promote safe swallowing (beneficence) and minimize harm (non-maleficence) against the patient's choices (autonomy). In dysphagia management, ethical conflicts can occur if there is a mismatch between the clinician's goal for swallowing safety and the patient's choices. That is, the clinician is working to protect the patient's health at all costs while the patient may be questioning the need for the intervention. Patients may refuse interventions (e.g., feeding tubes) or are non-compliant with diet changes (Maloney & Walshe, 2019). At some point, SLPs may eventually question whether it is ethical to continue services for patients who are rejecting recommendations and requesting diets that are believed to be harmful.

How do SLPs manage ethical conflicts in dysphagia, particularly with the CLD population? It is helpful to start by understanding the link between cultural values and/or perceptions of health risks associated with eating/drinking on patients' choices regarding treatment. Think of cultural values as the belief systems of a person or society. In general, the individualistic American culture values individual rights over society's. The tenants of freedom and individualism are ideals that the American Founders set forth and sought to establish when they drafted the Declaration and the Constitution and created a country in which the individual's rights to life, liberty, property, and the pursuit of happiness were to be recognized and protected (Younkins, 1998). In health care, this is seen in patient autonomy which is held sacrosanct; the patient has the ultimate right to make decisions regarding their treatment (i.e., individualism). However, for the majority of cultures worldwide, the rights and interests of the group supersede that of the individual (i.e., collectivism). Here, the views of the group have precedence; treatment decisions are made by the family, rather than the individual (Battle, 2002).

Understanding the individualistic-collectivism dimension of culture, and that it exists in some degree in any culture, help the SLP avoid ethical conflicts. First, it allows for understanding that autonomy may be interpreted differently by different cultures. Autonomy may mean that decisions regarding patient care are made by the family, not necessarily the patient, and represent what is best for the group. Second, SLPs can consider the wider health benefits associated with exercising food choice against the fear of aspiration (Leslie & Coyle, 2010). Thickening liquids does not necessarily eliminate aspiration risk and that not everyone with dysphagia who aspirates will develop pneumonia (Robbins et al., 2008). There are many other factors that predict aspiration pneumonia including respiratory status, strength of cough, management of secretions, voice quality (i.e., wet vs clear), tongue strength, oral hygiene, method of feeding, and patient mobility (Langmore et al., 1998). This is not to imply that patients who make educated decisions in opposition to SLPs' recommendations are not at risk for negative health consequences. Low and colleagues (2001) found that patients who did not comply with recommendations for thickened liquids were more likely to have chest infections and die from aspiration pneumonia than those who did (Low et al., 2001). Rather, it is important that the SLP fully explain the risks and consequences of the patient/family's choices and document these discussions in the medical record.

The perceptions of health risks associated with dysphagia and the strong diverse values associated with eating are sources of ethical conflicts in CLD populations. The conflicts can reflect a lack of understanding of the need for dysphagia intervention (Garcia, Chambers, & Molander, 2005), belief that the intervention is not effective (DiMatteo, 1994) and misperception of the swallowing severity (Leiter & Windsor, 1996). The misunderstandings do not necessarily reflect a language barrier, although this factor should be considered in the CLD population. Instead, the patient may have different cultural views of illnesses and how they should be treated. For example, in traditional Chinese culture, illness is believed to be caused by an imbalance in the opposites yin (negative, dark, cold, weak, feminine) and yang (positive, light, warm, masculine). Treatment is wholistic and taking specific treatments or medications are thought to be aversive. Hence, treatments/medications may be taken only until symptoms are relieved or not at all if the symptoms are not obvious (Koidou et al.,2013). In the Hispanic culture, illness is viewed as an imbalance of "hot" and "cold" conditions (Bledsoe, 2009). Medical problems manifesting from 'hot' conditions are treated with cold and vice versa. Thus, the patient's cultural beliefs of dysphagia treatments may clash with SLP's expectations for treatment.

Religious beliefs may shape the way individuals approach therapy and health care in general. For example, Hispanics may combine home remedies (*remedies casero*) or the use of folk healers (*curanderos*) with Western health care practices (Bledsoe, 2009; Keegan, 2000). Spiritual and religious influences also play a major role in defining illness, and hence dysphagia, which may be accepted as part of a Divine plan. Prayer and spiritual healing are reportedly used by the majority of Mexican Americans to treat heath conditions (Koidou, Kollias, Sdravou, & Grouios, 2013). Again, it would be an overgeneralization to assume that every member of the Hispanic population adopts these belief systems. However, becoming aware that these systems exist will help the SLP understand different cultural perspectives and approaches to health care thereby avoiding an ethnocentric perspective. Specifically, SLP's ascribing to the Western cultural view of illness as something to be treated at all costs may create treatment goals that do not align with the CLD patient's view of treatment outcomes (Battle, 2012). These are just some examples of how different cultural views shape how illnesses are perceived and may provide the SLP a more culturally sensitive framework for patient and family education.

Although it is not possible to know all aspects of every culture, it remains the SLP's responsibility to seek information as needed to provide culturally competent services. Communication with the CLD patient and family is key. Riquelme (2004) suggested the following to support culturally competent services:

- Recognize that values and beliefs vary among and within different cultures.
- View values and beliefs from different cultures within cultural, spiritual, and religious contexts.
- Learn about the language, customs, beliefs and values of cultural groups, prior to seeing the CLD patient.
- Be alert to and try to understand the nonverbal communications of various cultures such as personal space preferences, body language, style of hair and clothing.
- Asks questions to learn about the patient's culture and beliefs, participation in alternative medicine, and views of Western medical treatment.
- Have the patient/family explain problems from their own perspective.
- Expand the definition of culture to include not only patients who are ethnically diverse, but those who may belong to different religious groups, follow a different lifestyle, etc.
- Consider how culture influences all activities of daily living including participation in traditions.
- Be aware of family roles and how they vary.
- Consider modeling recommendations, in addition to supplying appropriately translated materials.
- Determine who should be involved in treatment recommendations (the patient vs extended family).
- Be flexible in allowing family members to participate in sessions. Broaden the concept of family to include extended family (cousins, uncles/aunts) and non-traditional families (non-married heterosexual or gay/lesbian couples).

Finally, it is essential that professional interactions are not biased by the SLP's personal values and cultural norms (Leslie & Coyle, 2010). Riquelme (2013) urges SLPs to understand their own personal biases and prejudices through self-evaluation and correction. This is necessary in order to counter any imbalance in the patient/clinician dynamic. While minimizing risk of aspiration may be paramount to the clinician, it may be of lesser importance to the patient who would rather accept the risk of pneumonia and retain the food/drink of choice that is culturally meaningful to them. SLPs must take care not to interject their own values and respect the patient/family's choices. This does not free the SLP from responsible, ethical care, but it allows the SLP to respect the informed decisions made by the patient/family. A culturally responsive view honors the decisions of a patient/family as "reasoned choices" rather than "non-compliance" (Riquelme, 2004).

Strategies to Promote Shared Decision Making

In order to provide culturally responsive management of dysphagia, the SLP must accommodate variability found among people from different cultural groups to ensure that the information gained during assessment is unbiased and the treatment plans reflect shared decisions. Gathering information to complete a dysphagia assessment and plan intervention for culturally diverse patients starts with an interview. The traditional approach is to frame questions to the patient in order to receive specific responses ("Do you cough when you drink?"). Conversely, a conversational approach with spontaneous questions and participation of all family members is often more suitable for diverse populations and typical of ethnographic interviewing (Hyter & Salace-Provance, 2019). The aim of ethnographic interviewing in dysphagia management is to learn about the patients' beliefs, values, customs, rituals, behaviors, and health concerns surrounding deglutition derived from their cultural, socioeconomic, and religious framework. Finally, it is important to consider each patient and family as unique individuals with their own distinctive set of beliefs and behaviors surrounding food, regardless of their cultural background. The following are specific strategies for ethnographic interviewing and establishing a dynamic of shared decision making within the context of cultural humility.

- **Frame the Interview**: Start by explaining the purpose of the dysphagia assessment avoiding professional jargon. Set aside personal biases and assumptions in order to establish a trusting relationship with the patient and family. This is done by calibrating attitudes and perspectives with the patient. Setting aside personal cultural beliefs and biases about food will allow the clinician to understand the patient's behaviors and experiences from a different cultural perspective (Westby, Burta, & Mehta, 2003).
- **Determine the Patient's View of Dysphagia:** Explore how a patient's culture influences their understanding of their swallowing problem by asking the following questions adapted from Kleinman and colleagues (1978):
    - What do you call your swallowing problem?
    - What do you think caused the problem?
    - Why do you think it started when it did?
    - What does your swallowing problem do to you? How does it work?
    - How severe is your swallowing problem? How long do you expect it to last?
    - What do you fear most about your swallowing problem?
    - What are the biggest problems that your swallowing problem has caused for you?
    - What kind of treatment do you think you should receive? What are the most important results you hope to receive from treatment?
- **Use Broad, Descriptive, Open-Ended Questions**: Questions that are broad ("Tell me about how you eat?" or "Describe the trouble you are having with eating.") will elicit more information that is important to the patient rather than questions that only elicit a yes or no response ("Do you have trouble chewing food?").

- **Asking for Specific Information**: Some specific information may need to be explored. Use prompts such as "Tell me more about how the food that gives you trouble" or "I'd like to get a better understanding of what happens when you try to drink." By asking the patient descriptive questions that target specific information, the clinician is in a better position to negotiate with the patient and family as an ally in treatment planning (Tomoeda & Bayles, 2002). It is important to understand specifics about mealtime rituals. Asking "When, where, and with whom do you eat?" is better framed as "I'd like to know more about what eating is like for you. Tell me about the meals you have in a typical day." Using this style of questioning, the SLP can inquire further about:
    - Groups they identify with (cultural, spiritual, generational, other)
    - Medical or traditional healing treatment and/or advice they are receiving
    - List of food preferences and dislikes
- **Ask One Question at a Time**: Questions that are asked too quickly can be overwhelming and turn a friendly interview into a formal interrogation. Instead, uses pauses to allow time for the patient or family member to add more information. The clinician should also restate and summarize what the patient has said. This will ensure that the patient's responses have not been interpreted from the clinician's perspective which may inaccurately represent the patient's beliefs.
- **Avoid the "Clip Board Barrier"**: Body language can engage or disrupt an interview. Mirror the patient's body language by leaning forward with eye contact or sitting back allowing more personal space and less direct intensity. Avoid taking copious notes of the patient's responses on a clip board. Instead, take minimal notes or use audio recording with permission, if possible, to maintain a conversational tone. The best approach is to put the clip board away and simply have a friendly conversation while listening to the patient. Nod to signal understand and encouragement to talk more. Go slowly, and at the very end of the interview, repeat specific questions and take notes.

For treatment plans to be successfully implemented, decisions must be made jointly through mutual respect of the patients' needs and understood in the realms of their culture and belief systems. Central to this is establishing a bond of trust and understanding of the patient and family members' point of view. Using language and terminology that matches the patient/family's level of understanding while listening to the patient/family's perspective gives the clinician information to help promote change. The clinician and the patient/family must inform each other and decide jointly how to proceed. These successful interactions are the basis of shared decision making. Recall that if the SLP has effectively educated the patient and family, then decisions made that deviate from a treatment plan can be viewed as a reasoned or "educated" choice rather than "non-compliance".

Working with Interpreters

Over 350 different languages are spoken in the United States with Spanish being the most often used second language (Hyter & Salas-Provance, 2019). Language differences have been identified as major barriers to quality and safety of patients in health care (Schyve, 2007). For swallowing evaluation and treatment, the consequences of miscommunication between the SLP and patient/family can lead to negative health outcomes and injury, misdiagnosis, or misunderstanding of the treatment plan and recommendations. In one landmark case, a patient was withheld treatment for an intracerebral hemorrhage because of the physician's misinterpretation of the word *intoxicado* used by the family to describe the patient's symptoms. While the family was referring to a general illness, the physician misinterpreted the meaning of this word to imply an overdose of drugs/alcohol and did not order brain scans. The outcome of this miscommunication was that the patient suffered life-long quadriplegia (Price-Wise, 2008). This case clearly illustrates the legal and ethical ramifications of failure to provide interpreter services. The use of an interpreter is no longer an option in health care, but a culturally responsive and necessary practice (Hyter & Salas-Provance, 2019). The key concepts that underlie the use of interpreters are:

- All patients have the right to request free interpreter services and must be made aware of this service.
- When possible, use professional, trained interpreters and avoid family members if possible. Do not use children to interpret for the patient.
- Brief the interpreter prior to the session regarding the key vocabulary used and meaning.
- Speak slowly and directly to the patient, not the interpreter, and allow sufficient time for successful interpreting.
- Use repetition and elicit confirmation from the patient (through the interpreter) that the information relayed was accurate. Family members especially may withhold information or filter messages to protect the patient. Similarly, the information from the patient interpreted to the SLP may biased to family member's view. The SLP needs to be aware of these caveats when using family members as interpreters.
- Adult family members or friends who the patient identifies as their preferred interpreter must be aware of HIPAA compliance standards.
- Recognize that it is unnatural, and difficult at times, to control the length and amount of information provided to the interpreter who then communicates to the patient and then reverse translates back to in English.

DYSPHAGIA CASE STUDY

The case study illustrates the importance of ethnographic interviewing, cultural awareness, and shared decision making in dysphagia management of CLD populations. This case is based on an actual patient seen by the author. Although some details have been altered to protect her identity, the course of treatment and outcomes presented reflect a realistic, rather than idealized, journey of an elderly Hispanic woman with dysphagia following a left hemisphere subcortical stroke receiving services from a monolingual (English) SLP in a skilled nursing facility. This case study highlights the course of treatment relating only to dysphagia and does not present details regarding her right hemisphere disorder or dysarthria for which she also received treatment.

Clinical and Social History

HL is an 84 year-old female who presented to the emergency room (ER) on 4/1/20XX, approximately two days after symptoms began, complaining of slurred speech, right facial drooping, and difficulty walking and swallowing. Medical history was significant for hypertension, hyperlipidemia, and gastroesophageal reflux disease. There was no history of stroke, dysphagia, cognitive, or communication problems. She was functionally independent for all activities of daily living (ADLs). Her weight on admission was 160 lbs. and body mass index (BMI) = 29. Current medications include clonidine (Catapres®), omeprazole (Prilosec®), atorvastatin (Lipitor®), and Bendroflumethiazide (Aprinox®).

HL immigrated from Mexico City to live with her son, daughter-in-law, and their children (ages 6, 10, and 16) in North Carolina (NC) 8 years ago and recently obtained permanent residency/citizenship. When she arrived, she communicated primarily in Spanish but after living in NC for the past 8 years, HL's English for simple conversations improved, but not to the point where she fully understood conversations regarding her medical needs without an interpreter present which was typically her son. Prior to her admission, HL enjoyed caring for her grandchildren. She did not drive but frequently took the city bus to church. Other pastime activities included watching daytime drama shows in Spanish and gardening.

Upon examination in the emergency room HL demonstrated weakness in the right upper limb (0/5) and lower limb (2/5), right facial droop, slurred speech, confusion, decreased tone, and altered sensation. A head CT revealed subacute densities in the left thalamic and internal capsule regions. Tissue plasminogen activator (tPA) was not administered. She was given aspirin therapy then monitored for intracranial edema and neurological status. NPO status was prescribed by nursing. An MBSS (see results that follow) was performed on Day 2 after admission and she was placed on NG tube feedings. On Day 5, the NG was removed, and HL began a pureed diet with honey thick liquids. The following day she was discharged to a SNF for rehabilitation.

Upon admission to the SNF the SLP gathered information from chart review, nursing, and dietary consultations. The family is concerned that HL is not eating the 'baby food' or drinking enough. HL takes her medications crushed in pudding with no problems but is refusing thickened liquids. HL has not eaten since her late arrival the day before and the dietician asked if the diet could be upgraded to increase oral intake. At this time, it is unclear how the decision was made to discontinue NG tube feedings and initiate a puree/HTL diet. The medical records from the hospital were incomplete and provided only a brief summary of HL's MBSS results:

Reduced lingual movements resulted in premature spillage of liquids into the pharynx prior to initiation of the swallow response. Reduced laryngeal closure resulted in consistent aspiration of thin (PAS 4/8) and nectar thick liquids (PAS 2/8). Asymmetric transit of puree bolus through the right pyriform sinus with mild right pharyngeal residue. Labored mastication of soft solid, difficulty forming and transporting a cohesive bolus. Recommend primary enteral support with trial oral feedings by SLP.

Recent lab work and dietary notes stated that HL is "at risk for dehydration; push fluids." Current medications are unchanged except for the addition of aspirin. HL's current weight is 156 lbs. representing a potential 4 lbs. loss since her initial presentation to the ER.

Next, HL was seen at bedside for a clinical swallowing evaluation (CSE) at lunchtime. The SLP carried in HL's lunch tray to be used for the CSE and attempted to reposition HL in bed at which point HL waved her hand in protest and declared "No!". The SLP explained the reason for the visit using simple English but HL refused to communicate with the clinician or accept any puree or HTL liquids offered. The SLP asked if HL would like to drink some 'good' water to which HL brightened "Yes, *please*. Please give me water. No honey!" The SLP assisted HL with thorough oral care and offered 4 ounces of cold water from a cup with patient controlled sips. A strong cough was noted after the third cup sip. The SLP presented the water protocol to HL using a natural and engaging communication style avoiding professional jargon and supplementing the information with pantomime and gesture. HL signaled apparent understanding with head nods and saying "Yes, wait for my son."

Table 1.

SLP: *(to the group) I'm sorry to interrupt dinner but I'm glad you all are here. I'm Kellyn one of the rehab therapists. I came by earlier to help Mrs. HL start drinking water again. Can I come in and talk to you? (to HL) I'd like to get to know more about what happened and the problems you're having.*	**HL:** They say I had a stroke. I don't know. (pause) Maybe I did. They took my food away and now they're making me starve. **Son:** We're really concerned that all she gets is baby food now and she absolutely won't eat it or drink that thick stuff. That's why we brought in McDonalds for dinner tonight. She's got to eat and drink something or she won't get strong enough to come home.
SLP: *Can you tell me more about why you're getting baby food?*	**HL:** No reason! They took me down for a swallow test and when I came back the nurse put a tube in my nose and took all of my food away. **Son:** They're afraid of pneumonia so they put that feeding tube in. Camden (the name of the SNF) won't accept patients on feeding tubes so they took it out the day before we got here and started her on that stuff. You can't even call it food. Mom won't eat it. We thought if we all came and ate together that might help.
SLP: *Sounds like this whole thing has been tough for all of you and you want to figure out what can be done. I'd like to ask you a few questions about what you've noticed, and then we'll move on to figuring out what we can do. Does that seem OK with you?*	**HL:** no response **Son:** Yeah, I think she's just lonely at meals. She never eats alone at home. Plus, they serve them so early here. She usually doesn't eat lunch until late afternoon and dinner's even later, like 8:00. She seems to be fine with drinking water though so thank you for that.
SLP: *I'm glad to hear she's drinking water. Let me tell you about the water protocol and how it works.*	(SLP explains the water protocol procedures, rationale and need for oral care).
SLP: *Can you tell me more about the food and drinks that are giving you trouble?*	HL: I don't have any trouble. Son: She's always had trouble with some meat but now when she drinks it makes her cough sometimes. HL (in English): Yes, but I can eat meat if it's softer. I do cough a little on the soda. Just a little but it sometimes chokes me. It's a lot better though.
SLP: *Why do you think this is happening?*	Son: They said the stroke affected her right side and so the food goes down the wrong pipe. Her biggest problem isn't eating, it's walking. HL (in English): I don't have my back teeth. The soda is too cold. I need hot tea instead to unblock the food.
SLP: *What else do you think can help?*	Son: She's been praying a lot. That helps. HL: What cannot be healed must be put up with. DIL: If someone's with her when she eats to remind her to take small bites and go slow, can got back to normal food? We've been sneaking in some of her favorite food and she does fine.
SLP: *I understand, good to know.* (to the DIL) *Tell me more about the foods she likes to eat.* (to HL) *Do you have trouble with things that break apart easy like rice or beans?*	HL: I don't eat rice or beans. DIL: She likes fish, French fries, spaghetti, anything tasty. GD: She really likes pancakes with butter and syrup. I make that a lot for us. DIL: and scrambled eggs, mashed potatoes with gravy, stuff like that. Sometimes I'll make enchiladas. She likes that. She doesn't cook much anymore but she really likes to eat (smiles). She really eats anything I cook for the family.
SLP: *Is there anything else I need to know?*	Son: She takes medicine for the reflux and really it doesn't seem to be a problem. That's pretty much it. The big job is to get her walking so we can get her home.
SLP: *I understand. It sounds to me like your swallowing might have gotten better since you first went to the hospital. You really don't like the pureed diet or the thickened liquids but might need softer foods that are easier to chew. Drinking water between meals and after you've cleaned your mouth seems to be going well but those thin drinks like soda gets a bit tricky and makes you cough. Your family really wants to help you find ways to eat safely so food and liquids don't get into your lungs and cause pneumonia and prevent you from going home. Does that sound right?*	HL: No, I don't want pneumonia. I want to go home. Son: Yes, that sounds right. We will be with her every day and can help her with whatever she needs. DIL: I'll be here in the mornings until GD gets here. My husband will be with her in the evenings but we all will probably come too. Son: She won't want an interpreter. She thinks they lie (all laugh). Her English is pretty good though for the everyday stuff, right Mamá? HL (in English): Yes, yes. (HL smiles at the SLP) I'm just listening.
SLP: *Well that's good to know! (smiling) I'm really looking forward to working together to figure out what we can do. I want to get an idea of what foods and drinks you like and also talk about that swallowing study. First I have some things to do that will help us get a better idea of some options for you to consider. I'd like to ask some more questions and then take a closer look at how you swallow. After that I want to look at how the muscles in your mouth are working. Does that sound okay to you?*	HL: (looks at son who nods then HL responds in English) Yes, that will be fine.

Clinical Evaluation

Upon returning to complete the CSE, the SLP found the entire family beginning a meal together brought in from a fast-food restaurant. The SLP explained the reason for the visit through her son who interpreted and discussed them with her to form responses. HL appeared disinterested and SLP redirected questions directly to her son. The following is a sample from the interview. HL's replies are labeled 'HL" and were interpreted from Spanish unless otherwise noted. All family replies are labeled as 'Son', daughter-in-law (DIL), or oldest granddaughter (GD).

The interview continued and concluded with a list HL's preferred foods/liquids. The patient participated in a CSE using the food items provided by the family and supplemented by the SLP. The SLP returned later to complete the cranial nerve/oral mechanism exam. The summary of the results of the assessment as written in the medical record are presented in Appendix 1. The results of the MBSS from the hospital and possible therapy approaches were presented.

Questions for the Reader

1. Why do you think HL appeared disinterested during the initial interview with the SLP? How could the SLP have made this first encounter more appropriate for HL?
2. How did the SLP build rapport given the language barrier and establish shared decision making throughout the initial assessment? What could have been improved?
3. Why was it important to begin the assessment with the CSE followed by the oral mechanism exam? What could the SLP do better to prepare HL for this evaluation?
4. How can the SLP information from the MBSS summary be used to plan for the clinical assessment? What other information is needed to help the SLP prepare for working with this CLD patient?
5. How can the SLP justify upgrading the diet without an objective assessment? Is this something that she is doing just because HL is from a CLD background?

Discussion of Questions for the Reader

1. *Why do you think HL appeared disinterested during the initial interview with the SLP? How could the SLP have made this first encounter more appropriate for HL?*
    a. HL simply may have been tired of the entire process surrounding the management of her dysphagia. Her disinterest could also be a sequalae of her brain injury. More likely, a cultural influence is at play. The oldest male (direct relative) holds the greatest position of power in most Hispanic families and is often the one who makes the health decisions for others in the family (Hyter & Salas-Provance, 2019). HL may have been recognizing her son's role in decisions regarding her health care. The SLP should have asked HL this directly for clarification. Also, the SLP failed to alert HL or her family that free professional interpreter services were available to them. Instead, the SLP assumed that HL would continue to use her son as her interpreter as stated in the hospital records. The SLP relied on the son to provide factual, unbiased, and correct information. The SLP should have met with the son prior to the evaluation to explain the important information that was needed from the meeting. Having native proficiency in Spanish does not necessarily prepare her son for accurate interpretation of HL's responses to questions regarding her health care.

2. *How did the SLP build rapport and establish shared decision making throughout the initial assessment? What could have been improved?*
   a. The SLP framed the interview by stating the purpose and what was going to occur. Broad, open ended questions were used to determine the family's perspective of dysphagia. The SLP showed that she was listening to the family's concerns and not judging their decision to bring in food for HL by stating "*I understand.*" The reflection statement made by the SLP ("*Sounds to me like this whole thing has been tough on you…*") signals understanding and compassion. Summarizing what was said and then asking if it was correct allowed HL and her family to make additions or express their feelings. The patient/family were asked about their views of dysphagia, what caused it, and what might help. By providing a rationale for what was going to happen next, and asking permission to continue, the SLP invited HL and her family to build a partnership where decisions regarding therapy would be made jointly.
   b. One area that needed improvement was the assumption of the SLP regarding the food HL preferred foods. She assumed that HL would prefer the traditional food in a found in typical Mexican diets (rice and beans). By applying this "text-book" knowledge, the SLP overgeneralized and asked if HL was having trouble with these foods. The SLP failed to consider the level of assimilation that may have occurred for HL living in the U.S. for the past 8 years. Recall that the family stated that they were bringing in her favorite foods. The SLP could have explored this more and through opened ended questions. Also, the SLP asked questions in succession, not allowing time for the patient or family to respond.
3. *Why was it important to begin the assessment with the CSE followed by the oral mechanism exam? What could the SLP do better to prepare HL for this evaluation?*
   a. By starting the clinical assessment with a friendly conversation, the SLP began the important first step in establish trust with the patient and her family. Although not ideal, moving the oral mechanism/CN exam to the end allowed the clinician to develop rapport with the patient prior to the more physically intrusive oral mechanism exam.
   b. The family had brought in dinner to eat with her. The CSE was performed first so that the family could finish their meal together.
   c. The SLP did not explain that part of the evaluation involved touching her face and neck. Explaining the procedures, why the information is important, and asking permission to touch the patient are important, especially when working with CLD patients.
4. *How can the information from the MBSS summary be used to plan for the clinical assessment? What other information is needed to help the SLP prepare for working with this CLD patient?*
   a. It can be assumed that the pharyngeal swallow was triggered at the level of the valleculae due to premature spillage caused by reduced tongue movements. The distinctions among premature spillage, delayed pharyngeal swallow trigger, and variations of normal swallowing events in the elderly (presbyphagia) are important to make. The trigger of the pharyngeal swallow can take place later and lower in the elderly, even to the level of the pyriform sinuses, and still be considered normal (Humbert & Robbins, 2008). Some laryngeal penetration can be normal in the healthy elderly, especially for liquid boluses (Daggett, Logemann, Rademaker, & Pauloski, 2006). Lingual pressures driving the bolus through the pharynx to the esophagus can also be reduced in healthy elders. This may cause mild residue in the pharynx after the swallow that is normal. Healthy elders accommodate these changes in swallowing function and continue to eat safely. However, symptoms of presbyphagia can become pathologic if

exacerbated by illness or disease. A stroke causing weak tongue movements, reduced airway closure, and increased pharyngeal residue, threatens airway protection. A closer examination of the lingual movements and the cranial nerves responsible for them, can be explored during the oral mechanism/CN exam. The information from the summary was helpful in alerting the SLP to what to look for. It is also important that the SLP be aware of cultural considerations regarding touching before beginning the CSE. The SLP cannot assume that because the CSE is a medical procedure that HL will be comfortable with an oral mechanism inspection. The SLP needs to fully explain what HL can expect in the following CSE and ask permission to touch her face, neck, etc.

b. Reduced laryngeal closure was identified on the MBSS so the SLP should check for adequacy of vocal fold closure during a voluntary cough and listen for voice quality changes after a swallow.

c. HL scored a 4/8 on the penetration/aspiration scale (PAS) for thin liquids. Scores of 1-5 are considered "penetration" and 6-8 are "aspiration" because the material is now in the lower airway. For HL, the liquid contacted the vocal folds but was ejected or coughed out with no residue remaining. Ultimately she protected her lower airway. HL was sensitive to the penetration, suggesting that the superior laryngeal nerve branch of CN X (Vagus) was intact, which is good! This information taken from the MBSS summary are positive prognostic indicators for HL's tolerance of aspiration. Even though she is aspirating thin liquids, her sensitivity to the aspiration and ability to eject it suggests a reduced risk of developing aspiration pneumonia. In planning for the CSE, the SLP should look for other risk factors associated with aspiration pneumonia including respiratory status, strength of cough, voice quality (i.e., wet vs clear), tongue strength, oral hygiene, and management of secretions.

d. The summary did not provide all the information that is important for treatment planning. For example, why was laryngeal closure incomplete? Many factors affect laryngeal closure during the swallow, including hyolaryngeal elevation and base of tongue retraction. There was no information regarding upper esophageal segment opening or pharyngeal contractions that might help explain the pharyngeal residue. Finally, understanding the rationale behind the recommendation for primary enteral support (tube feedings) would have been useful information. The SLP should contact the hospital and request that the full MBSS report be faxed to the facility.

5. *How can the SLP justify upgrading the diet without an objective assessment?*

A clinical swallow evaluation cannot objectively measure tongue movements, timing of the swallow response, presence of aspiration, laryngeal closure, or any of the pharyngeal stage components. Because HL just had an MBSS, a FEES was chosen as the most appropriate study to follow. The typically turnaround time for a FEES to be ordered and completed in the HL's SNF is 4-6 days. In the meantime, the family, nursing, and dietician were asking for modifications to HL's diet orders. Regardless, given HL's performance on the CSE and tolerance of soft solids, her diet upgrade to IDDSI level 7 regular/easy to chew is justified. Also, given her current respiratory health (good), ability to detect and clear aspiration (per MBSS), and her improvement in general medical status over the past week, upgrading her liquids to NTL was made and documented. Ideally, a FEES would have been performed prior to any diet upgrades and is still indicated.

Treatment Considerations

The SLP documented the patient's and family's understanding of the results of the swallowing assessments, need for strategies, and risks of health consequences associated with chronic aspiration. The son was consulted regarding the therapy plan and asked if HL could pray before each session. The family was encouraged to pray and be present at evening meals. They were also asked to bring in condiments from home. HL and her family members were trained in the use of compensatory strategies and swallowing exercises. She was seen 2x time per day (30 minute sessions). The SLP worked directly with HL on swallowing exercises during the first visit and family education/training during the second visit. The SLP presented the therapy exercises as "something to put up with" which HL agreed to. The compensatory strategies that HL consistently used were alternate consistencies and volitional/effortful swallow. After one week the family requested HL's diet upgraded to IDDSI level 7 regular/easy to chew with thin liquids. Orders were written for HL to be out-of-bed for meals. The family was intent on getting HL home as soon as possible. Their primary concern was her overall mobility and return to a normal diet. The oldest granddaughter took charge of HL's daily swallowing exercises.

Outcomes

A FEES was performed on the day before her discharge from the facility on day 26 post admission. The FEES revealed no aspiration of thin liquids, mild pharyngeal reside, and recommended an IDDSI 7 regular/easy to chew with thin liquids diet. The patient was discharged to home with follow-up home health physical and occupational therapy.

Additional Questions for the Reader

1. How could HL's cultural background impact her compliance in therapy and eating in general?
2. In what ways did the SLP capitalize on the HL's cultural background/beliefs to improve her meal intake and swallowing function?
3. What were the culturally sensitive approaches used to improve HL's success in dysphagia treatment?
4. Is it ethical to continue therapy when HL refused thickened liquids and requested diet change to thin?

Discussion of Questions for the Reader

1. *How could HL's cultural background impact her compliance in therapy and eating in general?*
    a. HL did not understand why she was put on an NG tube or why her diet was changed to the 'baby food'. She and the family did not come to the SNF fully understanding her deficits or course of treatment. This could represent a language barrier or, if interpreters were used at the hospital, a mistrust of the information presented. If HL did not understand the severity of her swallowing problems or that therapy would help, and/or understand the reason for the diet changes, then it was unlikely that she would comply with recommendations.
    b. The son commented twice that HL's primary problem was walking. HL looks to the son for guidance and understanding. If the son did not amplify the importance of working on swal-

lowing goals or acceptance of diet changes then there was probably very little the SLP could say to convince her of their importance.

c. HL's comment "what cannot be healed, has to be put up with" is a common saying in the Mexican culture suggesting that she accepted her condition as static and therapy will not work.

d. Meals at the SNF are a factor. The time of day meals are served are not what she was used to at home. She was also taking her meals alone in bed, which was unusual for her. The kinds of foods she was receiving at the SNF, not just the consistency, were likely very different from what she was used to which could affect her willingness to eat.

2. *In what ways did the SLP capitalize on the HL's cultural background/beliefs to improve her meal intake and swallowing function?*

a. HL and her family typically ate meals together. Encouraging this to continue resulted in HL eating and drinking more at meals. The SLP trained the family members to assist HL with compensatory strategies and swallowing exercises to maximize her recovery.

b. Menu orders were calibrated through dietary services to try to match HL's food preferences with menu choices. The family was encouraged to supplement with food and preferred condiments from home.

c. The SLP was sensitive to HL's beliefs and made the case that the swallowing strategies used (i.e., chin tuck, alternate consistencies, etc.) were what she could do to "put up with" what "cannot be healed."

d. Recognizing the son as the major decision maker for HL regarding treatment and getting him his input on the treatment plan increased the chances that HL would fully participate.

e. Praying for healing, asking others to pray for healing, is common among Mexican Americans. The SLP encouraged HL and her family to use prayer prior to therapy sessions.

3. *What were the culturally sensitive approaches used to improve HL's success in dysphagia treatment?*

a. It is important to understand how HL views the cause of her illness. Traditional medicine practices in Mexico are based on a view of health as a balance between hot and cold. Illness is due to an imbalance of these and the correction is by eating of foods or herbs of the opposite quality. *Emacho* (indigestion) is considered a 'hot' disease that is treated by drinking herbal tea will to "unblock" the food causing the problem. This kind of information regarding HL's beliefs, as well as the family's, can help the SLP negotiate certain foods or treatments that align with these beliefs. An example would be using HL's herbal tea in therapy to teach chin tuck and perform effortful swallow exercises.

b. It is important to respect HL's strong spiritual beliefs and their role in her recovery. Recall that prayer and spiritual healing are used by the majority of Mexican Americans to treat heath conditions. Although it is not known if HL was seeking these interventions, it may explain her reference to herbal tea as a treatment for her dysphagia. The SLP should point out the natural cause of the dysphagia and why the prescribed treatment strategies can be beneficial. But it is equally important to be consider and respect HL's alternate views for therapy.

c. Written instructions for swallowing precautions and exercises should be translated in Spanish and include pictures. The SLP can consider giving the Spanish version of the MD Anderson Dysphagia Inventory (MDAI) to measure QOL factors (Montes-Jovellar, Carrillo, Muriel, Barbera, Sanches, & Cobeta, 2018). By reading the MDAI questionnaire in her native language, HL may actually view it as an alternate authoritative source of information about dysphagia. This could lead her to a better understanding of dysphagia and the value of/need for SLP services. Goals and decisions regarding treatment should be made jointly. HL's illness impacts the entire family. Her strong family support and the roles each member plays in supporting decisions need to be fully understood by the SLP.

d. It's also important to pay close attention to body language, lack of response, or expressions of anxiety that may signal that HL or her family is in conflict with therapy but hesitant to communicate it. In the traditional Mexican culture orthodoxy, codes of behavior, and rules are highly valued. Innovations, unorthodox, or unfamiliar behaviors and/or ideas are not easily tolerated and can be a source of anxiety. The best approach is to provide detailed explanations of what to expect when introducing therapy activities to allow HL to a chance to feel secure. This is especially true if physical contact is required as a part of therapy. The SLP should ask permission before touching HL as part of assessment or therapy.

4. *Is it ethical to continue therapy when HL refused thickened liquids and requested diet change to thin?*
   a. Yes. It is unethical to for an SLP to refuse treatment to patients who need our services most! The SLP must educate HL and her family so that they can make informed decisions.
   b. As health care providers SLPs are ethically obligated to act in the patient's best interests. Best interests, though, do not only apply necessarily only to medical best interests. It extends to what is best for the patient. The SLP must respect what the patient/family thinks best supports their needs and what they value.

KEY POINTS

- Culturally responsive dysphagia therapy is more than offering culturally appropriate foods as a part of therapy. The SLP must understand the client's health beliefs and cultural perspective. There are many factors involving food that are unique to the individual as well as their cultural group. The patient's cultural milieu must be fully integrated into the clinical process.
- Goals for swallowing safety must be balanced with the patient's goals for QOL. Ethical challenges may represent a cultural mismatch between the clinician's priorities and patient's values. The SLP needs to adopt an attitude of cultural humility and understand the patient's culture in general and culture surrounding food as it relates to QOL.
- Management of dysphagia must extend beyond simply providing evidence-based interventions to ensure adequate and safe nutrition (beneficence), recommending the "safest" diet (nonmaleficence), for all patients (justice). It means providing non-biased, evidence-based information that allows the patient to make informed choices that respect cultural norms for making decisions (autonomy) that are essential for shared-decision making.
- Shared decision making is key to success. This requires good communication between the SLP and the patient/family. It is important to learn about the language, customs, beliefs and values of cultural groups, prior to seeing the CLD patient. It is also important ask questions about the patient's unique cultural perspectives and be careful not to assume or make overgeneralizations. Ethnographic interviewing techniques allow the SLP to gather insights about the patient/family's cultural perspective.
- Whether the patient comes from a similar or a different cultural background from the SLP, the culture surrounding food practices and beliefs must be viewed through an ethnographic lens for all patients in order to support culturally responsive practice.

REFERENCES

American Speech-Language-Hearing Association. (n.d.). *Adult Dysphagia*. Retrieved October 8, 2019 from http://www.asha.org/Practice-Portal/Clinical-Topics/Adult-Dysphagia/

Battle, D. (2002). Communication disorders in a multicultural and global society. In D. E. Battle (Ed.), *Communication disorders in multicultural populations* (3rd ed.; pp. 2–19). Boston: Butterworth-Heinemann.

Bhattacharyya, N. (2014). The prevalence of dysphagia among adults in the United States. *Otolaryngology - Head and Neck Surgery*, *151*(5), 765–769. doi:10.1177/0194599814549156 PMID:25193514

Bledsoe, B. (2009). Understand folk medicine's role in prehospital care of many Mexican Americans. *Journal of Emergency Medical Services*, *12*(34). Retrieved from https://www.jems.com/2009/11/30/understand-folk-medicines-role/

Brussel, S. A., & González-Fernandez, M. (2011). Racial disparities in the development of dysphagia after stroke: Further evidence from the Medicare database. *Archives of Physical Medicine and Rehabilitation*, *92*(5), 737–742. doi:10.1016/j.apmr.2010.12.005 PMID:21457943

Cichero, J. A. Y., Lam, P., Steele, C. M., Hanson, B., Chen, J., Dantas, R., ... Stanschus, S. (2017). Development of international terminology and definitions for texture-modified foods and thickened fluids used in dysphagia management: The IDDSI framework. *Dysphagia*, *32*(2), 293–314. doi:10.100700455-016-9758-y PMID:27913916

Daggett, A., Logemann, J., Rademaker, A., & Pauloski, B. (2006). Laryngeal penetration during deglutition in normal subjects of various ages. *Dysphagia*, *21*(4), 270–274. doi:10.100700455-006-9051-6 PMID:17216388

Davis-McFarland, E. (2008). Family and cultural issues in a school swallowing and feeding program. *Language, Speech, and Hearing Services in Schools*, *39*(2), 199–213. doi:10.1044/0161-1461(2008/020) PMID:18420523

Dennis, M. S., Lewis, S. C., & Warlow, C. (2005). FOOD trial collaboration. Effect of timing and method of enteral tube feeding for dysphagic stroke patients (FOOD): A multicentre randomised controlled trial. *Lancet*, *365*(9461), 764–772. doi:10.1016/S0140-6736(05)17983-5 PMID:15733717

DiMatteo, M. R. (1994). Enhancing patient adherence to medical recommendations. *Journal of the American Medical Association*, *271*(1), 79–83. doi:10.1001/jama.271.1.79 PMID:8258895

Faigle, R., Bahouth, R., Urrutia, V. C., & Gottesman, R. F. (2016). Racial and socioeconomic disparities in gastrostomy tube placement after intracerebral hemorrhage in the United States. *Stroke*, *47*(4), 31–36. doi:10.1161/STROKEAHA.115.011712 PMID:26892281

Feldman, P.H., McDonald, M.V., Eimicke, J., & Teresi. (2019). Racial and ethnic health disparities a vulnerable post-stroke home care population. *Journal of Racial and Ethnic Health Disparities, 6*(3), 525-535. https://doi-org.libproxy.uncg.edu/10.1007/s40615-018-00551-y

Garcia, J. M., Chambers, E. T. IV, & Molander, M. (2005). Thickened liquids: Practice patterns of speech-language pathologists. *American Journal of Speech-Language Pathology*, *14*(1), 4–13. doi:10.1044/1058-0360(2005/003) PMID:15962843

Gillman, A., Winkler, R., & Taylor, N. F. (2017). Implementing the free water protocol does not result in aspiration pneumonia in carefully selected patients with dysphagia: A systematic review. *Dysphagia*, *32*(3), 345–361. doi:10.100700455-016-9761-3 PMID:27878598

González-Frenández, M., Kuhlemeirer, K. V., & Palmer, J. B. (2008). Racial disparities in the development of dysphagia after stroke: Analysis of the California (MIRCal) and New York (SPARCS) inpatient databases. *Archives of Physical Medicine and Rehabilitation*, *89*, 1258–1359. PMID:18586139

Humbert, I. A., & Robbins, J. (2008). Dysphagia in the elderly. *Physical Medicine and Rehabilitation Clinics of North America*, *19*(4), 853–866. doi:10.1016/j.pmr.2008.06.002 PMID:18940645

Hyter, Y. D., & Salace-Provance, M. (2019). *Culturally responsive practices in speech, language, and hearing sciences*. San Diego, CA: Plural Publishing.

Kenny, B. (2015). Food culture, preferences, and ethics in dysphagia management. *Bioethics*, *29*(9), 646–652. doi:10.1111/bioe.12189 PMID:26481206

Kleinman, A., Eisenberg, L., & Good, B. (1978). Culture, illness, and care: Clinical lessons from anthropologic and cross-cultural research. *Annals of Internal Medicine*, *88*(2), 251–258. doi:10.7326/0003-4819-88-2-251 PMID:626456

Koidou, I., Kollias, N., Sdravou, K., & Grouios, G. (2013). Dysphagia: A short review of the current state. *Educational Gerontology*, *39*(11), 812–827. doi:10.1080/03601277.2013.766518

Langmore, S. E., Terpenning, M. S., Schork, A., Chen, Y., Murray, J. T., Lopatin, D., & Loesche, W. (1998). Predictors of aspiration pneumonia: How important is dysphagia? *Dysphagia*, *13*(2), 69–81. doi:10.1007/PL00009559 PMID:9513300

Leiter, A. E., & Windsor, J. (1996). Compliance of geriatric dysphagic patients with safe swallowing instructions. *Journal of Medical Speech-Language Pathology*, *4*, 289–299.

Leslie, P., & Coyle, J. (2010). Complex decisions involving gastrostomy feeding tubes: When you're never right or wrong. *Perspectives on Gerontology*, *5*(2), 42–47. doi:10.1044/gero15.2.42

Low, J., Wyles, C., Wilkinson, T., & Sainsbury, R. (2001). The effect of compliance outcomes for patients with dysphagia on videofluoroscopy. *Dysphagia*, *12*(2), 123–127. doi:10.1007004550011002 PMID:11305222

Maloney, J., & Walsh, M. (2019). Managing and supporting quality-of-life in dysphagia: A survey of clinical practice patterns and perspectives in the UK, Ireland, and South Africa. *International Journal of Communication Disorders*, *54*(1), 41–49. doi:10.1111/1460-6984.12429 PMID:30362200

Marik, P. E., & Kaplan, D. (2003). Aspiration pneumonia and dysphagia in the elderly. *Chest*, *124*(1), 328–336. doi:10.1378/chest.124.1.328 PMID:12853541

Montes-Jovellar, L., Carrillo, A., Muriel, A., Barbera, R., Sanchez, F., & Cobeta, I. (2019). Translation and validation of the MD Anderson Dysphagia Inventory (MDADI) for Spanish-speaking patients. *Head & Neck, 41*, 122–129. doi:10.1002/hed.25478 PMID:30549341

Padilla, A. H., Palmer, P. M., & Rodriguez, B. L. (2019). The relationship between culture, quality of life and stigma in Hispanic New Mexicans with dysphagia: A preliminary investigation using quantitative and qualitative analysis. *American Journal of Speech-Language Pathology, 28*(2), 1–16. doi:10.1044/2018_AJSLP-18-0061 PMID:31136241

Panther, K. (2005). The Frazier free water protocol. *Perspectives on Swallowing and Swallowing Disorders (Dysphagia), 14*(1), 4–9. doi:10.1044asd14.1.4

Pollan, M. (2009). *Food rules: An eater's manual.* New York, NY: Penguin.

Price-Wise, G. (2008). Language, culture, and medical tragedy: The case of Willie Ramirez. *Health Affairs Blog*. Retrieved from https://www.healthaffairs.org/do/10.1377/hblog20081119.000463/full/

Riquelme, L. (2004). Cultural Competence in Dysphagia. *ASHA Leader, 9*(7), 8–22. doi:10.1044/leader.FTR5.09072004.8

Riquelme, L. (2013). SIGnatures: Evolving Expressions of Culture. *ASHA Leader, 18*(11), 52–55. doi:10.1044/leader.SIGN.18112013.52

Robbins, J., Gensler, G., Hind, J., Logemann, J. A., Lindblad, A. S., Brandt, D., ... Miller Gardner, P. J. (2008). Comparison of 2 interventions for liquid aspiration on pneumonia incidence. *Annals of Internal Medicine, 148*(7), 509–518. doi:10.7326/0003-4819-148-7-200804010-00007 PMID:18378947

Rosenbek, J., Robbins, J., Roecker, E., Coyle, J., & Woods, J. (1996). A penetration-aspiration scale. *Dysphagia, 11*(2), 93–98. doi:10.1007/BF00417897 PMID:8721066

Schyve, P. M. (2007). Language differences as a barrier to quality and safety in healthcare: The Joint Commission perspective. *Journal of General Internal Medicine, 2*(S2), 360–361. doi:10.100711606-007-0365-3 PMID:17957426

Tomoeda, C. K., & Bayles, K. A. (2002). Cultivating cultural competence in the workplace, classroom, and clinic. *ASHA Leader, 7*(6), 4–17. doi:10.1044/leader.FTR1.07062002.4

U.S. Census Bureau. (2012). *U.S. Census Bureau projections show a slower growing, older, more diverse nation a half century from now*. Retrieved from https://www.census.gov/newsroom/releases/archives/population/cb12-243.html

Westby, C., Burda, A., & Mehta, Z. (2003). Asking the right questions in the right ways. *ASHA Leader, 8*(8), 4–17. doi:10.1044/leader.FTR3.08082003.4

Younkins, E. (1998, Jan). *Individualism and freedom: Vital pillars of true communities*. Retrieved from http://fee.org/freeman/detail/individualism-and-freedom-vital-pillars-of-true-communities

ADDITIONAL READING

Andersen, U. T., Beck, A. M., Kjaersgaard, A., Hansen, T., & Poulsen, I. (2016). Systematic review and evidence based recommendations on texture modified foods and thickened fluids for adults (^{3} 18 years) with oropharyngeal dysphagia. *e-SPEN Journal*, *8*(4), 127–134. doi:10.1016/j.clnme.2013.05.003

Hyter, Y. D., & Salace-Provance, M. (2019). *Culturally responsive practices in speech, language, and hearing sciences*. San Diego, California: Plural Publishing.

Kenny, B. (2015). Food culture, preferences, and ethics in dysphagia management. *Bioethics*, *29*(9), 646–652. doi:10.1111/bioe.12189 PMID:26481206

Riquelme, L. (2004). Cultural competence in dysphagia. *ASHA Leader*, *9*(7), 8–22. doi:10.1044/leader.FTR5.09072004.8

KEY TERMS AND DEFINITIONS

Assimilation: A process whereby an individual changes following exposure to a different culture. In assimilation, individuals of differing heritages and cultures acquire the basic attitudes, habits, and way of life of the dominant culture.

Collectivism: A societal view that places the needs of the group before the individual. Decisions made are for the benefit of the group.

Hispanic: Someone from a Spanish-speaking country. Hispanic is not a term that refers to a race of people but only refers to individuals with cultural ties to Spain. A person is any individual living inside the U.S. who Mexican, Puerto Rican, Guatemalan, Cuban, or Caribbean.

IDDSI: An international standardized framework for labeling texture-modified foods and thickened liquids. Level 1 = thin liquids; Level 2 = slightly thick liquids; Level 3 = mildly thick liquids; Level 4 = moderately thick liquids; Level 4 = extremely thick liquids/pureed; Level 5 = minced & moist foods; Level 6 = soft & bite-sized foods; Level 7 = regular foods.

Individualism: A societal view that places the needs of the individual as the priority. Decisions made are to benefit the individual.

Latino: An umbrella term to refer to all people from a Latin American countries or a U.S. citizens of Latin American descent. Latinos (or Latina for females) are from Spanish-Speaking countries including Cuba, Puerto Rico, the Dominican Republic, Mexico, and Central and South America. All Mexicans are also Latinos. Not all Latinos are Mexicans.

Nasogastric Tube: A feeding tube that runs from the nasal cavity to the stomach to deliver liquid nutrition.

Penetration Aspiration Scale (PAS): A scale to identify the level of penetration and aspiration in the airway. Level 1 = no penetration; Level 2 = material enters vestibule and is ejected with the swallow; Level 3 = material enters the vestibule and remains; Level 4 = material contacts the vocal folds and is ejected (coughed out); Level 5 = material contacts vocal folds and is not detected/coughed out; Level 6 = material crosses below the vocal folds and is cough out; Level 7 material crosses below the vocal folds, is detected but not cough out, despite effort; Level 8 = material passes below the vocal folds and is not detected (silent aspiration).

Tissue Plasminogen Activator (tPA): A drug used to dissolve blood clots causing strokes if given within 6 hours of the event.

Water Protocol: A protocol that allows patients who are NPO or on thickened liquids to receive regular water and ice chips following oral care between meals.

APPENDIX

Table 2. Summary of the results of the CN/oral mechanism examination and CSE

Cranial Nerve/Oral Mechanism Examination: Inspection of oral cavity reveal partial dentition with R/L mandibular molars missing. Poor oral hygiene noted with xerostomia suspected secondary to mild tongue fissures. No pooling of secretions or drooling. Hard/soft palate were WNL. Posture and respiration were assessed through observation. Pt leaning slightly to right, normal breathing pattern, Sp02 = 90%, nasal patency appeared WNL. CN VII: Slightly reduced facial tone on right side with right corner of the lips slightly depressed. Jaw position at rest was WNL. No ptosis noted. Lips were slightly dry with normal shape/size. Puff cheeks with air hold against resistance was reduced on right. Symmetrical brow wrinkle. Lip retraction and closure reveals slightly reduced ROM on right. Pt denies changes in smell/taste but did not discriminate salt/lemon flavors on right side of anterior 2/3 of tongue. CN V: Reduced bulk and bulge of masseter tone during jaw clenching to palpation on right. Symmetric mouth opening and resistance to closure. Jaw moves side-to-side symmetrically. Pt passed a sensory screening for all 3 facial quadrants. Reduced sensory awareness on right side of the anterior 2/3 of tongue with 2-point discrimination testing. CN IX/X: Volitional cough was strong, voice quality WNL. Gag reflex was not assessed. Laryngeal elevation appeared adequate during swallow assessed through palpation. CN XII: The tongue was assessed for symmetry and range of motion. Size of tongue for oral cavity was WNL. No evidence of fasciculations. Tongue deviated slightly to right on protrusion with lateral resistance to tongue bladed slightly reduced suggested right sided tongue weakness. Otherwise, tongue ROM appeared with WFL for protrusions, retraction and lateralization in all planes of movement. CN V, IX & X: Symmetric soft palate retraction noted with uvula midline at rest. Resonance appeared WNL.
CSE: The patient was seen for during a meal with a range of liquid/solid consistencies trialed and included a fish sandwich, french fries, pudding, applesauce, chocolate chip cookies, a vanilla shake, nectar thickened apple juice, and water. Respiratory rate at the beginning of the meal was 22 bpm and SpO_2 was 92%. Voluntary cough was strong suggesting good vocal fold closure. Oral preparation to swallow was mildly impaired due to reduced oral preparation of a cohesive bolus for IDDSI level 7 regular solids (chocolate chip cookie). Prolonged mastication and reduced bolus manipulation may be related to xerostomia and slightly reduced lingual movements. Unmasticated regular solids remained in the right lateral sulci after the swallow and the patient required digital assistance to clear material. Oral prep for patient controlled bite of IDDSI level 7 easy to chew (fish sandwich) was WFL. Adequate bolus formation and manipulation suspected with no residue remaining in the oral cavity after the swallow. Oral preparation for all other consistencies test appeared WNL (IDDSI levels 4-6). Oral containment for all consistencies was WNL. Cervical auscultation during oral intake of IDDSI level 2 mildly thick (i.e. NTL) and IDDSI level 1 slightly thick liquids (milkshake) revealed no changes in respiratory sounds after the swallow. No coughing, throat clearing or change in voice quality noted. Coughing occurred x1 immediately after oral intake of 1 tsp of IDDSI level 0 thin liquid water. No coughing during ingestion of thin liquids with use slight neck flexion across 5 trials. Voice quality remained clear and $Sp0_2$ levels remained stable (92%) at the end of the meal. This suggests that the respiratory workload for coordinating swallow/breathing pattern was not taxed over the course of eating a meal. Recommend upgrade diet to IDDSI level 7 easy to chew food from patient's preferred food list and level 2 drinks (NTL) with the following precautions: 1) small bites/sips 2) slight neck flexion (chin tuck) when swallowing thin liquids 3) volitional swallow for liquids 4) alternate food consistencies 5) multiple and effortful swallows to clear potential pharyngeal residue. Recommend FEES to objectively rule out aspiration, effectiveness of strategies to reduce aspiration, and assess airway protection/pharyngeal clearance. Swallowing rehabilitation exercises should include 1) CTAR; 2) effortful swallow; and 3) lingual strengthening. Water protocol should be continued.

Chapter 12
Healthcare Considerations for the Hispanic Population

Leslie W. Johnson
https://orcid.org/0000-0002-6651-4763
North Carolina Central University, USA

EXECUTIVE SUMMARY

The Hispanic community has both positive and negative health indicators related to their Hispanic culture. This chapter details aspects of the Hispanic culture that can influence healthcare prevention, diagnosis, and intervention, including traditional healthcare beliefs and practices. Additionally, various health disparities associated with the Hispanic population are discussed, particularly related to neurological disorders. The chapter concludes with a case study presentation based loosely upon an actual event from a young man with neurocysticercosis. This section details how the patient's Hispanic culture influenced lifestyle choices, which increased risk for this disease, while also detailing how his culture impacted certain aspects of his medical intervention.

INTRODUCTION

Members of the Hispanic population in the United States (U.S.) include people drawn from an increasingly diverse mix of countries, comprising native born U.S. Hispanics, and immigrants from other countries, namely ones in Latin America. By 2016, this population had reached nearly 58 million and currently continues to be the primary driver of U.S. population growth, accounting for half of the national population growth, since 2000 (Flores, 2017). From 2000 to 2050, it is expected that the Hispanic population will expand by 273% (Passel & Cohn, 2009). As the Hispanic population grows within the U.S., speech-language pathologists (SLPs) are seeing the number of patients from this cultural group increase within their caseload. It is important for SLPs to learn about the many intricacies of the Hispanic culture that may affect the healthcare of this population. Notably, given the high number of neurological conditions prevalent on SLPs' caseloads, it is imperative to understand how the Hispanic culture may influence specific neurological disorders.

DOI: 10.4018/978-1-7998-2261-5.ch012

Hispanics have both positive and negative health indicators associated with their culture. As a whole, demographically Hispanics are a younger population when compared to non-Hispanics (American Community Survey, 2008). Nearly one-half of the Hispanic population in the US is comprised of immigrants, with most national health indices suggesting that they are healthier than native-born Americans (Argeseanu, Ruben, & Narayan, 2008; Smith & Bradshaw, 2006). Turran and Goldman (2007) reported that Hispanic immigrants report overall fewer chronic conditions, spend fewer days out from work because of illness, and have lower mortality rates than U.S. born non-Hispanics. Despite having a lower income than non-Hispanics, Hispanics live longer, with an average life-expectancy of 75.1 years for men and 82.6 years for women (U.S. Census Bureau, 2008). Interestingly, Hispanic populations display other positive health indicators in terms of dietary choices, lifestyle choices including low levels of smoking and illicit drug use, and strong family structure; however, the longer each generation makes their home within the U.S., the more these positive indicators tend to depreciate (National Alliance for Hispanic Health, 2004).

Conversely, Hispanics are also faced with several negative indicators that likely affect their overall health. That may, in part, be a result of Hispanics having the highest uninsured rates (32%) of any racial or ethnic group within the U.S., with 20.6% of Hispanics under age 65 not having health insurance coverage (Centers for Disease Control and Prevention [CDC], 2017). Indeed, they are twice as likely as the overall U.S. population (15%) to lack health insurance coverage (Pew Hispanic Center, 2010). Other factors, such as decreased rates of immunization, lower socioeconomic status, less years of education, and fear of government authority among new immigrants may have negative consequences related to health outcomes. They may also have lower paying jobs, or be without health insurance or benefits essential for optimal healthcare, such as vision or dental insurance. Because Hispanics may lack full healthcare coverage, they may be less likely to regularly visit their primary care physician, and may be more likely to visit the emergency room for routine healthcare needs (Hough et al., 1987; Smith, 2000). Parangimalil (2001) suggested that the acculturation struggle may become a source of stress leading to conflicts among family and friends, potential breakdown of the family unit, and possible health problems. It seems acculturation among new immigrants, their children, and subsequent generations to follow may weaken the positive health factors indicative of the Hispanic culture and lead to the adoption of negative practices from mainstream U.S. culture, contributing to the declining health status of later generations.

Traditional Health Beliefs and Common Practices

Hispanic culture, like most other cultures, has several traditional belief systems explaining what causes illness, how it can be treated or cured, and who should be involved in the process. Though these beliefs may represent larger themes within the culture, the meaning of health, wellness, and illness does vary among individuals as cultural groups are not homogeneous even though they may share many beliefs and practices. For example, some may believe that health results from good luck, or is a reward for good behavior; whereas, others may believe illnesses may have either natural, organic causes or potentially supernatural, mystical causes. Additionally, for many in the Hispanic community, issues related to morbidity, or disability, rather than mortality, or death, are of great concern. This may mean that contracting a disease or illness and subsequently living with it and the ramifications associated with it are of high importance. The following are examples of common Hispanic beliefs related to overall health.

Beliefs Related to Illness

There are several health beliefs related to etiology of illness, or healing practices that may be common for many people within the Hispanic culture. For example, in general, physical and mental illness may be thought to result from an imbalance between a person and their environment, oftentimes referred to as humoral imbalance. These conditions are generally expressed as either "hot" and "cold", or "wet" and "dry" (Kemp & Rasbridge, 2004). These refer to intrinsic properties of various substances and conditions. The four humors contained in the body include blood (hot and wet), yellow bile (hot and dry), phlegm (cold and wet), and black bile (cold and dry). To correct an imbalance, people ingest foods, liquids, or herbs with the opposite quality, for example "cold" conditions are treated with "hot" interventions or medications.

Another example of a cultural belief related to illness is *empacho*. Illness can also result from a disruption of function within different parts of the body. *Empacho* is an example of this type of dislocation, or something getting "stuck" somewhere within the body. It may include indigestion caused by eating too much of the wrong food, or eating undercooked food. It may also refer to generalized intestinal obstructions characterized by abdominal pain, vomiting, constipation, anorexia, or gas and bloating. The most common treatment is drinking herbal teas, rubbing the stomach or back with essential oils, or pinching or aggressively massaging the spine.

Often referred to as the "Evil Eye", *mal de ojo*, is caused when someone looks at another person with admiration or jealousy. This may then cause the person who is looked upon to experience negative symptoms, such as fatigue, malaise, or even severe headache. This illness is believed to mainly affect infants and is felt to be a result of adults showing too much admiration to a child. *Mal de ojo* can be avoided by touching the infant's arm or leg when admiring it. A traditional Hispanic remedy for this includes saying a prayer while moving an egg over the victim's body. The victim then sleeps with the egg in a bowl underneath them overnight. Conversely, others believe that the most effective form of management is having the person who caused the *mal de ojo* provide treatment and care for the victim.

Another cultural health belief is *envidia*, or envy, which may cause illness and/or bad luck. Envy may be triggered by the success of others and subsequently can result in misfortune and illness, especially for the person who is envied or is envious of another. This illness is typically neutralized by physically touching the person who is envious or envied.

Susto, meaning 'scared' in Spanish, is sometimes referred to as fright sickness and can arise from a traumatic or frightening experience. This is thought to cause soul loss, whereby the soul leaves the body and wanders freely. The soul may not feel safe, or feels too scared to return to the physical body. Symptoms include anxiety, depression, insomnia, irritability, lethargy, and anorexia and may be acute or chronic in nature. *Susto* affects women more often than men.

Traditional beliefs, like the aforementioned ones, likely lead to traditional practices which have been passed down from generation to generation. Traditional practices related to these beliefs include some of the previously listed examples, or using home remedies, such as drinking herbal teas, and seeking care from relatives, neighbors, or other community members. Amulets may be worn, perfumes or sprays may be used, pictures and statues may be displayed, and candles or incense may be burned as well to promote healing. Some may depend on these customary healing systems not only because it is culturally approved, but also because this option may be much more financially viable. Expensive modern medical care may be unaffordable for many, and Hispanics who cannot afford Western medical care may only have the option to resort to customary healthcare practices (Livingston & Kahn, 2009).

Of note, many Hispanics may choose to combine culturally based health practices with Western medicine. They may seek medical care from a Western physician only after exhausting family or community resources, or they may combine traditional herbal remedies with standard Western pharmaceuticals. Furthermore, because some medications sold only in prescription form in the U.S., such as antibiotics, can be purchased easily without a prescription from Mexican pharmacies, some Mexicans living in the U.S. may make regular trips to Mexico to purchase medications at a lower cost, and may do so regardless of their health insurance status (Becker, Garcia, & Ellertson, 2004). It is not uncommon for someone who is ill to use a combination of prayer, herbal remedies, prescription medication obtained from a family member or friend, and/or prescription medications prescribed by a healthcare provider. It is also not uncommon for some Hispanics to not report the use of traditional or herbal remedies to their Western medicine practitioners (Rivera, Ortíz, Lawson, & Verma, 2002). This mixture of combining healthcare beliefs and practices is an example of many Hispanic's journey of assimilation. According to Sonderup (2010), it is important to understand that although many Hispanics are assimilating to the mainstream U.S. culture, they will likely never be fully assimilated. Rather, their path may likely be a continuum of acculturation, a process of integrating native or traditional immigrant cultural values with dominant cultural ones.

Familism/Collectivism

Familism is the valuing of family considerations over individual or community needs. It is reflected in many Hispanics' collectivistic culture. The collectivistic nature of the Hispanic culture can also influence healthcare beliefs and practices. For example, the well-being of the group may prevail over individual needs, or group activities may be more common. The family or community assigns mutual responsibility for any and all actions or consequences, and accountability is combined throughout the family or community organization. Because of this, group cooperation tends to be accentuated compared to individualistic responsibility and function (Gudykunst, 1998). This collectivist nature allows many individuals within the community to look to one another for opinions and previous experiences. Therefore, it is common for some Hispanics to share their medications with their social networks. The traditional Hispanic family structure tends to be patriarchal and follow a rigid hierarchical organization. This patriarchal structure often grants the father or oldest male relative the greatest authority in decision making, especially related to medical care (Kemp & Rasbridge, 2004). Men are often expected to provide for and be the head of their households. Publicly, women may be expected to demonstrate the upmost respect, or even submission, for the patriarch; though privately some women may hold a greater degree of influence over decisions. Women are likely to be the primary caregiver in instances of illness or taking care of aging family members, and may be responsible for most of the parenting. Oftentimes, women are expected to hold the family and home together through their domestic work, their knowledge of family history, and their understanding of cultural principles.

Religion/Spirituality

In the Hispanic culture, spiritual and religious influences oftentimes play a major role in daily life, especially related to health, illness, and healing. Culturally competent clinicians should consider the influence of religion and spirituality when providing care from people from diverse populations. Many Hispanics are Roman Catholics, though the influence of protestant evangelical churches is increasing. Like many other groups, Hispanics may turn to their religion or spirituality to understand and work through thoughts, feelings, or practices related to illness and/or healthcare. King and Bushwick (1994) reported that 77% of hospitalized patients thought that their physicians should consider their spiritual needs throughout the intervention process. These spiritual needs may be related to healing, faith in a power higher than the medical providers, coping mechanisms for suffering or end of life processes, or practices related to prayer. Other behaviors, such as making the sign of the cross or looking toward heaven may also be noted during various interactions. Inquiring about a patient's religious beliefs may have substantial clinical benefits, ranging from an increased understanding of the patient's perceptions on the cause of illness, establishing rapport by demonstrating respect for what the patient sees as important, and appropriately referring to clergy or pastoral care in a timely manner (Lujan, 2010). Prayer is an important aspect of many religious and spiritual experiences. Hispanic individuals may pray for various saints to intercede on their behalf with each saint specializing in a particular health related function. For example, St. Peregrine is the patron saint for patients with cancer. Rosary beads, crucifix or religious photographs may also be common within the Hispanic culture. Religion and spirituality play other important roles in healthcare for the Hispanic community related to important rites, such as the baptism of infants and the anointing of the sick, especially in life threatening situations. Many people within the Hispanic culture may take great comfort in clergy or chaplain visits. Positive health outcomes may be maximized when healthcare providers provide culturally competent care that includes respectful acknowledgement of these religious and spiritual influences.

Health Disparities Associated with the Hispanic Community

Health disparities are differences related to various populations which are deemed "unnecessary and avoidable", as well as "unfair and unjust" according to the World Health Organization. There is a health disparity in the Hispanic population related to both morbidity, the level of illness or disability a disease may cause, and mortality, the likelihood of a disease to cause death. This is likely related to social and economic marginality, and associated lifestyle adaptations and environmental exposures (Vega, Rodriguez, & Gruskin, 2016). There is additional research to suggest increasing morbidity and mortality rates among U.S.-born Hispanics compared with foreign-born Hispanics, with accelerating morbidity and mortality rates in post-immigrant generations of Hispanics (Argeseanu et al., 2008; Smith & Bradshaw, 2006). The CDC (2002) reported there is no viable evidence to support a genetic explanation for these outcome differences in the Hispanic population, and suggests that these disparities may be due to inadequate disease detection and/or management, stemming from lifestyle and environmental factors, as well as healthcare access options.

Lifestyle and Environmental Factors

Some have suggested that Hispanics have a greater exposure to multiple lifestyle factors that may negatively affect their overall health. These include greater occupational hazards, higher rates of cumulative adversity, and exposure to adverse residential-environmental conditions over the course of life (Vega, Rodriguez, & Gruskin, 2016). Work-related injuries continue to be increased in the Hispanic population, with rates of 5.0 per 100,000 for Hispanics and 4.0 per 100,000 for all workers, and these numbers are likely underreported (CDC, 2008). Injuries, even those that are life-threatening, are less likely to be reported by informal labor contractors and smaller employers, as well as less likely to be treated. There are disincentives to reporting injured workers related to immigrant documentation and increased vulnerability of detection and potential deportation. In many industries where Hispanic laborers are concentrated, such as manufacturing, construction, and agricultural work, there may be hazardous work environments, inadequate use of safety equipment and toxic exposures, and decreased training on preventing injuries (Silverstein, 2008). Regardless of having relatively stable employment rates, 76.9% for Hispanic men and 55.7% for Hispanic women in 2018, there remains a disproportionate poverty discrepancy within the Hispanic population, with 22% living below the poverty line, as compared with 10% of white non-Hispanics (US Department of Labor, 2018; Ramirez, 2004). Despite the vast differences in wealth and demographic structure, Hispanic immigrants tend to have superior longevity, with death rates falling over a 15-year period between 1990 and 2005 (National Center for Health Statistics, 2008). Still, the health of the Hispanic population is not static and is continually being reshaped by demography, secular trends in disease, and social forces (Zsembik & Fennell, 2005).

Access to Healthcare

Hispanics have a lower likelihood of seeking and receiving healthcare services than the total US population. This is likely related to lower access to and receipt of healthcare due to lower health insurance coverage and language barriers (CDC, 2002). Significantly, Hispanics have the highest rates of uninsurance compared to other racial and ethnic groups within the US. In 2015, 19.5% of the Hispanic population was not covered by health insurance, as compared to the 6.3 percent of the non-Hispanic white population (US Department of Health and Human Services, 2016). Barriers as a result of no or minimal health insurance, may contribute to fewer referrals for procedures, decreased preventive care, late detection of disease, poor chronic disease management, and lack of consistent care for the elderly (Vega, Rodriguez, & Gruskin, 2016). Others have reported Hispanics are less likely to obtain healthcare from a primary and consistent source, and do not routinely receive up to date evidence-based healthcare interventions or recommendations. Interestingly, a survey conducted by Livingston, Minushkin, and Cohn (2008), reported that lack of a regular healthcare provider for Hispanic respondents was not related to the cost of healthcare, or assimilation practices. Rather, when asked about why they lacked a usual provider, many respondents provided the principal reason was that they were seldom sick. Disparities in healthcare utilization can contribute to worse outcomes, including both morbidity and mortality.

Neurological Conditions with Associated Health Disparities

The Hispanic population has several prominent health disparities, related to both morbidity and mortality, across several specific diagnoses. For example, health disparities have been noted related to diabetes mellitus, cancer, liver disease, human immunodeficiency virus, homicide, and work-related injuries (Vega, Rodriguez, & Gruskin, 2016). We also see these disparities in neurological conditions, such as stroke, dementia, and neurocysticercosis (NCC). Given that SLPs are typically very involved with neurological patients on their caseloads, it is important to review some of the most common neurological conditions within the Hispanic community and review how these conditions affect people in this culture in unique ways.

A stroke is a medical emergency and occurs when there is decreased blood flow to an area of the brain or when there is bleeding from a cerebral artery onto the brain. Hispanics are disproportionately affected by stroke with prior population-based studies showing higher incidence rates in Hispanics and an increased likelihood of having a secondary stroke (Sheinart, Tuhrim, Horowitz, Weinberger, Godman, & Godbold, 1998; White & Atmar, 2002). Additionally, minority groups, including Hispanics, have been reported to suffer from greater neurological impairment, poorer functional outcomes, and higher mortality rates after stroke (as cited in Martinez et al., 2015). Interestingly, Hispanics have different risk factors for stroke compared to non-Hispanic whites. The average age for a stroke among non-Hispanic whites is 80, but among Hispanics living in the United States, it is 67 (CDC, 2017). Perhaps this is related to Hispanics' increased risk for high blood pressure, diabetes, and being overweight or obese.

Alzheimer's Disease (AD) is the most common type of dementia among individuals 65 or older. It is a progressive disease, characterized by its debilitating loss of memory with eventual deterioration of both cognitive and physical abilities. While advancing age is the greatest risk factor for development of AD, researchers have noted additional demographic factors that have contributed to the rise of AD. One such factor is associated with the relatively increased prevalence of AD within the Hispanic population (Vega, Rodriguez, & Gruskin, 2016). This is likely due to a combination of both health and genetic factors associated with AD. The Hispanic community is estimated to be 1.5 times more likely to develop AD than white non-Hispanics (Vega, Rodriguez, & Gruskin, 2016). Moreover, given the fast paced growth of the Hispanic population, the number of Hispanics living with AD is projected to increase nine-fold by 2060, reaching 3.5 million, and therefore posing a significant social and economic burden (Wu, Vega, Resendez, & Jin, 2016). Some have attributed this rise in AD within the Hispanic community to metabolic syndromes, vascular disorders, and genetics.

Neurocysticercosis (NCC) is more common in the Hispanic population than any other race or ethnic group. Cysticercosis is one of two forms of infection caused by the tapeworm, *Taenia solium. Taenia solium* is a parasite of both humans and pigs, and requires both species to complete its life cycle. People who eat pork containing *T. solium* cysts (cysticerci) develop an intestinal infection with the adult tapeworm, called taeniasis. This tapeworm passes its eggs through the person's feces. When these eggs are consumed by a pig, the eggs hatch in the intestine, releasing larvae that migrate and encyst in tissues. Cysticercosis occurs when people ingest tapeworm eggs directly, and as in pigs, the larvae migrate out of the intestine and into muscle and other organs and tissues. NCC occurs when larvae form cysticerci in the brain. NCC is the most common parasitic disease of the central nervous system. It can cause headaches, signs of intracranial hypertension, and psychiatric disturbances. Seizures are the most frequent manifestation of NCC, though cognitive changes have also been reported (Shandera, White, Chen, Diaz, & Armstrong, 1994). NCC affects males and females equally and manifests predominantly in young adults, with a peak occurrence between 25 and 35 years of age; however, infection (which does not necessarily lead to eventual disease) probably occurs much earlier in life (5-15 years of age) (Garcia, Gonzalez, Tsang, & Gilman, 2006).

Although commonly considered a disease of the developing world, NCC has been increasingly diagnosed in the US as the number of immigrants entering the U.S. has increased (White & Atmar, 2002). Regulations and food animal husbandry practices have dramatically reduced the parasite from the commercial pork industry, though new cases of NCC are reported annually. NCC cases diagnosed in the US have been mainly among immigrants from Mexico and Latin America. NCC is a disease that appears to be widely distributed and highly prevalent in Hispanic populations, and even within specific regions of the US (Ong et al., 2002). With NCC being on the rise in Southwest regions of the US, healthcare workers and epidemiologists are highlighting the relevance of NCC as a public health problem.

Case Study/ Clinical History

Antonio had been complaining of a headache, that would come and go, for the last 4 weeks. It was uncharacteristic of him to consistently complain of such things, because as a rather fit 27-year-old, he had relatively minimal health concerns. Antonio lived with his girlfriend, Maria, and they both were active in their surrounding Hispanic community. Antonio would work long days at his construction job, then come home and find time to take online courses through the local community college. He was taking additional classes in business and finance to aid him in starting his own construction company one day. Unfortunately, over the last several weeks, it was getting harder for him to concentrate for long periods of time to complete his online classes. Antonio spoke with both Maria, and his mother about his headache, who both suggested he drink peppermint tea at night when he felt the most pain and fatigue.

Antonio's headache persisted. One day on the job, Antonio had a seizure and was taken to his local hospital by an ambulance. The seizure lasted several minutes and included uncontrollable jerking movements of Antonio's arms and leg, with eventual loss of consciousness. Antonio awoke in the hospital unaware of what had occurred. He was in a strange place and had many wires connected to his head for electroencephalography (EEG) monitoring. Maria was there and reassured him he was safe and filled him in on what had happened. Antonio remained in the postictal state (a time of fluctuating consciousness and changes in mental status) for several hours after arrival to the hospital. During this time, he remained confused and with decreased arousal. Antonio was started on Keppra, a medication used in the treatment of seizure activity. In addition to continued EEG monitoring to evaluate for additional seizure activity, Antonio's physicians also performed a head computed tomography (CT) examination to see if it would show a cause of Antonio's seizure.

Two days after the onset of his seizure, Antonio's medical team determined he was ready for discharge from the hospital. There had been no additional seizure activity noted on Antonio's EEG readout, despite attempts to trigger another seizure. Antonio's head CT was limited by motion artifact, but demonstrated no acute intracranial changes. In a relatively healthy individual with no conclusive findings on head CT neuroimaging, the physicians determined Antonio's seizure was likely idiopathic in nature and supposed it could have been attributed to generalized dehydration or electrolyte imbalance, which may have caused his ongoing headache as well. Antonio was sent home with a 4 week follow up appointment with a neurologist, a prescription for continued use of Keppra, recommendations to drink plenty of fluids, and clearance to return to work after another week of rest.

Over the next few weeks, Antonio's headache continued, but it was generally managed with ibuprofen. He noticed continued difficulties concentrating both at work, and during his online night classes. Maria noted that Antonio seemed forgetful, irritable, and had difficulties doing tasks that previously had been very easy for him, such as making dinner for them. Antonio's employer noted similar characteristics, and eventually gave him less responsibilities on the job site. Holding true to the nature of his Hispanic culture, Antonio was reluctant to go back to his physician for his continued health problems, believing it would get better over time, or could be managed by traditional Hispanic treatments. He sought healing from a curandero he knew from his church, who specialized in the use of herbs in healing. Four weeks after his initial seizure, 2 days before his follow up appointment with a local neurologist, Antonio had another seizure, similar in presentation to his first one. This time he was at home with Maria preparing for bed. Maria called 911 and requested the first responders to transfer Antonio to the larger, level I hospital the next town over.

CLINICAL EVALUATION

Neuroimaging Evaluation

When Antonio reached the hospital, he was sedated by medications the first responders had given him upon their arrival to his house. Although his seizure activity had subsided, he remained confused and lethargic in the postictal state. Given his recent neurological complaints (i.e., seizure activity, headache, attention and memory difficulties), Antonio was taken to have a head CT immediately upon his hospital arrival. Because Antonio was unable to fully participate in a neurological examination when he first arrived, it was the results of the head CT that ultimately guided the medical team through the process of making a definitive diagnosis.

The results of Antonio's head CT identified multiple areas of cysts, some of which were racemose (appearing like a cluster of grapes), with mild areas of edema surrounding some of the larger cysts. The cystic lesions were generally located within the subarachnoid space, filling areas within the suprasellar cistern, one was proximal to the anterior cerebral artery, and another inferior to the gyrus rectus. There was a small infarction around 2 cysts noted in the subarachnoid space superior to the left frontal lobe. There were lesions located next to the right fusiform gyrus and occipital horn of the ventricular system, which were likely parenchymal rather than subarachnoid. No midline shift was appreciated.

The findings of the head CT were congruent with NCC, likely subtype subarachnoid-cisternal, given the location of the various cysticerci. A magnetic resonance imaging evaluation was recommended should further classification be needed, or should Antonio's clinical presentation decline. These results were immediately relayed to Antonio's neurology team.

Neurological Examination

Antonio came out of the postictal state the following morning. At that time, his neurology team was able to perform a full neurological examination to assess his neurological function, including testing his muscle strength, range of motion, and sensory abilities. Antonio was alert and oriented to person, place, and time. He had relatively poor sustained attention, which could have been due to the recent administration of pain and sedation medications. He was able to follow simple commands and answer simple questions. He scored a 26 on the Mini-Mental State Exam (MMSE) (Folstein, Folstein, & McHugh, 1975). Antonio's cranial nerve examination and reflex testing were both grossly unremarkable. He scored 4/5 muscle strength for both upper and lower extremities. Drift was noted on both arms. Regarding coordination and gait, these were both decreased mildly, as observed while Antonio walked from his room to the nurses' station. Sensory examination revealed mildly decreased right-sided sensation.

Overall, Antonio's neurological examination revealed mild cognitive, motor, and sensory impairments. Combined with the results from Antonio's head CT, the neurology team felt strong in their diagnosis of NCC. Given the results of Antonio's neuroimaging, they classified the NCC into active subarachnoid-cisternal. Based on Antonio's fluctuating mental status and ongoing clinical symptom presentation, they determined Antonio was in the colloidal vesicular stage of NCC. During this stage, the cyst membrane begins to break down, leading to an inflammatory response in the adjacent tissues, sometimes leading to edema (swelling due to increased amounts of fluid) and gliosis (a nonspecific, hypertrophic change of the brain's glial cells).

Cognitive Linguistic Evaluation

Given Antonio's initial symptom complaints and current clinical presentation, the neurology team consulted their SLP to perform a cognitive linguistic evaluation. The SLP performed a battery of subtests taken from standardized assessments which targeted all necessary components of cognition and language. Antonio was awake and alert upon the SLP's arrival to complete the cognitive linguistic evaluation. The SLP was able to gain vital background information on Antonio related to his educational, employment, and social history. In a conversation with Antonio and Maria, the SLP noted Antonio had a high school diploma and was currently taking online college-level classes. She confirmed his responsibilities at his construction job, which mainly were related to carpentry work after the initial residential frame was in place. Antonio lived with Maria, they had no children together, but often kept their nieces and nephews overnight. They were very active in the Hispanic community in their town, including religious and social functions. Antonio's native language was Spanish, which he continued to speak at home, at work, and in many of his social engagements with friends. Antonio learned English as a young boy when he started school, was fluent in this language, and used it primarily in his education and everyday interactions outside the Hispanic community.

On cognitive linguistic testing, the SLP noted overall mild to moderate cognitive impairments. Antonio had the greatest difficulties with executive function, short term recall, and higher level attentional tasks. She noted relatively good insight into these deficits, but minimal ability to self-correct many of the errors made throughout the examination. Antonio's comprehension and expression language abilities were intact despite completing the assessment in English. Antonio was motivated to get better and eager to start therapy. His goals were to get better and return to work and school within the next several weeks.

Questions for the Reader

1. Why was Antonio's NCC not identified upon his first hospitalization?
2. What other neurological impairments can present like NCC and how is NCC differentiated from those?
3. What do you think caused Antonio's NCC?
4. What aspects of the Hispanic culture likely put Antonio at an increased risk for contracting NCC?
5. What aspects of the Hispanic culture may have influenced Antonio's healthcare seeking behaviors?
6. From reading the results of Antonio's head CT, what difficulties should the SLP have anticipated?
7. What aspects of Antonio's neurological examination are most pertinent to the SLP?
8. Antonio scored a 26 on his MMSE. What does this likely indicate to the SLP?
9. What is/are the next step(s) for the SLP in the cognitive linguistic intervention for Antonio?

Discussion of Questions for the Reader

1. *Why was Antonio's NCC not identified upon his first hospitalization?* Given that Antonio initially presented to the hospital with a single seizure, this heavily guided his neurologist's medical work up. The neurology team is almost always going to start with a head CT to look for intracranial changes. More often than not, seizures are not identifiable on head CT's though there may be something noted on the head CT that is causing the seizure (i.e., a brain tumor or a brain injury). At that time, perhaps the cysticerci lesions were not large enough to be identified through radiographic imag-

ing, or there was minimal edema associated with them, therefore they were not readily identified. This head CT may also have been influenced by motion artifact, meaning that Antonio had too many movements in the CT scanner to get an accurate radiographic image. Antonio's other clinical symptoms (his headache, concentration issues), could all have been secondary to dehydration, or electrolyte imbalance, as his neurology team assumed at the time of his initial presentation. NCC is often a complex disease process, and therefore a complex diagnostic process as well because its presentation depends on the locations of the lesions, the number of the lesions, the person's immune response, and the person's symptom complaints.

2. *What other neurological impairments can present like NCC and how is NCC differentiated from those?* Clinically, NCC can present similar to other neurological impairments, including traumatic brain injury, stroke, brain abscess, hydrocephalus, or encephalopathy. NCC can be differentiated from those by an astute radiologist upon review of the patient's neuroimaging, typically the head CT. NCC can also be confirmed via histological demonstration of cysticerci, or positive antibodies found in cerebrospinal fluid or serum.
3. *What do you think caused Antonio's NCC?* NCC develops by means of fecal-oral contamination, and is acquired by the ingestion of the pork tapeworm's *Taenia solium* eggs, which have been shed in the stools of a person carrying the tapeworm in their gut. Unbeknownst to him, Antonio likely accidentally acquired these eggs during a meal. Moreover, it is likely unknown when this contamination occurred as the eggs and cysts can remain dormant in the host's body for many years after initial infection. Not until those cysts begin to break down or become too large do symptoms start appearing.
4. *What aspects of the Hispanic culture likely put Antonio at an increased risk for contracting NCC?* NCC is typically considered a disease of the developing world, and disproportionately affects impoverished and underrepresented minority populations (Serpa & White, 2012). The rise in the number of cases of NCC in developed countries, like the U.S., and in certain populations within the U.S., i.e., within the Hispanic community, has been well documented (White & Atmar, 2002). For example, some areas in the Southwestern U.S. which have large Hispanic populations, have reported the incidence of NCC among Hispanics to be at least 8 to 10 per 100,000 per year with 1000 new cases of NCC diagnosed each year (Serpa & White, 2012). There may be several explanations for this, ranging from significant travel between disease-endemic areas in Mexico, to immigrants acquiring the tapeworm prior to immigration, to persons with the adult tapeworm being asymptomatic and not aware of the potential risk to themselves or to others. Other at risk factors for Antonio to acquire NCC include his age and gender. NCC has been noted more frequently in males, and is most common in 24-35 year olds (Wallin & Kurtzke, 2004).
5. *What aspects of the Hispanic culture may have influenced Antonio's healthcare seeking behaviors?* Antonio may have been influenced by his Hispanic culture in seeking healthcare. Males may be more likely to wait until the last minute to obtain care (Parangimalil, 2001). He had previously sought help from other community resources, so perhaps he was waiting for those to decrease his symptoms before turning to typical Western medicine. Additionally, financial or insurance matters may have complicated his situation.

6. *From reading the results of Antonio's head CT, what difficulties should the SLP have anticipated?* The results of Antonio's head CT indicated several lesions in left frontal lobe, with larger ones noted on the left side. Other areas affected were parts of the limbic and ventricular systems, as well as the right temporal-occipital lobe. These are fairly diffuse and widespread lesions. The SLP may have anticipated difficulties related to executive functioning and memory (frontal lobe), expressive language (left frontal lobe), emotional processing and memory (limbic system), visuospatial processing or calculations (temporal-occipital lobe), or a variety of neurocognitive changes related to the functioning of the ventricular system.
7. *What aspects of Antonio's neurological examination are most pertinent to the SLP?* SLPs should familiarize themselves with all aspects of the neurological examination; however, some are more pertinent to their work than others. For example, important information from Antonio's neurological exam was that he was oriented times three (to person, place, and time), he scored a 26 on his MMSE, and the neurologists noted relatively good language abilities. Additionally, Antonio's cranial nerve exam was grossly unremarkable, which is important information related to Antonio's swallowing abilities.
8. *Antonio scored a 26 on his MMSE. What does this likely indicate to the SLP?* The MMSE is a commonly used cognitive screen that many neurologists use to screen for dementia. Administration is quick, requiring relatively little supplies, or training. While a general indicator of severe cognitive impairment, it lacks sensitivity to mild cognitive impairment. Also, it can be impacted by several demographic factors, including age and education. Antonio is a high school graduate, therefore given his education level he surpasses the MMSE cut off score of 24 or below, and may be presumed competent. But this score may not be reflective of his true baseline cognitive abilities, i.e., how he was before the onset of his initial headache, before his first seizure, and before his diagnosis of NCC. Although a Spanish translation of the MMSE was released in 2010, it is unlikely this was normed within the Hispanic population. Therefore, there may be cultural biases associated with the standardization of the MMSE that impacted Antonio's score. Any individual scoring a 26 or above may be presumed competent, though the high score for the test is 30. A score of 26 should indicate to the SLP, and the neurologist, that something on the test was difficult for Antonio and further cognitive assessment is warranted.
9. *What is/are the next step(s) for the SLP in the cognitive linguistic intervention for Antonio?* The SLP has already performed a formal cognitive linguistic assessment and should develop Antonio's treatment plan based off those results, with input from Antonio and his family as to what goals are of particular importance to them. The SLP is likely to target cognitive skills over linguistic ones, with the most emphasis on executive function, memory, attention, and metacognition. Depending on Antonio's wishes, and accessibility of interpreters at the SLP's facility, the intervention sessions could be conducted in either English or Spanish. Antonio's medical treatment is likely to impact his cognitive abilities and the SLP should discuss with the neurologist what changes may be expected and in what timeframe. As Antonio's overall medical status improves (i.e. he receives treatment for his NCC and he gets better from a medical standpoint), the SLP should anticipate general improvements in Antonio's cognition and his ability to participate in therapy.

Treatment Considerations

From a medical standpoint, the neurology team treated Antonio with several medications. These included the antiparasitic drug, albendazole, to eliminate the tapeworm infection. They continued Antonio's Keppra, an anticonvulsant medication, to manage his seizure activity. While still alive, most larvae cysts do not cause an inflammatory reaction in their host because their cyst wall stays intact and does not interfere with the host's blood-brain barrier. In Antonio's case, the neurology team believed that some of the cysts were beginning to degenerate, thus causing an acute inflammatory response in Antonio's brain. This was noted by edema on Antonio's head CT report. To target this, the neurology team started Antonio on a corticosteroid, aimed at reducing the edema located around some of the intracranial cysticerci. Antonio remained in the hospital for a total of 3 weeks. Eventually, as the cysts begin to degenerate, by natural processes, or as a result of the antiparasitic drug therapy, they may calcify. This causes an additional inflammatory response from the host, though the process of why and how this occurs is not fully understood (CDC, 2017). Therefore, the neurology team recommended Antonio follow up with them regularly after his discharge from the hospital for the next 4-6 months.

The SLP picked Antonio up for treatment while he remained acutely hospitalized. She saw him for 30-40 minute sessions, and he received treatment 2-3 times a week. Therapy was conducted in English and focused on executive function, memory, and higher level attention tasks. Executive function tasks included sequencing job function steps related to Antonio's construction work and planning an organized day to optimize Antonio's success in his home, work, and school environments. Memory tasks were related to the use of compensatory strategies, such as setting alarm reminders on his phone and using repetition and rehearsal to aid in working memory and short term memory tasks. Attention tasks primarily consisted of alternating and divided attention tasks geared towards activities that were typical of Antonio's job needs. A major portion of each session also emphasized metacognitive skills. Metacognition refers to the ability to think appropriately about one's thinking skills. It refers to the processes of planning one's steps, monitoring one's performance, understanding what went well and what needed work, and correcting those actions to ensure improved performance in the future. Antonio had good insight into many of his deficits, but lacked the ability to self-correct these breakdowns. Therefore, the SLP also targeted problem identification and problem solving. Finally, the SLP included educational information related to Antonio's diagnosis of NCC, the causes and treatment of it, and why it had caused cognitive changes for Antonio (relating the site of his lesions, back to noted impairments in function). The SLP was able to incorporate much of this information into recall tasks for Antonio. At his time of discharge, Antonio felt he was at his baseline cognitive function and that he no longer had any cognitive related changes associated with his NCC. The day before discharge, the SLP repeated her cognitive linguistic assessment, which demonstrated improved abilities across all cognitive domains, but persistent executive function and memory deficits that the SLP did not believe were indicative of Antonio's baseline abilities. The SLP recommended continued speech therapy services as an outpatient. Antonio was reluctant to commit to this, but the case worker put a prescription for outpatient speech therapy services in Antonio's discharge paperwork packet.

Outcomes

By the time Antonio was discharged from the hospital, the neurology team categorized him into the granular nodular stage, indicating that his clinical symptoms had largely resolved, and that his intracranial cysticerci were slowly degenerating, forming coarse, mineralized granules in their place. They continued to monitor Antonio for clinical changes, which may indicate that he had transitioned into the final stage of NCC, the nodular calcified stage. This is characterized by the calcification of the cysticerci within the brain, meaning they are no longer in an active stage. Antonio filled the prescription for the antiparasitic, corticosteroid, and anticonvulsant medications his doctors had recommended, but did not refill them as prescribed. Antonio did keep two follow up appointments with his neurology team, but cancelled the others believing they were no longer needed. He again visited his community curandero, who recommended a new herbal rub and tea mix to facilitate Antonio's overall healing and restore his humoral balance. Antonio's friends and family agreed that he was back to his usual self and agreed with him that he probably did not need any more speech therapy sessions or neurology appointments.

Maria provided care for Antonio during his first 2 weeks after discharge, and his extended family and friends brought over meals to fill the refrigerator and freezer. They brought various candles to be burned and offered prayers of healing and support. Antonio made it a point to tell each of them about his diagnosis of NCC and how they too may be at risk for the same disease. He reviewed the risk factors associated with NCC, likely symptoms of NCC, the course of his hospitalization, and how the disease affected his thinking skills. Much of this information he recalled was from his work with his SLP. Despite his openness about his diagnosis of NCC, he hid a growing fear related to the consumption of foods containing any type of pork. Any dishes his family or friends brought containing pork, he politely accepted but immediately trashed upon their departure. He said prayers and lit candles to various patron saints in an attempt to alleviate this growing anxiety.

Four weeks after returning home, Antonio resumed work at his construction job. He was unable to re-enroll in his academic coursework until the start of a new semester. Shortly after his return to work, he again noted a headache at the end of the day. Maria noted he was more frustrated and easily agitated while at home. His supervisor reported he seemed forgetful at work and again was having difficulties keeping up with all the tasks required of him. Antonio had already cancelled his 6-week follow up neurology appointment and he did not want to return to urgent care or the emergency department to seek medical advice. Rather, he found the prescription for outpatient speech therapy in his hospital discharge packet and made an appointment. Upon reviewing Antonio's chart and listening to Antonio's current complaints, the SLP agreed to repeat a cognitive linguistic assessment to determine if Antonio still qualified for treatment. She reinforced with Antonio that he needed to call his neurologist's office and make a follow up appointment with them as well.

Additional Questions to the Reader

1. Why do you think Antonio chose not to refill his treatment prescriptions?
2. What likely influenced Antonio's decision to not follow through with his follow up neurology appointments?
3. Why do you think Antonio noted difficulties only upon his return to work?
4. What do you think the SLP was likely to find upon a repeat assessment of Antonio's cognitive linguistic abilities?
5. What do you think is Antonio's prognosis related to his NCC and related to his cognitive function?

Discussion of Additional Questions to the Reader

1. *Why do you think Antonio chose not to refill his treatment prescriptions?* Antonio may have chosen not to refill his prescriptions for a variety of reasons. It may be related to lack of prescription drug health insurance coverage, or the additional out-of-pocket financial burden for those specific medications may have been too great for Antonio to manage. As Antonio was starting to feel better, perhaps he felt that he no longer needed the medications and therefore did not need to fill the subsequent doses. Or perhaps Antonio felt he could be better served looking to a more traditional healing method, such as using therapeutic herbs or oils. Not quite as likely, though still plausible, may be that Antonio simply forgot to refill the medications given the noted memory changes documented by the SLP.
2. *What likely influenced Antonio's decision to not follow through with his follow up neurology appointments?* Again, Antonio's lack of extended follow up with his neurology team may have been related to insurance coverage concerns, or due to ongoing financial distresses related to additional co-payments, additional tests recommended, or additional prescription medications to purchase. Furthermore, once Antonio returned to work, he likely did not feel he could take any more time off given he had already been out on medical leave for an extended period. Location may have also influenced Antonio's ability to follow up with the neurologist. Perhaps he lived in a remote location and travel to the appointment was too far, he might not have had means of transportation, or may not have had the extra money to pay for the expenses associated with the trip. Oftentimes, when people feel they are medically healed, or at least on the road to recovery, they chose not to keep recommended follow up medical appointments given the added inconvenience those appointments may bring.
3. *Why do you think Antonio noted difficulties only upon his return to work?* Many patients with cognitive impairments do not readily notice the difficulties these impairments may have on their day to day activities while they remain hospitalized. This is likely because while they are in the hospital they are not working or are not in school, they are not involved in routine household chores like cleaning and cooking, they are told what they need to do and when they need to do it, and they have assistance with many of their activities of daily living. Oftentimes, breakdown can occur once the patient is discharged and returns back to their home and/or work life responsibilities. They find it harder to manage many tasks, especially as they now have much more independence. During his first few weeks at home, Maria offered a good deal of assistance and supervision for Antonio. Many cultures place greater importance on the family unit than the individual, and it may be very likely that rather than carrying out tasks independently, there may be a strong cultural pull for family members to offer assistance whenever any signs of struggle may be noted. In the early days of being home, perhaps Maria offered so much help that Antonio did not feel the full brunt of his cognitive difficulties until he returned to work and was faced with managing things by himself. Additionally, mental fatigue and decreased physical stamina may have limited Antonio in the work environment, thus putting increased strain on his cognitive function. Ultimately, higher level cognitive impairments, like Antonio's, likely added to Antonio's increased difficulties upon his return to work.

4. *What do you think the SLP was likely to find upon a repeat assessment of Antonio's cognitive linguistic abilities?* The SLP who repeated Antonio's cognitive linguistic assessment was likely to find similar difficulties related to executive function and memory as noted previously. Perhaps there may have been some level of continued cognitive improvement associated with continued medical recovery; however, it is unlikely that Antonio's cognition would have tested within normal limits, especially given the increased difficulties he reported upon return to work. The SLP may also have noted the use of compensatory strategies related to memory and problem solving that may have helped Antonio score better on certain measurements. If so, these were likely due to Antonio implementing these strategies as taught to him by his previous SLP.
5. *What do you think is Antonio's prognosis related to his NCC and related to his cognitive function?* Despite not refilling his prescription medications and noting an increased struggle upon return to work, Antonio likely has an overall good prognosis related to both his NCC and his cognitive abilities. He has several positive prognostic indicators, including his age, social support, and motivation to improve. He does need to take certain precautions to ensure continued improvement, both related to his NCC and his cognitive function, including continuing to actively participate in speech therapy sessions and likely need to follow up with his neurologist to ensure medical stability of the NCC.

KEY POINTS

There are both positive and negative health indicators associated with the Hispanic culture. They may comprise of such things as:

- Positive:
    - Relatively healthy lifestyles with decreased instances of obesity, lower levels of smoking and illicit drug use
    - Decreased reports of chronic conditions and decreased mortality rates
    - Strong family structures
- Negative:
    - Increased rates of no or minimal insurance
    - Lower immunization rates and lower socioeconomic status
    - Decreased use of primary care practitioners and increased emergency room visits
    - Acculturation may lead to the adoption of negative health or lifestyle practices, which may over time decrease the noted positive behaviors

The Hispanic culture has several traditional healthcare beliefs and common practices that clinicians should be aware of, including:

- Common belief systems related to humoral imbalance, empacho, mal de ojo, envidia, and susto
- Familism/Collectivism
- Religion/Spirituality
- Using home remedies or traditional practices prior to or in conjunction with Western medicine
- Seeking care from relatives or other Hispanic community members

There are several health disparities that contribute to increased morbidity and mortality for many within the Hispanic community. These disparities include:

- Lifestyle and environmental factors related to education, employment, or socioeconomic status
- Access to healthcare- ranging from insurance status to prevention and intervention disparities
- Increased risk factors for certain neurological diseases, including stroke, Alzheimer's dementia, and NCC
- Aspects of Antonio's case study may be specific to the Hispanic culture, as well as his diagnosis of NCC, but some of these principles can also be applied to other culturally diverse groups. This may include the specific culture's beliefs related to:
- When and how to utilize standard Western medicine
- Sharing of experiences with other community members
- Adherence to physician recommendations

Remember that the Hispanic culture is rich in traditional beliefs and practices. These likely influence most aspects of the individual's lifestyle including their opinions about healthcare. This can impact how the person views illness, how apt they are to seek intervention from traditional customs or from Western focused practitioners, and how they communicate with their healthcare providers. Relating to the patient on these culturally sensitive aspects of their life can be crucial to providing appropriate healthcare intervention.

REFERENCES

American Community Survey. (2008). *Selected population profile in the United States –Hispanic or Latino (1-year estimates).* Washington, DC: U.S. Census Bureau.

Argeseanu, C. S., Ruben, J. D., & Narayan, K. M. (2008). Health of foreign-born people in the US: A review. *Health & Place*, *14*(4), 623–635. doi:10.1016/j.healthplace.2007.12.002 PMID:18242116

Becker, D., Garcia, S., & Ellertson, C. (2004). Do Mexico City pharmacy workers screen women for health risks when they sell oral contraceptive pills over-the-counter? *Contraception*, *69*(4), 295–299. doi:10.1016/j.contraception.2003.11.014 PMID:15033404

Centers for Disease Control and Prevention. (2002). Access to healthcare and preventive services among Hispanics and non-Hispanics. *Morbidity and Mortality Weekly Report*, *53*(40), 937–941.

Centers for Disease Control and Prevention. (2008). Work-related injury deaths among Hispanics—United States, 1992–2006. *Morbidity and Mortality Weekly Report, 57*(22), 597–600. PMID:18528315

Centers for Disease Control and Prevention. (2017). *FastStats: Health of Hispanic or Latino Population*. National Center for Health Statistics.

Flores, A. (2017). How the US Hispanic population is changing. *Pew Research Center*. Retrieved from https://www.pewresearch.org/fact-tank/2017/09/18/how-the-u-s-hispanic-population-is-changing/

Garcia, H. H., Gonzales, A. E., Tsang, V. C., & Gilman, R. H. (2006). Neurocysticercosis: Some of the essentials. *Practical Neurology, 6*(5), 288–297. doi:10.1136/jnnp.2006.101253

Gundykunst, W. B. (1998). *Bridging differences: Effective intergroup communication*. Newbury Park, CA: Sage.

Hough, R. L., Landsverk, J. A., Karno, M., Burnam, M. A., Timbers, D. M., Escobar, J. I., & Regier, D. A. (1987). Utilization of health and mental health services by Los Angeles Mexican Americans and non-Hispanic whites. *Archives of General Psychiatry, 44*(8), 702–709. doi:10.1001/archpsyc.1987.01800200028005 PMID:3632245

Kemp, C., & Rasbridge, L. A. (2004). Mexico. In *Refugee and immigrant health: A handbook for health professionals*. Cambridge, UK: Cambridge University Press.

King, D. E., & Bushwick, B. (1994). Beliefs and attitudes of hospital inpatients about faith healing and prayer. *The Journal of Family Practice, 39*(4), 349–352. PMID:7931113

Livingston, G., & Kahn, J. R. (2002). An American dream unfulfilled: The limited mobility of Mexican Americans. *Social Science Quarterly, 83*(4), 1003–1012. doi:10.1111/1540-6237.00129

Livingston, G., Minushkin, S., & Cohn, D. (2008). Hispanics and healthcare in the US: Access, information, and knowledge. *Pew Research Center*. Retrieved from https://www.pewhispanic.org/2008/08/13/hispanics-and-health-care-in-the-united-states-access-information-and-knowledge/

Lujan, J. (2010). Meeting religious needs of Hispanic clients to provide culturally competent care. *The Internet Journal of Allied Health Sciences and Practice, 8*(2), 4.

Martinez, O., Wu, E., Sandfort, T., Dodge, B., Carballo-Dieguez, A., Pinto, R., ... Chavez-Baray, S. (2015). Evaluating the impact of immigration policies on health status among undocumented immigrants: A systematic review. *Journal of Immigrant and Minority Health, 17*(3), 947–970. doi:10.100710903-013-9968-4 PMID:24375382

National Alliance for Hispanic Health. (2004). *Delivering preventive health care to Hispanics: A manual for providers*. US Department of Health and Human Services, Health Resources and Services Administration.

National Center for Health Statistics. (2008). *Trends in the health of Americans*. Department of Health and Human Services, National Center for Health Statistics. Retrieved from https://www.cdc.gov/nchs/data/hus/hus08.pdf

Ong, S., Talan, D. A., Moran, G. J., Mower, W., Newdew, M., Tsang, V. C. W., & Pinner, R. W. (2002). Neurcysticercosis in radiography imaged seizure patients in US emergency departments. *Emerging Infectious Diseases*, *8*(6), 608–612. doi:10.3201/eid0806.010377 PMID:12023918

Parangimalil, G. J. (2001). Latino health in the new millennium: The need for a culture-centered approach. *Sociological Spectrum*, *21*(3), 423–429. doi:10.1080/027321701300202064

Passel, J. S., & Cohn, D. V. (2009). *A portrait of unauthorized immigrants in the United States. Pew Hispanic Center Report*. Washington, DC: Pew Research Center.

Pew Hispanic Center. (2010). *Country of origin profiles- Hispanics in the United States.* Retrieved from http://pewhispanic.org/data/origins/

Ramirez, R. R. (2004). *We the people: Hispanics in the US. (Census 2000 special reports).* Washington, DC: Bureau of the Census, US Department of Commerce.

Rivera, M., Ortíz, M., Lawson, M. E., & Verma, K. M. (2002). Evaluation of the use of complementary and alternative medicine in the largest Southwest United States Mexico border city. *Pharmacotherapy*, *22*(2), 256–264. doi:10.1592/phco.22.3.256.33543 PMID:11837563

Serpa, J. A., & White, A. C. (2012). Neurocysticercosis in the United States. *Pathogens and Global Health*, *106*(5), 256–260. doi:10.1179/2047773212Y.0000000028 PMID:23265549

Shandera, W. X., White, A. C. Jr, Chen, J. C., Diaz, P., & Armstrong, R. (1994). Neurocysticercosis in Houston, TX: A report of 112 cases. *Medicine*, *73*(1), 37–52. doi:10.1097/00005792-199401000-00004 PMID:8309361

Sheinart, K. F., Tuhrim, S., Horowitz, D. R., Weinberger, J., Godman, M., & Godbold, J. H. (1998). Stroke recurrence is more frequent in blacks and Hispanics. *Neuroepidemiology*, *17*(4), 188–198. doi:10.1159/000026172 PMID:9701833

Silverstein, M. (2008). Getting home safe and sound: Occupational safety and health administration at 38. *American Journal of Public Health*, *98*(3), 416–423. doi:10.2105/AJPH.2007.117382 PMID:18235060

Smith, A. (2000). *Ethnomed: Mexican cultural profile*. Retrieved from http://ethnomed.org/ethnomed/cultures/mexican/mexican_cp.html

Smith, D. P., & Bradshaw, B. S. (2006). Rethinking the Hispanic paradox: Death rates and life expectancy for US non-Hispanic White and Hispanic populations. *American Journal of Public Health*, *96*(9), 1686–1692. doi:10.2105/AJPH.2003.035378 PMID:16380579

Sonderup, L. (2010). Hispanic marketing: A critical market segment. *Advertising & Marketing Review.* Retrieved from https://www.cdc.gov/healthcommunication/pdf/thisjustin/tji_1_201108.pdf

Turran, C. M., & Goldman, N. (2007). Socioeconomic differences in mortality among US adults: Insights into the Hispanic paradox. *The Journals of Gerontology. Series B, Psychological Sciences and Social Sciences*, *63*(3), S184–S192. doi:10.1093/geronb/62.3.S184 PMID:17507594

U.S. Census Bureau. (2008). Washington, DC: Population Estimates – Hispanic or Latino.

U.S. Department of Health and Human Services, Office of Minority Health. (2016). *Profile: Hispanic/ Latino Americans*. Retrieved from https://minorityhealth.hhs.gov/omh/browse.aspx?lvl=3&lvlid=64

U.S. Department of Labor. (2018). *TED: The Economics Daily*. Bureau of Labor Statistics. Retrieved from https://www.bls.gov/opub/ted/2018/76-point-9-percent-of-hispanic-men-employed-january-2018.htm?view_full

Vega, W. A., Rodriguez, M. A., & Gruskin, E. (2016). Health disparities in the Latino population. *Epidemiologic Reviews*, *31*(1), 99–112. doi:10.1093/epirev/mxp008 PMID:19713270

Wallin, M. T., & Kurtze, J. F. (2004). Neurocysticercosis in the United States: Review of an important emerging infection. *Neurology*, *63*(9), 1559–1564. doi:10.1212/01.WNL.0000142979.98182.FF PMID:15534236

White, A. C., & Atmar, R. L. (2002). Infections in Hispanic immigrants. *Clinical Infectious Diseases*, *34*, 1627–1632. doi:10.1086/340620 PMID:12032899

Wu, S., Vega, W. A., Resendez, J., & Jin, H. (2016). *Latinos & Alzheimer's disease: New numbers behind the crisis*. Retrieved from: https://health.ucdavis.edu/latinoaging/news/pdf/Latinos_and_AD_USC_UsA2-Impact-Report.pdf

Zsembik, B. A., & Fennell, D. (2005). Ethnic variation in health and the determinants of health among Latinos. *Social Science & Medicine*, *61*(1), 53–63. doi:10.1016/j.socscimed.2004.11.040 PMID:15847961

ADDITIONAL READING

Blanchard, J., & Lurie, N. (2004). R-E-S-P-E-C-T: Patient reports of disrespect in the health care setting and its impact on care. *The Journal of Family Practice*, *53*(9), 721–730. PMID:15353162

Livingston, G., Minushkin, S., & Cohn, D. (2008). Hispanics and healthcare in the US: Access, information, and knowledge. *Pew Research Center*. Available at https://www.pewhispanic.org/2008/08/13/hispanics-and-health-care-in-the-united-states-access-information-and-knowledge/

Serpa, J. A., & White, A. C. (2012). Neurocysticercosis in the United States. *Pathogens and Global Health*, *106*(5), 256–260. doi:10.1179/2047773212Y.0000000028 PMID:23265549

KEY TERMS AND DEFINITIONS

Cognition: Cognition the mental action or process of acquiring knowledge and understanding through thought, experience, and the senses.

Cognitive-Linguistic Impairment: Cognitive-linguistic impairments impact a person's thinking skills and communication skills. Areas of cognition that may be impacted include executive function, memory, attention, and visual spatial skills. Areas of communication that may be impacted can be related to both linguistic and paralinguistic abilities.

Dementia: Dementia is a neurological condition characterized by a decline in cognitive abilities, such as memory, attention, language, and problem solving. Alzheimer's dementia is the most common type of dementia.

Health Disparity: A health disparity is a preventable difference in the burden of disease, injury, violence, or opportunity to achieve optimal health. Not all differences between groups may be considered disparities, but rather only differences which systematically and negatively impact less advantaged group.

Neurocysticercosis (NCC): NCC is a preventable parasitic infection caused by larval cysts of the pork tapeworm. These cysts can infect various parts of the host's neurological system, causing a variety of neurological changes depending on the location and severity of the infection.

Outcome: A medical outcome includes clinical end points; physical, social, and role functioning in everyday living; patients' perceptions of their general health and well-being; and satisfaction with treatment.

Stroke: A stroke occurs when a blood vessel that carries oxygen and nutrients to the brain is either blocked by a clot or ruptures. When that happens, part of the brain cannot get the blood (and oxygen) it needs, so it and brain cells die.

Chapter 13
Traumatic Brain Injury in Culturally Diverse Populations:
Navigating Healthcare Intervention for Adults

Leslie W. Johnson
https://orcid.org/0000-0002-6651-4763
North Carolina Central University, USA

EXECUTIVE SUMMARY

This chapter highlights traumatic brain injury (TBI) and various health disparities within this population, particularly gaps related to patients from culturally diverse backgrounds. A review of three main health disparities is included, related to increased risk for sustaining a TBI, intervention barriers related to TBI, and long-term outcome after TBI. This chapter also evaluates how culture influences aspects of TBI intervention by exploring cultural considerations apparent in diverse populations. The chapter concludes with an examination of a case study based on an actual patient who sustained a TBI and details how his Native American culture impacted his healthcare choices and how his healthcare providers adapted intervention strategies given cultural influences unique to his clinical presentation.

INTRODUCTION

Traumatic brain injury (TBI) can have a negative impact on cognitive, behavioral, and/or emotional function. These changes may make it difficult for some individuals with TBI to maintain and develop social relationships, return to pre-injury employment, or fully re-integrate back into their communities (Olver, Ponsford, & Curran, 1996). As the United States becomes increasingly diverse, healthcare providers, including speech-language pathologists (SLPs) and audiologists are more frequently working with culturally and linguistically diverse (CLD) individuals as part of their typical caseload. This is evident across various populations, including the neurologically impaired one. Existing intervention models have

DOI: 10.4018/978-1-7998-2261-5.ch013

not generally been adapted to adequately meet the needs of patients from culturally diverse backgrounds (Uomoto & Wong, 2000).

There is a growing body of evidence related to how clinicians interact with patients from CLD backgrounds. Within this literature, there are some studies that focus on how clinicians can interpret the behaviors of patients from CLD backgrounds, and consequently adjust their interactions throughout the assessment and rehabilitation periods. Applying a more culturally appropriate clinical model may help the patient engage more thoroughly in the intervention process, which may in turn improve treatment outcomes. Ultimately, this may contribute to minimizing the health disparity gaps associated with TBI in CLD populations. Clinical experiences can drive future studies by identifying problematic issues not adequately addressed in the literature to date. Much of this section reviews the health disparities related to TBI in CLD populations. This section concludes with the presentation of a case study that is based on an actual patient's experience with acute TBI and how the patient, his family, and his medical team including the SLP, worked to learn and adapt their behaviors accordingly to facilitate intervention based on his cultural preferences.

HEALTH DISPARITIES RELATED TO TBI IN CLD POPULATIONS

There is evidence to suggest that health disparity gaps are prevalent in the TBI population (Lequerica & Krch, 2014; Niemeirer & Arango-Lasprilla, 2007). These disparities demonstrate that people from CLD backgrounds are at a greater risk for sustaining a TBI (Heffernan et al., 2011). Moreover, people from CLD backgrounds often face barriers that impact sufficient and appropriate intervention after TBI leaving them at an increased risk of poorer long-term outcome (Gao, Kumar, Wisniewski, & Fabio, 2018; Meagher, Beadles, Doorey, & Charles, 2015). These health disparities are multi-faceted, with a variety of driving issues, likely related to "mistrust of healthcare professionals, racism, environment barriers impacting accessibility, quantity and quality of education, lack of bilingual professionals, as well as the lack of culturally relevant assessment and intervention tools" (Lequerica & Krch, 2014, p. 645). The following section explores these three specific health disparities noted in patients experiencing TBI within CLD populations.

Increased Risk for Sustaining a TBI

Gender, socioeconomic status, and ethnic origin are all significant risk factors in the occurrence of TBI. Men are up to three times more likely than women to sustain a TBI (Chase, Ratcliff, Vernich, Al-Sukhni, Yasseen, & Colantonio, 2012). Furthermore, younger men are more likely to sustain a TBI (Stein, 2001). Lower socioeconomic status has been associated with increased risk for brain injury (Ivins et al., 2003). Some have postulated that individuals with lower socioeconomic status are more vulnerable to a spectrum of adverse mental and physical health outcomes which may make them more susceptible to TBI (Nguyen, Evans, & Zonderman, 2007; Smith, 2004). Others have noted that minorities are more likely than Caucasians to be residents of inner cities, earn lower wages, work longer hours per week, and have a prior history of a TBI (Jarder, Weiss, Cohen & Pepe, 2000). In the United States, African Americans have higher rates of brain injury than other groups (Langlois, Rutland-Brown, & Thomas, 2004). Some have noted that African Americans and Caucasians have a similar incidence of TBI, but African Americans are more likely to die from their TBI (Kraus & McArthur, 1996). Interestingly, Kisser and colleagues (2017) reported that elderly African Americans were more likely to experience TBI than other age groups within that race (Kisser, Waldstein, Evans, & Zonderman, 2017). In examining other races, Blackmer & Marshall (1999) reported that Native Americans are more likely to experience a TBI than non-Native Americans, and that alcohol is more likely to be involved. Others have noted that people from CLD backgrounds are more likely to sustain their TBI from acts of violence and automobile vs. pedestrian crashes (Burnett, Kolakowsky-Hayner, Slater, Stringer, Bushnik, Zafonte, & Cifu, 2003). This increased risk for sustaining a TBI may predispose certain people from CLD populations for the additional health disparities that follow.

Intervention Barriers

In general, people from CLD groups are more likely to experience barriers to access of healthcare services, ranging from emergency room attention to outpatient and community-based clinics. This is often attributed to minorities with brain injury who face socioeconomic and insurance status barriers that impact whether or not they receive inpatient rehabilitation or outpatient services. Demographic factors relevant to CLD minority groups, such as lower levels of preinjury education and employment, or lower socioeconomic status, may prevent access to and utilization of healthcare services (Sherer et al., 2003). For patients with a TBI who are seen in the emergency department, minorities wait longer to see a physician, are three times more likely to receive care from a resident, and are less likely to be sent back to their referring physician after discharge (Bazarian, Pope, McClung, Cheng, & Flesher, 2003).

Socioeconomically disadvantaged populations, such as the uninsured or underinsured, have been reported to undergo fewer operative procedures, receive fewer therapy sessions, and have higher mortality rates after trauma (Haas & Goldman, 1994; Haider, Chang, Efron, Haut, Crandall, & Cornwell, 2008). Additionally, studies have shown that African Americans and Hispanics are less likely to receive the highest quality emergency room care, less likely to be discharged to rehabilitation centers for further treatment, and less likely to receive additional and more intensive rehabilitative therapies (Gary, Arango-Lasprilla, & Stevens, 2009). Others have demonstrated that people from CLD populations overall receive fewer minutes of physical therapy (PT), occupational therapy (OT), and speech therapy (ST) (Burnett et al., 2003). These intervention barriers likely contribute to the overall poorer long-term outcomes observed in culturally diverse populations.

Long-Term Outcome After TBI

Cross-cultural research in the area of outcome after TBI is lacking, with relatively little known about the experiences of individuals from CLD backgrounds (Saltapidas & Ponsford, 2007). Even among CLD populations who receive rehabilitation after TBI, health disparities persist and affect daily functioning in many aspects of life. Reasons for this are likely multifaceted based on specific cultural values. Some cultures may value reliance on the family community for support after an illness and be reluctant to follow up with post-discharge care and services from medical professionals. Additionally, the inability to follow up with such services may be limited by remote geographic location. For example, many patients do not have the gas money to travel to urban healthcare centers if they live in more rural areas. Outcome disparities after TBI related to disability, employment, and community reintegration have been noted for people from CLD backgrounds (see Niemeier & Carlos Arango-Lasprilla, 2007 for review). For example, minority populations have been noted to experience worse overall disability levels with decreased functional independence, which were notable up to 5 years post-TBI (Gary et al., 2009). Hispanic patients with TBI are more likely to be severely disabled 6 months after injury (Marquez de la Plata et al., 2007). People from CLD backgrounds have been noted to have decreased job stability, less receipt of vocational support services, and overall less successful terms of employment (Gary et al., 2009). Studies have shown that after TBI minorities are less involved in employment or other productive activities at one year post-injury compared to Caucasians and twice as likely to show unstable employment patters during the first few years after TBI (Kreutzer et al., 2003; Sherer et al., 2003).

In examining community reintegration, some researchers have noted that African Americans and Hispanics were more likely to experience social isolation up to 1 year post-TBI (Cavallo & Saucedo, 1995). Others have reported people from CLD backgrounds experience increased rates of depression and increased instances of post-traumatic stress following TBI (Gao et al., 2018). Jorge, Robinson, Starkstein, and Arndt (1994) reported minorities, when compared to Caucasians, have lower levels of social functioning and higher rates of alcohol abuse after TBI. African Americans are significantly more likely than Caucasians to report lower satisfaction with life and social integration after TBI (Sherer et al., 2003). All of this all can culminate into poorer long-term outcome after TBI for those patients most at risk, contributing to changes within their social structure, in employment options, community reintegration, and overall quality of life.

HOW CULTURE IMPACTS TBI INTERVENTION

Culture can influence both the patient and the clinician. The patient may have cultural influences related to symptom presentation, perception of diagnosis and related impairments, expectations for recovery, need for outside intervention services, and anticipated prognosis for short-term and long-term improvement. The clinician may have cultural influences related to interactions with the patient and family, overt and covert biases, or stereotypical prejudices. Relatively little is known about the experiences of CLD patients with TBI, including their beliefs about TBI, rehabilitation associated with TBI, and anticipated outcomes expected after TBI (Saltapidas & Ponsford, 2007).

Healthcare Factors

Currently, many healthcare workers and facilities follow a typically Western style of medical intervention. This may be an outdated model of rehabilitation not fitted to patients from CLD backgrounds. Historically, this has led to mistrust of healthcare workers from some cultures and potential biases on the behalf of healthcare workers concerning cultures other than their own. Seasoned clinicians know that developing a trusting relationship between the patient and the clinician is key to creating a successful intervention plan. Researchers have noted various minority populations may have developed a mistrust of healthcare providers over time (Benkert, Hollie, Nordstron, Wichson, & Bins-Emerick, 2009). This likely influences how the patient relates to and interacts with their healthcare provider. Cultural beliefs related to healing and the roles of the healer and the patient may vary across cultures.

In the acute inpatient rehabilitation setting, individuals from CLD backgrounds may have difficulties shifting roles from a more passive "patient" to a more active and interactive member of their treatment team. In this setting, patients are required to assume more responsibility for attaining their treatment goals. This may be different for an individual from a CLD background, who may view only the physician as an authority figure in the treatment plan, not themselves as well. Consequently, the patient-clinician dyad may be misunderstood or under-valued. Still, if given the opportunity, patients from CLD backgrounds have been noted to generally participate in rehabilitation programs to the same extent as patients from English speaking backgrounds (Saltapidas & Ponsford, 2007). This dyad may also be affected by healthcare workers, who may have either overt or covert biases related to people from CLD backgrounds. Increased prejudicial attitudes of healthcare staff can be related to decreases in intended helping behaviors, which has the potential to negatively impact an individual's recovery. Redpath and Linden (2004) reported that if the perception that an individual's behavior contributed to their injury was noted by healthcare workers, this may contribute to stigmatization and subsequent negative consequences for the patient. Linden and Redpath (2011) demonstrated that healthcare workers may have prejudicial attitudes towards their patients with TBI related to blame and social interaction, and unintentionally show fewer helping behaviors toward them. Together, these factors related to patient cultural preferences and potential clinician cultural biases can ultimately influence intervention after TBI.

Influence of Dominant Discourses

Dominant discourses refer to the typical, mainstream culture. In the United States, healthcare tends to follow a Western model, with mostly English-speaking practitioners. These perceived dominant discourses, related to language, race, and class, can impact the care patients receive after TBI. For example, individuals with limited English proficiency may feel more vulnerable and be less likely to self-advocate, ask relevant health questions, and express their basic needs (Ledger, 2002). Effective communication is essential in healthcare settings so that patients can fully benefit from services received, and so that they do not further injure themselves by not following misunderstood safety precautions. In addition to most healthcare practitioners speaking predominately English, much of the research conducted, and subsequent evidence-based practices, has been studied on English-speaking populations. Furthermore, many of the assessment tools used by practitioners, including neuropsychiatrists and SLPs in particular, are written in English and were standardized on predominately English-speaking populations. Straight translations into other languages, and even use of an interpreter to translate the standardized tests, still has many limitations, namely the cultural biases many of these tests possess. These biases are often directly related to culture, language, race, socioeconomic status, or educational level. Application to populations different from the population the test was standardized on makes the use of the standardized scores derived from these tests fairly meaningless. Lequerica and Krch (2014) suggested measuring the patient's level of acculturation, or the degree to which an individual assimilates to the language, customs, and world view of the majority society, as part of testing the cognitive abilities of people with TBI from CLD backgrounds. This may enable the clinician to informally assess how dominant discourses are influencing the intervention of their patient with TBI.

Interpersonal Influences

Psychological factors, motivation, social interaction, and pre-morbid life roles may all impact intervention after TBI. Different cultures have different beliefs related to reasons for illness and anticipated recovery, and coping styles after injury. For example, religion or spirituality differs among many cultures. It is common for people who have experienced a traumatic medical event to turn to their cultural religion or spirituality as a coping mechanism. There is likely a wide range of cultural influences related to religion and spirituality, ranging from such extremes as the person feels they have an illness because they are being punished for their sins to a person who may hold on to the faith that God will heal them through prayer. The latter patient may perceive that by participating in therapy, God may see this as a lack of faith in his healing power (Lequerica & Krch, 2014). There is minimal literature related to the specific coping styles that people from CLD backgrounds may employ after TBI. One study reported that African American caregivers report more time spent serving as caregivers compared to other racial groups and tend to opt for support from houses of worship rather than professional support (Meagher et al., 2015). Some studies have noted maladaptive coping styles, such as an increased reliance on drugs and alcohol, can be noted after TBI, though this has not been demonstrated specifically in populations of cultural diversity (Wolters, Stapert, Brands, & van Heugten, 2010). More information is needed related to specific ways burden of caregiver responsibility and need for social support systems change after TBI in minority populations.

Family Dynamics

The individual and the family may be viewed differently based on cultural values. Family support, family interactions, and family involvement are important in many aspects of healthcare, but is increasingly important as therapists work to help patients through the rehabilitation process. The cultural influence of family dynamics may affect patient behavior or clinician expectations. For example, understanding whether the patient comes from an individualistic culture versus a collective culture may be an important detail for therapists to consider. Many cultures place greater importance on the family unit than the individual, and it may be very likely that rather than carrying out tasks independently, there may be a strong cultural pull for family members to offer assistance whenever any signs of struggle may be noted. Others may feel they have brought shame to their family as a result of their TBI and may withdraw from participating fully in medical intervention and eventual post-discharge care. Understanding the hierarchy of the family structure, and who makes medical related decisions and how those decisions are made, is key in ensuring the success of any intervention program.

Outcome Measures

The Western practice of healthcare tends to value outcome measures indicative of returning to the patient's level of function before their injury. Oftentimes a goal of many healthcare providers is to have the patient with TBI reintegrate back into the community upon discharge. This typically relates to a patient's ability to return to work or school. However, this may not be an important goal for people from CLD backgrounds. For example, some individuals may value return to church activities as an essential goal after TBI. Studies have reported that when compared to Caucasians, African Americans and Hispanics value domestic activities, such as parenting, housekeeping, and cooking, as more important than return to full-time employment (Sander, Clark, & Pappdis, 2010). It appears these groups may place more value on their role within their family unit than their role within their larger community. If that is the case, it is likely that significant measurements of outcome vary from culture to culture and need to be discussed between the clinician and patient as part of goals of care planning and eventual discharge planning as well. This likely includes conversations related to caregiver support systems available at discharge and who will provide assistance or supervision for the patient related to physical and cognitive activities. Increased burden of care for family members has been noted after TBI, effecting stress, depression, anxiety, and overall unhealthy family functioning, though these outcomes have not been directly associated with specific cultures. More research is needed related to how people from diverse backgrounds view functional outcome after TBI related to both their functioning within the community and within their own family unit.

CASE STUDY/CLINICAL HISTORY

Jonas was 53 years old when he was in a severe motor vehicle collision. While driving to work, he was T-boned by an oncoming truck that ran a red light. Jonas was a restrained driver, but given the speed and location of impact, he still suffered considerable injuries. There was airbag deployment and prolonged extrication from the vehicle. When EMS arrived, they noted minimal responsiveness from Jonas and gave him an initial Glasgow Coma Scale (GCS) (Teasdale & Jennett, 1974) score of 6. The GCS is a standardized measure used to assess severity of TBI, and a GCS score is given to each patient with a TBI by the medical professional who first responded to the patient. He was also given a Rancho score of III. The Rancho Los Amigos Scale is a standardized way to assess individuals after TBI. It can be used by any medical professional and is based on the cognitive and behavioral presentations of the patient as they emerge from coma or other impaired levels of consciousness (Rancho Los Amigos National Rehabilitation Center, 2011). Jonas was intubated (placed on the ventilator by a long tube through his mouth, down his throat, and into his lungs) on the scene to maintain airway protection. Jonas was airlifted to the nearest Level I Trauma center.

Upon arrival to the hospital, the medical team noted multiple orthopedic injuries, including three broken ribs, a left anterior pneumothorax (collapsed lung), open book pelvic fracture, and bilateral clavicular fractures. Head computed tomography (CT) showed left frontal scalp hematoma, multiple bilateral frontal and temporal lobe punctate intraparenchymal hemorrhages, concerning for diffuse axonal injury, and left frontal subarachnoid hemorrhage. An approximate four mm left-to-right midline shift was noted, indicated swelling with Jonas' brain.

Given his injuries, Jonas was unable to provide his medical or social history upon arrival. Family arrived several hours after Jonas was admitted and were able to offer collateral information. Jonas' prior medical history included history of congestive heart failure and diabetes, both currently managed by medications. Jonas and his family are Native American and members of the Lumbee tribe. They live in a region of the state heavily populated by people from this cultural background. Prior to his injury, Jonas was employed full-time as a car mechanic and lives with his wife of 28 years, Julia. They have three children together, all of whom live independently, but close by, and are actively involved with the family.

Over the course of the next three weeks, Jonas went through many medical procedures including chest tube placement to heal his pneumothorax, pelvic embolization with eventual pelvic ring open reduction internal fixation (a surgery to repair his broken pelvis), bronchoscopy to assess for additional lung damage, left frontal craniotomy to drain the blood from around his brain, and Corpak tube placement (a feeding tube through the nose that provided nutrition). He remained intubated on the ventilator for 19 days. He was successfully extubated (removed from the ventilator with the tube which was down the throat into the lungs removed) and his oxygen requirements were weaned to 28% FiO2 via nasal cannula.

Clinical Evaluation

Once medically stable, the SLP was consulted to evaluate Jonas' cognitive linguistic abilities, as well as his swallowing function. During the SLP's chart review, she noted Jonas' prior medical and social history, reason for admission, medical progress to date, and recent radiographic studies. Jonas' most recent head CT was completed approximately one week before and revealed reduction in size of the left frontal scalp hematoma, and redemonstration of bilateral frontal and temporal lobe punctate intraparenchymal hemorrhages again concerning for diffuse axonal injury. It also noted surgical changes associated with the left frontal craniotomy. The most recent chest x-ray noted interim removal of the patient's endotracheal tube, low lung volumes, bibasilar opacities (left greater than right), with no pneumothorax appreciated.

Before initiating the evaluation, the SLP spoke with Jonas' nurse who stated Jonas remained on many medications, including acetaminophen (pain medication), docusate (stool softener), Pepcid (treats gastroesophageal reflux disease), labetalol (for high blood pressure), Keppra (an anticonvulsant used to treat or prevent seizures), insulin (as needed for diabetes), and Ativan (sedative) with a dose of fentanyl (treats severe pain) administered three hours ago due to increased facial grimacing likely due to pain associated with the patient's pelvic repair. The nurse also reported Jonas had only brief periods of wakefulness and did not follow commands with her. She noted several family members who had been with the patient since his accident, including his wife, three children and their spouses, four grandchildren, and various friends and extended family members. She also noted although the family respected the intensive care unit's policy of only two visitors at a time in the room, they frequently rotated family members throughout the day and into the evening to spend time with Jonas.

Jonah was seen by the SLP for a cognitive-linguistic assessment at the bedside. He was sleeping upon the SLP's arrival, so the SLP made introductions with the patient's wife, Julia, who was reading by the bedside. Julia reported her husband had a good night and had been resting for the last hour or so since his daughter left. Julia said in times of wakefulness, Jonas would make eye contact with her and follow her around the room if she moved. He would occasionally smile, and attempt to make verbalizations, which she reported were limited to grunting noises or single word utterances. The clinician explained the role of the SLP within the hospital setting, mentioning she had been asked by Jonas' physicians to evaluate his cognitive and language abilities, as well as his swallowing abilities as appropriate. Julia consented to allow the SLP to proceed with her examination.

The SLP attempted to arouse Jonas with a strong sternal rub, performed by a repetitive circular motion made by the SLP's palm to the patient's sternum. This elicited some moaning from Jonas and pulling away from the therapist. She then repositioned Jonas in a more upright position, maintaining precautions congruent with safety standards related to his pelvic repair. In this upright position, Jonas intermittently opened his eyes to both tactile and verbal stimuli, though for brief periods of time. During these brief periods of arousal, the SLP noted intermittent eye contact, short verbalizations of 'No', no simple command following, but awareness of his environment and himself. The SLP noted Jonas was inconsistent in his responses, with poor initiation and generally delayed reactions. With a cold washcloth to the forehead, Jonas was able to sustain arousal better and the SLP attempted to give him ice chips. She noted immediate lip movement and closure around the ice chip, which continued with each bolus presentation. Jonas was able to nod his head intermittently when asked if he wanted more. No overt signs or symptoms of aspiration were appreciated with any ice chip bolus presentation. Voicing after the swallow was noted one time on a yawn which sounded clear.

Questions for the Reader

1. What are relevant components from the chart review the SLP should note?
2. How do you think pain, or the use of pain medications, may be affecting Jonas' current clinical presentation?
3. How severe in nature do you believe Jonas' cognitive linguistic impairments are?
4. What Rancho level do you think the SLP gave Jonas?
5. What type of education can the SLP provide for Jonas and his family currently?
6. What are some general influences of the Native American culture that the SLP should consider?
7. What specific aspects of Jonas' Native American culture may impact the SLP's intervention with Jonas and his family moving forward?
8. What are the next steps for the SLP?

Discussion of Questions to the Reader

1. *What are relevant components from the chart review the SLP should note?* Important considerations for the SLP to note from a review of Jonas' chart include the following: his initial GCS score, the results of his head CT and need for craniotomy, social history, and current medication regimen. Jonas' initial GCS score indicates a severe level of brain injury. Not only has the initial GCS been used to determine injury severity, it has also been used as a predictor of prognosis (Balestreri et al. 2004). A low initial GCS score of 6 should indicate to the SLP that not only did Jonas sustain a severe TBI, but he also has a poorer prognosis given the extent of this injury. Another important consideration for the SLP should be the results of Jonas' head CT. All patients who arrive to the hospital with any neurological symptoms, such as headache, or seizure, or weakness, or numbness, receive a head CT. It is vital in determining if there is any life-threatening bleeding within the brain. Jonas' TBI was excessive enough to cause bleeding within the brain in multiple areas. This bleeding, and the subsequent pressure it was likely causing within the cerebrum, was so significant that the physicians felt neurosurgery was indicated to control it, therefore a craniotomy was performed. A craniotomy can take several forms, but generally involves some method of removing the blood that has collected on the brain. Moreover, Jonas' injury was so severe that diffuse axonal injury was suspected, which has long been associated with overall poorer prognosis after TBI (Paterakis, Karantanas, Komnos, & Volikas, 2000). Patients with diffuse axonal injuries tend to have more severe injuries and have an increased chance of remaining in a coma for longer periods after TBI. Important aspects of Jonas' social history to consider are his family support, employment prior to admission, and Native American culture. Additionally, review of Jonas' currently prescribed medications is important and discussed in response to the following question.
2. *How do you think pain, or the use of pain medications, may be affecting Jonas' current clinical presentation?* Although likely that Jonas' clinical presentation was impacted by his current pain medication regimen, much of his clinically noted impairments should be attributed to his significant TBI. He is on several types of pain medications or sedative medications, which may influence his clinical presentation. The use of these types of medications has been repeatedly shown to impact arousal and cognitive linguistic abilities (Dhingra, Ahmed, Shin, Scharaga, & Magun, 2015). The SLP should consider finding a time for her session when Jonas' pain is controlled, but also when the effects of the pain medications are not dramatically interfering with his participative abilities.

3. *Given the background information, how severe in nature do you believe Jonas' cognitive linguistic impairments are?* At this time, Jonas is presenting with severe cognitive linguistic deficits. He has decreased arousal and poor attention. He is showing some awareness of his environment and his self, for example, he interacts with caregivers and medical staff, pulls away from noxious stimuli, and has sleep/wake cycles. His communication and language abilities are poor as well, for example, he has good tracking abilities, is able to make eye contact, engages in some purposeful, but simple, verbalizations, and occasionally is able to follow simple commands. These responses are generally delayed in nature, and inconsistent, which is congruent with severe TBI.
4. *What Rancho level do you think the SLP gave Jonas?* The SLP gave Jonas a Rancho level of III. In this stage, the patient demonstrates a localized response, meaning they may respond to specific stimuli, such as a simple command, and likely has some awareness of the environment around them, such as watching someone walk around the room or reaching for a blanket if cold. Their responses are likely delayed and inconsistent.
5. *What type of education can the SLP provide for Jonas and his family currently?* The SLP initiated education for Jonas' family at her initial assessment. This included information related to both the role of the SLP and general TBI information. The SLP confirmed that she would be seeing Jonas as part of his routine medical plan of care, targeting the areas of swallowing and cognitive linguistic impairment. She provided information on Jonas' current level of cognitive linguistic functioning and offered additional information on the anticipated trajectory of recovery after brain injury, using the Rancho Scale as a reference frame. The SLP continued education related to things the family could be doing at this time for Jonas, including providing re-orientation information, keeping the room calm and quiet, limiting distractions, bringing in favorite belongings from home, giving him rest periods, allowing extra time for him to respond, keeping comments and questions short, and explaining what is occurring prior to doing it.
6. *What are some general influences of the Native American culture that the SLP should consider?* It is important to explore the beliefs concerning the causes and eventual treatment of illness within the lenses of an individual's culture. This information can ultimately help the provider better understand their patients and may help to plan culturally acceptable interventions and treatment strategies in a collaborative relationship with the patient and the family. Many Native Amcricans believe that illness is caused by an imbalance in the patient's spiritual, emotional, and/or social environment. Some tribes may believe that it is due to unwanted evil spirits, or due to the sins of the patient's ancestors. Healing in the Native American culture likely refers both to the physical healing and the emotional or spiritual healing of the patient. They believe the most important element of each person is the essence of one's being, or the individual's spirit, and for wellness to occur the spirit must be considered. Therefore, it is typical to see both medical and spiritual healing or treatment provided to Native American patients. Many Native Americans consider healing to be a sacred calling, a gift that has been provided to the healer for the purpose of helping others. Some Native Americans view death as part of life and talk about it openly, whereas others do not. Many believe that each person is put on the earth for a short time and for a purpose. When that purpose is accomplished, the person is then ready to leave this world, no matter what medical healing options may be offered. Appreciating the patient's cultural background related to health, illness, treatment, and death should provide an appropriate framework for intervention.

Other aspects of Native American culture that may influence healthcare is that many Native Americans, especially elderly ones, may exhibit a basic distrust of the Western healthcare system. This is based on the historical abuses and belief that this system is based on "greed" rather than care for the individual. Additionally, many Native Americans take a non-interference view of treatment, believing that the medical professional, or healer, knows best and therefore they may be hesitant to ask questions or engage in counseling or education conversations.

Respect is a key component of Native American culture. Respect can be shown to Native Americans by healthcare workers in a variety of ways, including talking softly, limiting physical touch, respecting a patient's modesty, and not looking the person straight in the eyes, especially elders. As the extended family is important and valued within the Native American culture, offering a place for the family to gather within the healthcare setting may be important. Deliberation over important decisions may be a time consuming process and decisions are very likely to be delayed if agreement cannot be reached in the Native American culture. Oftentimes, providing a private space for the family to discuss important matters will allow for conversations to be had that may facilitate everyone in the group coming to a suitable decision for the family.

7. *What specific aspects of Jonas' identification with the Native American culture may impact the SLP's intervention with Jonas and his family moving forward?* In the United States alone, there are more than 500 nations of Native Americans, each having their own separate customs, language, culture, set of beliefs, and religious practices (Mulkey, Lacock, & Scott, 2004). Jonas was a member of the Lumbee tribe. Although not living on tribal land since he was in his early 20s, Jonas and his family lived within a town where 89% of the population identified as Lumbee, according to the 2000 US Census report. Both of Jonas' parents were Lumbee, as is Julia, Jonas' wife. He considers his Native American culture to be one of the defining aspects of his life, though he has acculturated to mainstream Americanism with his language, dress, employment, and many social activities.

Jonas continues to maintain a strong sense of Native American spirituality and believes that healing most effectively occurs when combining both Native American medicine and herbal treatments with Western medicine and pharmaceuticals. He and his family strongly believe that a spiritual healer is essential in moving forward with Jonas' healing. In their culture, values, customs, and sacred traditions are passed on through oral traditions and ceremonies. These may include such things as dancing, singing, drumming, prayer, or feasting. Jonas and his family are eager to have prayer songs and a ritual sage smudging performed at Jonas' bedside as part of the healing process.

Jonas and his family value "doing" instead of "talking", so while Jonas has been in a medically induced coma, and even once he started regaining consciousness after his injury, his family has often questioned why the medical team continues to tell them what they are going to do and what the next steps of Jonas' recovery are going to be. They are looking for more action from the team, and less verbal information on Jonas' plan of care.

Finally, Jonas' elderly parents, his wife, his children, his grandchildren, his siblings and their spouses and children are all considered active participants and responsible for the care of Jonas. The family thrives when all together and although they remain compliant with the hospital's visitor policy, they question its value.

8. *What are the next steps for the SLP?* The SLP should speak directly with Jonas and his family about what aspects of their Native American culture are important to consider when providing ongoing intervention for Jonas, developing treatment goals, and determining measures of functional outcome. The SLP needs more information on how Jonas views his spiritual healing tied to his medical healing. It would be beneficial to know if there are any cultural influences related to diet the SLP needs to be aware of before proceeding with the swallowing evaluation. How involved does Jonas want his family in his intervention and who from the family can the SLP provide information? Finally, how can the SLP best establish a trusting relationship with Jonas and his family? Answers to these, and other pertinent questions, may help guide the SLP as she continues to assess Jonas' swallowing and cognitive linguistic abilities and establish an appropriate plan of care.

Treatment Considerations

Given the extent of Jonas' injuries, there are a variety of services the SLP can provide. Although many of the SLP's initial services were impacted by Jonas' level of alertness and attention, as well as his pain and pain medication regimen, there remain many important aspects of care to be targeted by the SLP. Much of the SLP's early assessment related to both dysphagia (disordered swallowing) and cognitive linguistic impairment consisted of test, re-test techniques. An example of a test, re-test technique would be the SLP assessing Jonas' ability to follow one step commands during each session because patients in the acute stage of their injury can change dramatically from one day to the next. For the next week, Jonas remained a Rancho level III. Given his lower level of consciousness, Jonas was a lower priority patient for the SLP, who saw him 1-2 times this week, for brief 15-20 minute sessions. At this time, the SLP continued to recommend NPO (nothing by mouth) except ice chips after oral care.

Approximately five weeks after his injury, Jonas had progressed to a Rancho level IV. At this point, Jonas pulled out his Corpak and the SLP was asked to re-assess his swallow function. After a Modified Barium Swallow Study, the SLP recommended a soft mechanical diet with thin liquids. He continued to improve from a cognitive linguistic standpoint, though sessions were often limited due to his frequent outbursts and increased agitation. The SLP provided redirectional cues often as she targeted tasks related to attention, memory, orientation, and language. Given his improved alertness and interaction, the SLP increased Jonas' frequency of treatment sessions to 2-3 times a week, with sessions lasting as long as Jonas could tolerate due to his periods of agitation and ongoing pain management difficulties.

The Rancho level IV stage was a difficult stage in Jonas' recovery for his family. He was most unlike his typical self at this point, with increased frustration, use of foul language, and yelling at his caregivers. At this point, highly concerned over his spiritual well-being, the family asked a spiritual healer from their community to come perform a healing ceremony. Although limited by hospital rules and regulations, the healer was able to perform a prayer song with a hand drum and shaker, as well as a sage and sweet grass smudging using oils rather than burned herbs. Within the week, Jonas had progressed out of the Rancho level IV stage to a level V.

From a medical standpoint, Jonas progressed nicely as his orthopedic injuries continued to heal and his pain became better managed. Increasingly, the SLP was able to focus her therapy sessions on improving Jonas' cognitive abilities related to orientation to his environment, improved attention, and basic safety awareness. Jonas continued to need aggressive services from the occupational therapist (OT) and physical therapist (PT), in addition to the services he was already receiving from the SLP. By this point, each therapist was able to see Jonas for 30-45 minute therapy sessions, 3-4 times a week. The medical team recommended Jonas be discharged to an acute inpatient rehabilitation (AIR) facility. The family took an additional week to deliberate between taking Jonas to AIR versus taking him home with them where he would receive home health therapy services. Ultimately, the family opted to have Jonas go to AIR to receive continued therapy before hopeful discharge home.

Outcomes

At his time of discharge from acute care, Jonas was eating and drinking a regular diet with thin liquids without difficulties. He was rated as a Rancho level VI. Jonas was discharged to an AIR within the same healthcare system as his acute hospitalization, so the SLP who worked with him in acute care was able to intermittently work with him in AIR as well. Jonas' speech therapy intervention in AIR focused on rehabilitation of Jonas' executive function, short term memory, and metacognitive skills. Although noting steady improvement in most areas, the SLP continued to report decreased initiation and slow response times for certain tasks. While these impairments are often evident in patients with TBI, Jonas appeared more deliberate about this, especially in tasks related to turn taking and conversational speech. Jonas' family did not appear highly concerned about this part of his journey to recovery, and asked the SLP to focus more on improving Jonas' short term recall. Similarly, when the SLP was targeting the metacognitive skill of insight into current deficits and difficulties this may pose upon Jonas' reintegration back into his community, Jonas' family conveyed they were not highly concerned about this and would rather the SLP focus treatment on something more "functional".

While in AIR, each patient receives intense therapies for three hours a day at least. Patients are seen by each discipline (OT, PT, and SLP) for hour long sessions, 6-7 times per week. During his first week of rehab, Jonas was noted to be increasingly more disgruntled with staff and caregivers. By the end of his day, he would lash out at his wife, and not want to participate in therapy. This change did not appear related to his recent change in environment, nor due to acute neurological changes. After discussions with his medical team and family, it was apparent that Jonas' pain was not being appropriately treated and he was having increased muscular pain due to his increased therapeutic activities. A change in medications remedied this situation and Jonas continued his rehabilitation without significant setbacks.

As part of his rehabilitation, the rehab team routinely dedicated a portion of Jonas' day to Jonas' spiritual healing, which was facilitated by members of Jonas' Lumbee community who took turns sharing oral traditions or leading prayer songs. Jonas and his family developed trusting relationships with the rehab team which facilitated buy-in to treatment tasks. Eventually generalization of therapy tasks learned inside the therapy room were noted in tasks outside of the therapy room as well. Jonas reported he enjoyed working with his therapists because they used active listening skills and incorporated Jonas and his extended family into the decision making process for establishing Jonas' goals of care.

After a 3-week AIR stay, Jonas was discharged home under his family's supervision. The case manager set up outpatient services for him for OT, PT, and SLP. He was provided information on a local TBI support group. Jonas discharged from AIR as a Rancho level VIII, a total of almost 11 weeks after the car accident that caused his injuries.

Additional Questions for the Reader

1. What was the role of the SLP in working with the patient and educating the family while Jonas was going through the Rancho level IV stage?
2. What were likely important considerations for Jonas and his family when deciding to go to AIR or to go home?
3. What aspects of Jonas' Native American culture may have been impacting what he and his family considered a priority in speech therapy sessions?
4. Why do you think Jonas was reluctant to relay to his medical team that his pain was not adequately controlled?
5. How did the medical team facilitate Jonas' need for both medical and spiritual healing?
6. Are there any additional considerations about Jonas' cultural background that may have influenced his intervention while hospitalized or upon discharge?

Discussion of Additional Questions for the Reader

1. *What was the role of the SLP in working with the patient and educating the family while Jonas was going through the Rancho level IV stage?* The SLP's role during this stage of recovery was to provide a safe environment for continued assessment and intervention related to SLP services. The SLP can continue to evaluate and treat dysphagia and cognitive linguistic impairments during this time, as is appropriate and tolerable for the patient. Much of the SLP's role during this time was also related to providing continued education to the patient and the family about TBI, the stages of TBI recovery, current recommendations, and anticipated prognosis. Functional information related to tasks the family could provide for their loved one at that time are also important. These may include reassuring the patient that they are safe, finding calm activities for the patient, redirecting the patient as needed related to agitation and confusion, offering frequent rest breaks, limiting the number of visitors, and keeping the environment calm and quiet.
2. *What were likely important considerations for Jonas and his family when deciding to go to AIR or to go home?* This was likely a difficult decision for Jonas and his family. After being in the hospital for 8 weeks, the idea of another three weeks was rather daunting. Discernment over continuing therapy in AIR versus continuing therapy at home likely involved consideration and deliberation amongst many family members. For many Native Americans, if agreement was not obtained quickly, it is highly likely that discussions continued until the entire family was able to reach an agreeable decision. Moreover, despite Western culture valuing the AIR experience as a means to more effectively treat TBI, that may not be a belief shared by some Native Americans who may value other things higher than medical intervention. Slow and deliberate consideration of treatment options may be very likely for Native Americans and the validation or approval of a spiritual leader may be helpful for some groups.
3. *What aspects of Jonas' Native American culture may have been impacting what he and his family considered a priority in speech therapy sessions?* Native American culture values contemplation and active listening. Listening and waiting to respond, as well as the accompanying pauses in conversation and potentially extended silences that may accompany this, are all considered valuable communicative exchanges. The direct expression of opinion, consistent with the Western "my turn to talk now" mentality, and potential for interruption may be seen as disrespectful to many Native

Americans. Therefore, the idea of treating Jonas' communication to quicken the pace, or have more aggressive verbal behaviors was not valued by Jonas nor his family.

Similarly, Jonas' Native American culture likely influenced the metacognitive skills the SLP was attempting to target in therapy. Most Native Americans maintain present orientation, without looking back towards the past or onward towards the future. The concept of planning for what may be difficult for Jonas at discharge given his new disabilities after the accident, was likely not congruent with Native American culture, which tends to show indifference towards future planning, believing if there is a future, it will take care of itself.

4. *Why do you think Jonas was reluctant to relay to his medical team that his pain was not adequately controlled?* Both acute and chronic pain is generally undertreated in Native American populations. Native Americans may be less likely to ask for pain medication, as traditionally they are taught to withstand pain as a skill for survival. Others may choose to not ask for pain medication as they may see it as a weakness, or that their body is failing them, something that they may have difficulty accepting.
5. *How did the medical team facilitate Jonas' need for both medical and spiritual healing?* The medical team facilitated Jonas' need for spiritual healing both in the acute and AIR setting. According to his family, the ritual ceremony of smudging with sage and sweet grass oils was a key feature in moving him out of the Rancho level IV stage. In the AIR setting, the team allowed for frequent chantings, shaker beats, and prayer song rituals to be performed. These were all done with certain modifications to meet hospital rules and regulations, but Jonas and his family were all satisfied with the results. For the Native American culture, the concept of healing is a broad term that combines religion, spirituality, herbal medicine, and rituals used to treat both medical and emotional conditions. Oftentimes, providing healing is more than providing medicine, treatments, or even a cure for a disease. Rather, it is more about healing the person as a whole.
6. *Are there any additional considerations about Jonas' cultural background that may have influenced his intervention while hospitalized or upon discharge?* Although this was not a factor in Jonas' intervention, there is a high incidence of alcohol and drug abuse for many Native American populations (Beauvais, 1998). Jonas did voice concerns over the need to develop appropriate coping strategies should his injuries impact his ability to reintegrate back into his community affect his mental health, so he would not be quick to turn to alcohol as some of his peers had previously.

It may have also been helpful to know what outcome measure Jonas would be measuring his success by. Was it return to work? Or community reintegration back into previously held tribal or religious role? Or perhaps success would be measured by level of independence in the home environment or ability to resume all pre-morbid household roles? Determining which of these outcome measures may be most indicative of success according to the Native American culture may have been helpful for Jonas' rehab team.

KEY POINTS

The following health disparities have been noted related to TBI within culturally diverse populations:

- Increased risk for sustaining a TBI
- Intervention barriers related to access of services across the continuum of care
- Poorer long-term outcome after TBI

Culture can impact TBI intervention by influencing both the patient and the clinician. A variety of cultural influences have been documented related to:

- Healthcare factors including distrust of healthcare professionals, thus affecting the patient-clinician dyad
- Influence of dominant discourses related to language and race, and the inherent biases of both assessment and therapy tools developed by dominant culture researchers
- Interpersonal influences related to psychological and motivational factors, as well as life role ideals
- Family dynamics, which can have both positive and negative affects related to intervention
- Outcome measures related to community reintegration and return to work

Aspects of Jonas' case study are specific to the Native American culture, but some of these principles can also be applied to other culturally diverse groups. This may include the specific culture's beliefs related to:

- Illness and healing
- Demonstration of respect and norms for social interaction
- Family dynamics and decision making

Given the health disparities related to TBI for people from culturally diverse backgrounds, it is apparent that "one size fits all" healthcare is not ideal for many patients. Healthcare providers can modify and adapt their service models, and their methods of interaction with patients to better accommodate people from culturally diverse backgrounds. This can be mutually beneficial to all parties involved. This still allows for the therapist to employ evidence-based practices, but within thc context of the patient's cultural belief system. This in turn can maximize patient compliance and motivation for intervention leading to improvements with the patient's engagement with therapy. Not only can providing culturally sensitive intervention likely improve outcomes after brain injury, it can also enrich the patient's healthcare experience, which may help to enhance future healthcare utilization for both that patient and potentially other members of that patient's cultural background.

REFERENCES

Arrastia, R. (2007). Ethnic differences in rehabilitation placement and outcome after TBI. *The Journal of Head Trauma Rehabilitation*, *22*(2), 113–121. doi:10.1097/01.HTR.0000265099.29436.56 PMID:17414313

Balestreri, M., Czosnyka, M., Chatfield, D. A., ... Pickard, D. (2004). Predictive value of Glasgow coma scale after brain trauma: Change in trend over the past ten years. *Journal of Neurology. Neurosurgery & Psychology*, *75*, 161–162. PMID:14707332

Bazarian, J., Pope, C., McClung, J., Cheng, Y., & Flesher, W. (2003). Ethnic and racial disparities in emergency department care for mild traumatic brain injury. *Academic Emergency Medicine*, *10*(11), 1209–1217. doi:10.1197/S1069-6563(03)00491-3 PMID:14597497

Beauvais, F. (1998). American Indians and alcohol. *Spotlight on Special Populations*, *22*(4), 253–259. PMID:15706751

Benkert, R., Hollie, B., Nordstron, C. K., Wickson, B., & Bins-Emerick, L. (2009). Trust, mistrust, racial identity and patient satisfaction in urban African American primary care patients of nurse practitioners. *Journal of Nursing Scholarship*, *41*(2), 211–219. doi:10.1111/j.1547-5069.2009.01273.x PMID:19538706

Blackmer, S. C., & Marshall, J. (1999). A comparison of traumatic brain injury in the Saskatchewan native North American and non-native north American populations. *Brain Injury: [BI]*, *13*(8), 627–635. doi:10.1080/026990599121359 PMID:10901690

Burnett, D. M., Kolakowsky-Hayner, S. A., Slater, D., Stringer, A., Bushnik, T., Zafonte, R., & Cifu, D. X. (2003). Ethonographic analysis of traumatic brain injury patients in the national model systems database. *Archives of Physical Medicine and Rehabilitation*, *84*(2), 263–267. doi:10.1053/apmr.2003.50091 PMID:12601659

Cavallo, M. M., & Saucedo, C. (1995). TBI in families from culturally diverse populations. *The Journal of Head Trauma Rehabilitation*, *10*(2), 66–77. doi:10.1097/00001199-199504000-00008

Chase, S., Ratcliff, G., Vernich, L., Al-Sukhni, E., Yasseen, B., & Colantonio, A. (2012). Preventive health practices and behavioral risk factors in women surviving traumatic brain injury. *Health Care for Women International*, *33*(7), 631–645. doi:10.1080/07399332.2012.673652 PMID:22681747

Dhingra, L., Ahmed, E., Shin, J., Scharaga, E., & Magun, M. (2015). Cognitive effects and sedation. *Pain Medicine*, *16*(1suppl 1), 37–43. doi:10.1111/pme.12912 PMID:26461075

Gao, S., Kumar, R. G., Wisniewski, S. R., & Fabio, A. (2018). Disparities in health care utilization of adults with TBI are related to insurance, race, and ethnicity: A systematic review. *The Journal of Head Trauma Rehabilitation*, *33*(3), E40–E50. doi:10.1097/HTR.0000000000000338 PMID:28926481

Gary, K. W., Arango-Lasprilla, J. C., & Stevens, L. F. (2009). Do racial/ethnic differences exist in post-injury outcomes after TBI? A comprehensive review of the literature. *Brain Injury: [BI]*, *23*(10), 775–789. doi:10.1080/02699050903200563 PMID:19697166

Haas, J. S., & Goldman, L. (1994). Acutely injured patients with trauma in Massachusetts: Differences in care and mortality, by insurance status. *American Journal of Public Health*, *84*(10), 1605–1608. doi:10.2105/AJPH.84.10.1605 PMID:7943478

Haider, A. H., Chang, D. C., Efron, D. T., Haut, E. R., Crandall, M., & Cornwell, E. E. (2008). Race and insurance status as risk factors for trauma mortality. *Archives of Surgery*, *143*(10), 945–949. doi:10.1001/archsurg.143.10.945 PMID:18936372

Heffernan, D. S., Vera, R. M., Monaghan, S. F., Thakkar, R. K., Kolzloff, M. S., Connolly, M. D., ... Cioffi, W. G. (2011). Impact of socioethnic factors on outcomes following traumatic brain injury. *The Journal of Trauma Injury Infection and Critical Care*, *70*(3), 527–534. doi:10.1097/TA.0b013e31820d0ed7 PMID:21610339

Ivins, B. J., Schwab, K., Warden, D., Harvey, S., Hoilien, M., Powell, C. O., ... Salazar, A. M. (2003). Traumatic brain injury in US army paratroopers: Prevalence and character. *The Journal of Trauma Injury Infection and Critical Care*, *55*(4), 617–621. doi:10.1097/01.TA.0000052368.97573.D4 PMID:14566111

Jarger, T. E., Weiss, H. B., Cohen, J. H., & Pepe, P. E. (2000). Traumatic brain injuries evaluated in US emergency departments, 1992-1994. *Academic Emergency Medicine*, *7*(2), 134–140. doi:10.1111/j.1553-2712.2000.tb00515.x PMID:10691071

Jorge, R. E., Robinson, R. G., Starkstein, S. E., & Arndt, S. (1994). Influence of major depression on 1 year outcome in patients with traumatic brain injury. *Journal of Neurosurgery*, *81*(5), 726–733. doi:10.3171/jns.1994.81.5.0726 PMID:7931619

Kisser, J., Waldstein, S. R., Evans, M. K., & Zonderman, A. B. (2017). Lifetime prevalence of TBI in a demographically diverse community sample. *Brain Injury: [BI]*, *31*(5), 620–623. doi:10.1080/02699052.2017.1283057 PMID:28326858

Kraus, J., & McArthur, D. (1996). Epidemiologic Aspects of Brain Injury. *Neuroepidemiology*, *14*(2), 435–450. PMID:8827181

Kreutzer, J. S., Marwitz, J. H., Walker, W., Sander, A., Sherer, M., Bogner, J., ... Bushnik, T. (2003). Moderating factors in return to work and job stability after traumatic brain injury. *The Journal of Head Trauma Rehabilitation*, *18*(2), 128–138. doi:10.1097/00001199-200303000-00004 PMID:12802222

Langlois, J., Rutland-Brown, W., & Thomas, K. (2004). Traumatic brain injury in the United States, emergency department visits, hospitalizations, and deaths. *Centers for Disease Control and Prevention*. Retrieved from https://www.cdc.gov/traumaticbraininjury/tbi_ed.html

Ledger, S. D. (2002). Reflections on communicating with non-English speaking patients. *British Journal of Nursing (Mark Allen Publishing)*, *11*(11), 773–780. doi:10.12968/bjon.2002.11.11.773 PMID:12070380

Lequerica, A., & Krch, D. (2014). Issues of cultural diversity in acquired brain injury (ABI) rehabilitation. *Journal of Neurologic Rehabilitation*, *34*, 645–653. PMID:24796439

Linden, M., & Redpath, S. (2011). A comparative study of nursing attitudes towards young male survivors of brain injury: A questionnaire survey. *International Journal of Nursing Studies*, *48*(1), 62–69. doi:10.1016/j.ijnurstu.2010.05.011 PMID:20965077

Meagher, A. D., Beadles, C. A., Doorey, J., & Charles, A. G. (2015). Racial and ethnic disparities in discharge to rehabilitation following traumatic brain injury. *Journal of Neurosurgery*, *122*(3), 595–601. doi:10.3171/2014.10.JNS14187 PMID:25415069

Mulkey, P., Lacock, M., & Scott, K. (2004). *Guidelines for Healthcare Providers Interacting with American Indian Patients and Their Families*. Chicago, IL: Metropolitan Chicago Healthcare Council.

Nguyen, H. T., Evans, M., & Zonderman, A. B. (2004). Poverty and self-reported mental disorders: Findings from the healthy aging in neighborhoods of diversity across the life span study (HANDLS). *Annals of Epidemiology*, *17*(9), 736. doi:10.1016/j.annepidem.2007.07.042

Niemeier, J., & Carlos Arango-Lasprilla, J. (2007). Toward improved rehabilitation services for ethnically diverse survivors of traumatic brain injury. *The Journal of Head Trauma Rehabilitation*, *22*(2), 75–84. doi:10.1097/01.HTR.0000265095.06565.7b PMID:17414309

Olver, J. H., Ponsford, J. L., & Curran, C. (1996). Outcome following traumatic brain injury: A comparison between 2 and 5 years after injury. *Brain Injury: [BI]*, *10*(11), 841–848. doi:10.1080/026990596123945 PMID:8905161

Paterakis, K., Karantanas, A. H., Komnos, A., & Volikas, Z. (2000). Outcome of patients with diffuse axonal injury: The significance and prognostic value of MRI in the acute phase. *The Journal of Trauma Injury Infection and Critical Care*, *49*(6), 1071–1075. doi:10.1097/00005373-200012000-00016 PMID:11130491

Rancho Los Amigos National Rehabilitation Center. (2011). *The rancho levels of cognitive functioning.* Retrieved from: https://web.archive.org/web/20110514024558/http://rancho.org/Research_RanchoLevels.aspx

Redpath, S., & Linden, M. (2004). Attitudes towards behavioral versus organic acquisition of brain injury. *Brain Injury: [BI]*, *18*(9), 861–869. doi:10.1080/02699050410001671838 PMID:15223739

Saltapidas, H., & Ponsford, J. (2007). The influence of cultural background on motivation for and participation in rehabilitation and outcome following traumatic brain injury. *The Journal of Head Trauma Rehabilitation*, *22*(2), 132–139. doi:10.1097/01.HTR.0000265101.75177.8d PMID:17414315

Sander, A., Clark, A., & Pappadis, M. R. (2010). What is community integration anyway? Defining meaning following traumatic brain injury. *The Journal of Head Trauma Rehabilitation*, *25*(2), 121–127. doi:10.1097/HTR.0b013e3181cd1635 PMID:20134333

Sherer, M., Nick, T. G., Sander, A. M., Hart, T., Hanks, R., Rosenthal, M., ... Yablon, S. A. (2003). Race and productivity outcome after traumatic brain injury: Influence of confounding factors. *The Journal of Head Trauma Rehabilitation*, *18*(5), 408–424. doi:10.1097/00001199-200309000-00003 PMID:12973271

Smith, J. (2004). Unraveling the SES: Health connection. *Population and Development Review*, *30*, 108–132.

Stein, D. G. (2001). Brain damage, sex hormones recovery: A new role for progesterone and estrogen? *Trends in Neurosciences*, *24*(7), 386–391. doi:10.1016/S0166-2236(00)01821-X PMID:11410269

Teasdale, G., & Jennett, B. (1974). Assessment of coma and impaired consciousness. A practical scale. *Lancet*, *2*(7872), 81–84. doi:10.1016/S0140-6736(74)91639-0 PMID:4136544

Uomoto, J. M., & Wong, T. M. (2000). Multicultural perspective on the neuropsychology of brain injury assessment and rehabilitation. In E. Fletcher-Janzen, T.L., Strickland, & C.R. Reynolds (Eds.), Handbook of cross-cultural neuropsychology (pp. 169-184). New York, NY: Kluwer Academics/Plenum Publishers. doi:10.1007/978-1-4615-4219-3_11

Wolters, G., Stapert, S., Brands, I., & van Heugten, C. (2010). Coping styles in relation to cognitive rehabilitation and quality of life after brain injury. *Neuropsychological Rehabilitation, 20*(4), 587–600. doi:10.1080/09602011003683836 PMID:20446171

ADDITIONAL READING

Tsai, J. (2016). A critique of cultural competency in health care. *In-Training: Stories from Tomorrow's Physicians, 2.* Retrieved from https://in-training.org/critique-cultural-competency-10456

KEY TERMS AND DEFINITIONS

Cognitive-Linguistic Impairment: Cognitive-linguistic impairments impact a person's thinking skills and communication skills.

Community Reintegration: Community reintegration is the process of integrating back into society following an injury. It is a broad term, encompassing the full participation of people back into community (home, work, church, neighborhood, etc.) life.

Diffuse Axonal Injury (DAI): DAI is a form of TBI, which occurs when the brain rapidly shifts inside the skull. During this time, the long connecting fibers in the brain called axons are sheared, rotated, and/or twisted as the brain rapidly accelerates and decelerates.

Health Disparity: A health disparity is a preventable difference in the burden of disease, injury, violence, or opportunity to achieve optimal health between groups of people.

Healthcare Barriers: Barriers to health services include high cost of care, inadequate or no insurance coverage, lack of availability of services, and lack of culturally competent care.

Healthcare Gap: Gaps in medical care refer to disparities in healthcare access, healthcare needs and medical services when comparing different populations that fall along racial, ethnic, or socioeconomic lines.

Outcome: Outcome is the probability that a consequence may occur. Outcome measures after TBI may be related to cognitive-linguistic abilities, physical abilities, community reintegration, and/or return to work/school.

Traumatic Brain Injury (TBI): A TBI occurs when there is sudden damage to the brain, typically caused by a blow or jolt to the head. Immediate or delayed symptoms may result, which can have a wide range of severity levels.

Chapter 14
Hearing Loss and Diabetes in an African American Adult

Diane M. Scott
https://orcid.org/0000-0002-7472-7208
North Carolina Central University, USA

EXECUTIVE SUMMARY

Research has linked hearing loss to other medical conditions such as diabetes. Studies have shown that hearing loss is more common in individuals who have diabetes than in those who do not. Hyperglycemia, or raised blood sugar, is a common effect of uncontrolled diabetes and over time leads to serious damage to many of the body's systems, especially the nerves and the blood vessels. Consequently, diabetes can affect the blood vessels of the inner ear and the vestibulocochlear (VIII cranial) nerve fibers. This case study examines the interrelationship between diabetes and hearing loss in an African American adult while examining the issues of the higher prevalence of diabetes in African Americans and the role of audiologists in the care of individuals with hearing loss and diabetes.

INTRODUCTION

Research has linked hearing loss to other disabling conditions in adults, such as diabetes, cognitive decline and dementia, clinical depression, cardiovascular disease, and other illnesses (Bainbridge, Hoffman, & Cowie, 2008; Lin & Ferruci, 2012; Mener, Betz, Genther, Chen, &, Lin, 2013). These linkages are referred to as "comorbidities," which refers to the presence of more than one disorder in the same person. Comorbidity is associated with worse health outcomes, more complex clinical management, and increased health care costs.

Hearing loss and diabetes are both chronic conditions that are similar and can co-exist in a patient. They are both invisible, progressive, often incurable, and treatable. Both require professional care as well as self-managed behavioral change for long-term success. There are racial/ethnic differences in the prevalence of hearing loss as well as in the prevalence of diabetes. For African Americans the prevalence rates are diametrically opposite. Hearing loss is less common in non-Hispanic African Americans

DOI: 10.4018/978-1-7998-2261-5.ch014

compared to non-Hispanic Whites, while diabetes is more common in African Americans than Whites. That can lead to a complicated relationship between hearing loss and diabetes.

Diabetes in Adults

Diabetes is a chronic disease that occurs either when the pancreas does not produce enough insulin or when the body cannot effectively use the insulin it produces. Insulin is a hormone that regulates blood sugar. Hyperglycemia, or raised blood sugar, is a common effect of uncontrolled diabetes and over time leads to serious damage to many of the body's systems, especially the nerves and the blood vessels. Diabetes can be a direct cause of death as well as high blood glucose.

The most common types of diabetes are type 1, type 2, and gestational diabetes. Type 1 diabetes (previously known as insulin-dependent, juvenile or childhood-onset) is characterized by deficient insulin production and requires daily administration of insulin. The cause of type 1 diabetes is not known and it is not preventable. Symptoms of the disease include frequent urination, increased thirst and/or hunger, sleepiness, weight loss, blurred vision, difficulty in concentrating, and slow healing of infections. These symptoms may occur suddenly.

Type 2 diabetes (formerly known as non-insulin-dependent or adult-onset) results from the body's ineffective use of insulin. Type 2 diabetes comprises the majority of people with diabetes around the world, and is largely the result of excess body weight and physical inactivity. Symptoms may be similar to those of type 1 diabetes, but are often less marked. As a result, the disease may not be diagnosed until several years after onset, once complications have already arisen.

Gestational diabetes develops in some women when they are pregnant. Most of the time, this type of diabetes goes away after the baby is born. However, if a woman developed gestational diabetes during pregnancy, she has a greater chance of developing type 2 diabetes later in life. Sometimes diabetes diagnosed during pregnancy is actually type 2 diabetes. Gestational diabetes often has no symptoms, or the symptoms may be mild, such as being thirstier than normal or having to urinate more often. Gestational diabetes is sometimes related to the hormonal changes of pregnancy that make the body less able to use insulin. Genes and extra weight may also play a role in the development of gestational diabetes.

In all types of diabetes, the end result is an elevation in blood sugar levels which must be managed. Diabetes is a leading cause of blindness, kidney failure, amputations, heart failure, and stroke (World Health Organization [WHO], 2019). Diabetes complications are divided into microvascular (damage to small blood vessels) and macrovascular (damage to larger blood vessels). Microvascular complications include damage to the eyes (retinopathy) leading to blindness, to the kidneys (nephropathy) leading to renal failure and to the nerves (neuropathy) leading to impotence, and diabetic foot disorders (which include severe infections leading to amputation).

Macrovascular complications are primarily diseases of the coronary arteries, peripheral arteries, and the cerebrovasculature leading to cardiovascular diseases such as heart attacks, strokes, and insufficiency in blood flow to the legs. Early macrovascular disease is associated with atherosclerotic plaque in the blood vessels supplying blood to the heart, brain, limbs, and other organs. Late stages of macrovascular disease involve complete obstruction of these vessels. Cardiovascular disease (CVD) is the major cause of morbidity and mortality in patients with diabetes (American Diabetes Association, 2015).

Diabetes is a global public health issue. In 2015, 30.3 million Americans, or 9.4% of the population, had diabetes. Of the 30.3 million adults with diabetes, 23.1 million were diagnosed and 7.2 million were undiagnosed. The percentage of Americans aged 65 and older with diabetes remains high, at 25.2%, or

12.0 million seniors (diagnosed and undiagnosed) (American Diabetes Association, 2018). There are also large numbers of Americans who are prediabetic. Prediabetes is a serious health condition where blood sugar levels are higher than normal, but not high enough yet to be diagnosed as type 2 diabetes. In 2015, 84.1 million Americans aged 18 and older had prediabetes. Of the 84 million individuals with prediabetes, 90% do not know they have it (American Diabetes Association, 2018).

Diabetes prevalence rates vary by race/ethnicity. The rates of diagnosed diabetes in adults by racial/ethnic background are:

- 7.4% of non-Hispanic Whites
- 8.0% of Asian Americans
- 12.1% of Hispanics
- 12.7% of non-Hispanic African Americans
- 15.1% of American Indians/Alaskan Natives (American Diabetes Association, 2018)

The prevalence rates of diabetes indicate that American Indians/Alaskan Natives, African Americans, and Hispanics are approximately twice as likely to be diagnosed with diabetes as non-Hispanic Whites. This in turn affects women of color in the following ways:

- American Indian/Alaska Native women have the highest rate of diabetes among all racial and ethnic groups in the United States. However, rates of diabetes are different in different regions of the United States. Rates are lowest in Alaska Native people and highest in people who are American Indian and live in certain areas of the Southwest (Centers for Disease Control and Prevention [CDC], 2017).
- Diabetes is almost twice as common in non-Hispanic African American women compared to non-Hispanic White women (CDC, 2017).
- Among Hispanic women in the United States, it may be more or less common for women from different countries of origin to be diagnosed with the disorder (CDC, 2017). For example, Mexican American women have almost twice the rate of diabetes diagnosis compared to White women, yet Cuban American women have a lower rate compared to White women (CDC, 2017).
- Diabetes is the fifth-leading cause of death for Asian/Pacific Islander women in the United States (CDC, 2018). However, it may be more or less common for women of different Asian groups to be diagnosed with the disorder. One in every 33 Chinese American women is diagnosed with diabetes compared to 1 in every 10 Asian Indian women (CDC, 2017).

Diabetes in African American Communities

Health disparities in diabetes and its complications and co-morbidities exist worldwide. As previously indicated, racial/ethnic minorities have a higher prevalence of diabetes than non-minority individuals. There are multiple factors that contribute to these disparities, including biological and clinical factors, and health system and social factors (Golden et al., 2012).

As the data in Table 1 indicate, the prevalence of diabetes is more common in African American women than in African American men and about 2 times higher than in non-Hispanic White women. In addition, African Americans are more likely to suffer complications from diabetes, such as end-stage renal disease and lower extremity amputations. According to the Office of Minority Health, in 2010,

Table 1. Age-adjusted prevalence of diagnosed diabetes per 100 population

	African Americans	White	African Americans/ White Ratio
Men	9.2	6.3	1.5
Women	9.9	5.3	1.9
Total	9.5	5.8	1.6

(Source: CDC 2016b United States Diabetes Surveillance System)

non-Hispanic African Americans were 4.2 times more likely to be diagnosed with end stage renal disease as compared to non-Hispanic Whites. Non-Hispanic African Americans were also 3.5 times more likely to be hospitalized for lower limb amputations as compared to non-Hispanic Whites and were twice as likely as non-Hispanic Whites to die from diabetes (Office of Minority Health, 2016).

Given the differences in diabetes prevalence rates, what steps can be taken to eliminate this health disparity? In a study investigating possible causal factors for the health disparity, Bancks, Kershaw, Carson, Gordon-Larsen, Schreiner, & Carnethon (2017) analyzed data from more than 4,200 participants in the CARDIA (Coronary Artery Risk Development in Young Adults) study. Study participants were recruited at ages 18 to 30 years from Birmingham, AL; Chicago, IL; Minneapolis, MN; and Oakland, CA. Approximately 49% of the participants were African American and 54% were women. The researchers collected information from the participants about various risk factors for diabetes for a period of over 30 years. Not surprisingly, the study found that the chance of developing type 2 diabetes was significantly higher for African American adults than White adults (about 66 more cases of diabetes per 1000 people). The difference was greatest between African American women and White women.

Bancks et al. (2017) used statistical analyses to determine which factors contributed to the rates of diabetes. They determined that biological risk factors accounted for most of the health disparity. The researchers observed that obesity is a major factor in creating these disparities. It is interesting to note that African American women have the highest rates of being overweight or obese compared to other groups in the U.S. About four out of five African American women are overweight or obese (Office of Minority Health, 2017). Based on the results of this study and others, lifestyle changes such as adopting a healthy nutrition plan and getting regular physical activity can lead to lasting weight loss, which in turn can reduce an individual's risk for developing diabetes.

Prevalence of Hearing Loss in Adults

The National Institute on Deafness and Other Communication Disorders (2015) provides the following statistics on the prevalence of hearing loss:

- One in eight people in the United States (13 percent, or 30 million) aged 12 years or older has hearing loss in both ears, based on standard hearing examinations.
- About 2 percent of adults aged 45 to 54 have disabling hearing loss. The rate increases to 8.5 percent for adults aged 55 to 64. Nearly 25 percent of those aged 65 to 74 and 50 percent of those who are 75 and older have disabling hearing loss.

Based on the National Interview Health Survey, 2012, approximately 15% of American adults (37.5 million) aged 18 and over report some trouble hearing (Blackwell, Lucas, & Clarke, 2014). Among adults aged 20-69, the overall annual prevalence of hearing loss dropped slightly from 16 percent (28.0 million) in the 1999-2004 time period to 14 percent (27.7 million) in the 2011–2012 time period (Hoffman, Dobie, Losonczy, Themann, & Flamme, 2017).

Age is the strongest predictor of hearing loss among adults aged 20-69, with the greatest amount of hearing loss in the 60 to 69 year old age group. In addition, men are almost twice as likely as women to have hearing loss among adults aged 20-69 (Hoffman, Dobie, Losonczy, Themann, & Flamme, 2016). Non-Hispanic White adults are more likely than adults in other racial/ethnic groups to have hearing loss, while non-Hispanic African Americans have the lowest prevalence of hearing loss among adults aged 20-69 (Hoffman, Dobie, Losonczy, Themann, & Flamme, 2017).

Hearing Loss and Diabetes

Given the prevalence of hearing impairment in the general population, what effect does the presence of diabetes mellitus have on the prevalence rate of hearing loss? Studies show that hearing loss is more common in people who have diabetes than in those who do not have the disease. Additionally, of the 84 million adults in the United States who have prediabetes, the rate of hearing loss is 30 percent higher than in those with normal blood glucose (American Diabetes Association, 2017). Bainbridge, Hoffman, and Cowie (2008) analyzed data from hearing tests of about 5,140 adults between the ages of 20 and 69 participating in the National Health and Nutrition Examination Survey (NHANES) from 1999-2004. The participants with diabetes were found to be more than twice as likely to have mild-to-moderate hearing loss than those without the disease. The occurrence of high frequency hearing loss (defined as the average of pure tone thresholds at 3000, 4000, 6000, and 8000 Hz) was more prevalent in diabetics (54%) than in non-diabetics (32%).

Several studies have examined the role of age, race/ethnicity, and sex in the development of hearing loss in individuals with diabetes. Diabetic subjects with hearing impairment have been found to be significantly older (56.9 years) than those without hearing impairment (51.2 years). Among those individuals with hearing impairment, a lesser proportion were non-Hispanic African Americans and Mexican Americans. No sex differences were observed in low/mid-frequency hearing impairment; however, a significantly higher percentage of male subjects had high frequency hearing impairment (Bainbridge, Hoffman, & Cowrie, 2011). Nearly all of the participants reported that they had type 2 diabetes.

A meta-analysis review of 13 studies involving 20,194 participants and 7,377 individual cases examining the relationship between hearing loss and diabetes revealed that the prevalence of hearing loss among individuals with diabetes was more than twice that of individuals without diabetes. The association between hearing loss and diabetes was stronger among individuals younger than age 60 and was independent of sex (gender) or chronic exposure to noise (Horikawa et al., 2013).

A certain degree of hearing loss is a normal part of the aging process, but it is often accelerated in patients with diabetes, especially if blood-glucose levels are not being controlled with medication and diet. Women between the ages of 60 and 75 with poorly controlled diabetes had significantly worse hearing than those whose diabetes was controlled (The Hearing Review, 2012).

Given the findings of research studies over the years, Bainbridge et al. (2011) concluded that diabetes may contribute to hearing loss by damaging nerves and blood vessels within the auditory system. In addition, the research findings support recommendations to monitor the hearing of patients with diabetes and those at-risk for developing diabetes on an annual basis.

Underlying Mechanisms on the Effects of Diabetes in the Peripheral and Central Auditory Systems

The underlying biological and physiological mechanisms in diabetes that can affect the function of the auditory system have been pinpointed. Kim and colleagues (2017) published a cohort study of over 253,000 adults with baseline hearing within normal limits who were followed from 2002-2014. Over 2,800 study participants developed hearing loss. After accounting for factors such as noise exposure, body mass index, smoking, alcohol use, and exercise, a hazard ratio for developing hearing loss was determined. A hazard ratio is a measure of how often a particular event happens in one group compared to how often it happens in another group, over time. A hazard ratio of one means that there is no difference between the two groups. A hazard ratio of greater than one or less than one means that a particular event happens in one group more than the other group(s).

The hazard ratio for developing hearing loss was 1.04 for those with pre-diabetes and 1.36 for those with diabetes. The researchers hypothesized that the vascular effects of diabetes damage the blood supply to the cochlea leading to sensorineural hearing loss. More specifically, high blood glucose levels may damage the blood vessels in stria vascularis and nerves impacting the biochemistry and neural innervation of the cochlea (Kim et al., 2017).

A visual depiction of the underlying mechanisms for the effects of diabetes on the auditory system is as follows:

As stated previously, hyperglycemia is a common effect of uncontrolled diabetes and over time leads to serious damage to many of the body's systems, especially the blood vessels and the nerves. As illustrated in Figure 1, hyperglycemia can lead to microangiopathy. Microangiopathy is a disease of the capillaries, in which the capillary walls become so thick and weak that they bleed, leak protein, and slow the flow of blood. Diabetes predisposes to the development of microangiopathy in many areas of the body (Dowd, 2019).

Oxidative stress plays a pivotal role in the development of diabetes complications. Oxidative stress is essentially an imbalance between the production of free radicals and the ability of the body to counteract or detoxify their harmful effects through neutralization by antioxidants. Oxidative stress can affect cochlear hair cells directly as well as damaging the stria vascularis in the peripheral auditory system and can cause neuropathy in the central auditory system (Dowd, 2019).

Histological studies have found changes in the cochlea associated with both type 1 and type 2 diabetes that form the bases for the description of the possible effects of hyperglycemia on the auditory system. Studies observed a thickening of the vessel walls of the basilar membrane and the vessels of the stria vascularis in all turns in type 1 diabetes mellitus patients (Fukushima et al., 2005). In addition, atrophy of the stria vascularis was located in all turns (Fukushima et al., 2005) with a loss of the outer hair cells (Fukushima et al., 2005; Lisowska, Namyslowski, Morawski, & Strojek, 2001). Moreover, a loss of spiral ligament cells was also found (Fukushima et al., 2005).

Figure 1. Flowchart on the effects of diabetes in the peripheral and central auditory systems

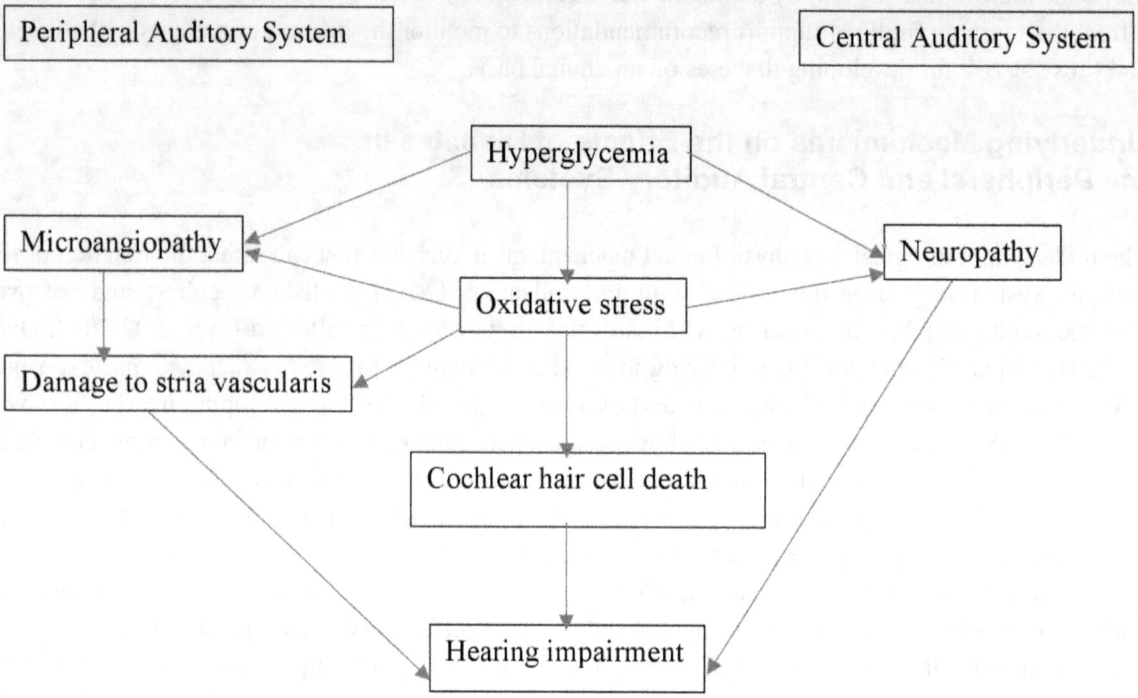

Several studies separated type 2 diabetes patients into those treated with insulin and those taking oral blood glucose-lowering agents, comparing them with a nondiabetic control group. In the group taking insulin, the vessel walls of the basilar membrane and stria vascularis vessels in all turns were significantly thicker than those of controls (Fukushima et al., 2006; Kariya et al., 2010). In the group on glucose-lowering agents, the walls of the stria vascularis vessels were also significantly thicker than in controls, mainly in the basal turn of the cochlea (Fukushima et al., 2006; Kariya et al., 2010). In addition to vascular changes, atrophy of the stria vascularis was observed in the lower basal, lower middle, upper middle and apical turns of the cochlea spiral in the insulin group, and mainly in the lower middle turn (no changes in the apical turn) in the group on glucose lowering agents (Fukushima et al., 2006). There was also a significant loss of outer hair cells, especially in the lower and upper basal turns, but no loss of inner hair cells (Fukushima et al., 2006).

When comparing type 1 and type 2 diabetes patients, significant cochlear vessel wall thickening was found in both type 1 and type 2 diabetes patients compared to control groups, with more pronounced thickening in type 2 than in type 1 diabetes. Likewise, vessel wall thickening was more pronounced in insulin-treated type 2 diabetes than in type 1 diabetes. The latter difference could be explained by the fact that type 2 diabetes patients treated with insulin have more advanced disease (Fukushima et al., 2006).

Hyperglycemia can affect small blood vessels and nerves throughout the human body; therefore, diabetes can impact hearing (the cochlea), balance (the vestibular system), and central processing for both (VIII cranial nerve). Hyperglycemia can have a two-prong effect in the vestibular system. First, it can affect the polyol pathway, which is a two-step metabolic pathway in which glucose is reduced to sorbitol, which is then converted to fructose. It is a strong candidate mechanism to explain, at least in part, the cellular toxicity of diabetic hyperglycemia. It has been found that the polyol pathway is the major contributor to oxidative stress in the lenses and nerves of diabetic mice (Chung, Ho, Lam, &Chung, 2003). Changes in the polyol pathway in turn lead to overproduction of extracellular matrix and increased lipid droplets and lysosomes in the connective tissue of the utricle and the saccule. These changes impair the diffusion of oxygen, nutrients, and waste, thus leading to the degeneration of type 1 hair cells (Dowd, 2019).

Secondarily, hyperglycemia can affect protein processing within myelin. The lysosomes digest large portions of the vestibulocochlear (VIII) nerve, which leads to myelin sheath thinning and reduced axonal fiber diameters (Dowd, 2019). The effects of the two prongs can lead to vestibular dysfunction with longer latencies and reduced amplitudes of vestibular evoked potentials (Dowd, 2019). As such, audiologists need to be concerned about vestibular problems in patients with diabetes.

Evidence supports the fact that hyperglycemia is an important risk factor for the development of diabetic microvascular complications. Studies have shown that racial/ethnic minorities with type 2 diabetes have worse glycemic control (Kirk et al., 2005). Most studies indicate that compared to non-Hispanic Whites, non-Hispanic African Americans and Mexican Americans have increased insulin resistance (Golden et al., 2012; Haffner et al., 1996) and augmented insulin secretion/hyperinsulinemia (Albu et al., 2005; Haffner et al., 1996) independent of being severely overweight or obese. These two groups have poorer glycemic control. At this point in time it is unclear what effects if any poorer glycemic control in racial/ethnic minorities may have on the peripheral or central auditory system.

In summarizing the relationship between diabetes and hearing loss, these facts should be noted.

- Hearing loss is twice as common in individuals who have diabetes than in individuals who do not have the disease. The hearing loss is more likely to be high frequency. The hearing loss is more likely to be found in males and non-Hispanic Whites; however, diabetes is more common in racial/ethnic minority groups especially for most racial/ethnic minority women.
- The effects of diabetes on the auditory system can be seen in both the peripheral and central auditory systems along with the vestibular system. The underlying culprit for the development of hearing loss associated with diabetes is hyperglycemia. Hyperglycemia can lead to serious damage to the body's systems, especially the blood vessels and the nerves. Diabetes predisposes the body to the development of microangiopathy, a disease of the capillaries, and to neuropathy.

Consider these facts in examining the following case study.

CASE STUDY

Background Information

ST, an African-American female, was in her mid-50s. She was divorced and lived alone. ST had 2 adult children and 5 grandchildren. She had not been feeling well for a while, but had difficulty pinpointing just what her medical problems were so that she would know where to get help. She often felt dizzy and disoriented. She also experienced frequent thirst. ST knew where every bathroom was in any place she went, which is not uncommon among women. However, she had to use the bathroom at least every hour. She also had high cholesterol levels and was overweight heading toward obese. She was supposed to be exercising more to lose weight. Her cholesterol levels and weight were among her reasons for not seeking immediate medical assistance.

One day, after 2 years of experiencing these symptoms, ST's children and grandchildren came for an extended visit. She was very busy enjoying her time with her children and grandchildren. She began experiencing flu-like symptoms one morning. She felt feverish, and her body ached. She thought she might have a virus and went to bed. Two hours later, she was feeling worse. Her family suggested that she go to an urgent care center. After performing a number of tests, the physician at the center came to see ST. In a no-nonsense tone of voice, he said, "You have type 2 diabetes." ST was in shock. She knew a little about diabetes but was unsure what type 2 diabetes meant. She was given no further information about diabetes but instructed to see her primary care physician as soon as possible. ST went to see a primary care physician and with her help and the assistance of a dietician, ST began taking control over her diabetes with medication (pills), diet, and exercise. However, ST had to deal with the realities that self-care for diabetes is a lifelong challenge, and getting things under control took some time. It took several months after her diagnosis for her to learn what she needed to know and feel somewhat comfortable managing her diabetes. Denial, anger, and sadness were some of her responses to the diagnosis of diabetes. ST had to learn to accept her situation and take personal responsibility for her health in order to regain her emotional balance. She needed assistance from professional counselors.

Given the presence of the diabetes, ST's primary care physician asked questions about her vision and any foot problems. ST had been wearing glasses for about 5 years mostly for reading and had not noticed any foot problems. Her primary care physician did not inquire about any hearing problems or examine any effects that her prescribed medications might have on the auditory system.

Clinical Case History/Clinical Evaluations

As time passed, ST noticed that she was occasionally having difficulty understanding speech in noisy environments. At times she felt embarrassed at social gatherings. She was being told by family and friends that she sometimes misunderstood words. She became uncomfortable knowing that she was missing important information in group gatherings. At first, she did not know what to do, but her daughter suggested she go see an audiologist. ST eventually went to see an audiologist, 2 years after her diagnosis of diabetes. On the case history form ST indicted that she had no history of noise exposure and her only chronic diseases were diabetes and high cholesterol. She took Metformin for the diabetes and Lipitor for high cholesterol. She was losing weight but was still classified as overweight. ST was employed full-time as an executive assistant to a state official. An audiological evaluation was conducted, which included pure tone air and bone conduction, speech, and immittance testing.

Test results indicated that ST had a bilateral high frequency sensorineural hearing loss. The high frequency hearing loss began above 2000 Hz with thresholds ranging from 30 to 50 dB HL from 3000 to 8000 Hz. Immittance testing revealed normal tympanograms with normal compliance (Type A tympanograms). Acoustic reflex thresholds were within normal limits suggesting the possibility of recruitment. Speech reception thresholds agreed with pure tone thresholds and speech recognition scores in quiet were 92% for the right ear and 90% for the left ear, both of which were within normal limits.

Questions for the Reader

1. What are the risk factors for hearing impairment among U.S. adults with diabetes?
2. What risks factors should an audiologist be concerned about given the presence of hearing impairment in an African American woman with diabetes?
3. What further baseline audiological testing should be conducted with individuals who have been diagnosed with diabetes?
4. Should an audiologist make any specific referrals for patients with diabetes?

Discussion of Questions for the Reader

1. *What are the risk factors for hearing impairment among U.S. adults with diabetes?* Among U.S. adults with diabetes, a higher likelihood of hearing impairment has been identified for those individuals who are older, non-Hispanic White, male, or who have lower income. Individuals with diabetes with low HDL (good cholesterol), a history of coronary heart disease, symptoms of peripheral neuropathy, or those who report poor health also exhibit a greater likelihood of hearing impairment (Bainbridge et al., 2011).

ST was 60 years old, overall her health was not poor, and she exhibited no evidence of peripheral neuropathy, except for the possibility of vision problems caused by diabetes because she was wearing glasses. She was taking medication for her cholesterol, and had a steady job. Audiologists should note the risk factors for the development of hearing impairment associated with diabetes but try to avoid assumptions based on risk factors alone.

2. *What risk factors should an audiologist be concerned about given the presence of hearing impairment in an African American woman with diabetes?* Hyperglycemia is an important risk factor for the development of diabetic microvascular complications. Microvascular complications can affect the stria vascularis. Several studies have shown that racial/ethnic minorities with type 2 diabetes have poorer glycemic control (Kirk et al., 2005). In addition, African American women have the highest rates of being overweight or obese compared to other groups in the U.S. ST's diabetes appeared to be under control through the use of medication, but she was still overweight. Maintaining a healthy weight and exercising is one of the major changes that individuals especially African Americans can make to control their diabetes.
3. *What further baseline audiological testing should be conducted with individuals who have been diagnosed with diabetes?* Research indicates that patients with diabetes are at a greater risk of developing hearing loss, therefore audiological tests to monitor auditory function should be a part of the comprehensive management care plan for patients with diabetes (Bainbridge, Hoffman, & Cowrie, 2008). The Audiology Project (TAP, 2019) was founded to promote the audiology-based medical management of patients with chronic diseases. One of TAP's goals for best audiological management is to have all persons with diabetes receive a baseline hearing test and a balance screening when they are first diagnosed with diabetes, and then regularly monitored. Dowd (2019), who is the CEO of TAP, has recommended that a baseline of auditory function be established by conducting otoacoustic emissions (OAEs), auditory brainstem responses (ABRs), and speech-

in-noise testing in addition to pure tone and speech audiometry in combination with immittance measures.

OAEs are sounds given off by the inner ear when responding to an external sound. Hair cells in the inner ear respond to that sound by vibrating. The vibration produces a very quiet sound that echoes back into the middle ear. If individuals have normal hearing, they will produce OAEs. If their hearing loss is greater than 25–30 decibels (dB), they will not produce OAEs. Distortion product otoacoustic emissions (DPOAE) are responses generated when the cochlea is stimulated simultaneously by two pure tone frequencies. The prevalence of DPOAEs is 100% in normal adult ears. Responses from the left and right ears are often correlated (that is, they are very similar). For subjects with normal hearing, women have higher amplitude DPOAEs. Aging processes have an effect on DPOAE responses by lowering the DPOAE amplitude and narrowing the DPOAE response spectrum (i.e., responses at higher frequencies are gradually diminishing) (Otoacoustic Emissions Portal, 2019).

Several studies have been conducted examining DPOAEs in patients with diabetes. A meta-analysis was conducted of research studies utilizing DPOAEs for the evaluation of auditory function in diabetics. The data from seven articles were analyzed. PTA thresholds were within normal limits in all patients with diabetes at low-middle frequencies. The mean DPOAE amplitudes of the patients with diabetes were significantly lower than those of the controls at 1, 2, and 4 kHz (Hao, Fu, Zhang, Zhang, Zhao, & Li, 2017). The test results imply that cochlear function is impaired even before pure tone thresholds are affected in individuals with diabetes.

In a study completed in China, the auditory function of 51 patients with type 2 diabetes, 55 patients with pre-diabetes, and 43 control subjects was evaluated. As assessed by pure tone testing (using the PTA), a significantly higher number of patients with type 2 diabetes (45.1%) were identified with hearing loss compared to patients with prediabetes (23.6%) and control subjects (25.6%). There was no significant difference in the PTA between the patients with prediabetes and control subjects. Mean DPOAEs amplitudes of the prediabetes patients were significantly lower than that of the control subjects at all frequencies tested (Li, Zhang, Fu, Bi, Li, & Liu, 2018). In this case, prediabetes was not necessarily associated with significant hearing loss; however, cochlear malfunction may have been present as indicated by the abnormal DPOAEs.

Auditory brainstem responses, which are used to test the integrity of auditory system and to make inferences about hearing, have been reported to exhibit either prolonged latencies or reduced amplitudes in individuals with diabetes. Using speech-evoked ABR, it has been reported that subcortical processing of speech is altered in individuals with diabetic mellitus (Gupta, Bhat, & Kumar, 2015). In the Hao et al. study (2017), ABR data were also analyzed. For the patients with diabetes, the latencies of waves I, III, and V were significantly later than those of the control subjects. In addition, the wave interval I-V was significantly longer in patients with diabetes. The elongated wave latencies and wave interval suggest retrocochlear damage in patients with diabetes.

Based on utilizing an audiological management plan recommended for individuals with diabetes, ST should undergo additional testing.

4. *Should an audiologist make any specific referrals for patients with diabetes?* The diagnosis of hearing loss in an individual with diabetes should lead to the creation of a hearing management plan involving a management team. Recommendations are that diabetes care should be managed by a multidisciplinary team that may include primary care physicians, subspecialty physicians,

> nurse practitioners, physician assistants, nurses, dietitians, pharmacists, dentists, podiatrists, optometrists, audiologists, and mental health professionals. Specific recommendations have been made that audiologists align themselves with pharmacists for otovestibulotoxic monitoring. Basically, audiologists should ask their patients, "Are you taking medications for diabetes and other health problems?" They should also align with optometry to monitor vision problems, dentistry to monitor loss of teeth and abnormal gum swelling, and podiatry to monitor the toes and feet (Dowd 2019).

ST was being treated for her diabetes by her primary care physician. None of the drugs she was taking had any known ototoxic or vestibulotoxic effects but any changes to her medications needed to be monitored. ST had been wearing glasses for over 5 years, so her vision definitely needed to be monitored. Diabetic retinopathy is 46% more prevalent in non-Hispanic African Americans than non-Hispanic Whites (Harris, Klein, Cowie, Rowland, & Byrd-Holt, 1998). Periodontal disease has been associated with poor glycemic control. ST was not asked about periodontal disease. At that time ST did not report any problems with her feet and toes. African Americans have high rates of at least two of the most serious complications from diabetes, amputation (usually of a toe or foot) and kidney failure.

Treatment

ST was informed of the results of her audiological evaluation. The relationship between hearing impairment and diabetes was also discussed with her along with providing her with educational materials and website information. She was scheduled for further testing to obtain DPOAEs, ABRs, and speech-in-noise scores as part of her baseline audiological data. Recommendations regarding a hearing aid were delayed until after the additional testing. ST was also provided with information on the relationship between diabetes and possible balance problems because the VIII cranial nerve serves both the auditory and vestibular systems. Vestibular issues should be analyzed in conjunction with vision, foot care, and fractures. The patient can be asked "Have you fallen, or do you have a fear of falling?" The audiologist specifically asked questions about her vision, foot care, dental care, and any additional medications.

Outcomes

The additional test results revealed DPOEs amplitudes that were of reduced amplitude at the low to mid frequencies and absent at the high frequencies. The ABR latencies of waves I, III, and V were significantly delayed compared to norms and the wave interval I-V was significantly longer.

The Quick Speech in Noise (SIN) (Etymotic Research, 2001) is an adaptive SNR (signal-to-noise ratio) test that was used to measure ST's ability to understand speech in noise. It consists of a series of IEEE sentences presented in a background of four-talker babble. In the QuickSIN, the intensity level of the sentences remains fixed while the noise level varies. Sentences are presented at either 75 or 80 dB HL while the CD automatically varies the SNR in 5-dB steps starting at +25 SNR. Five key words are scored in each sentence and one point is given for each key word repeated correctly. The number of correct key words is subtracted from the reference of 25.5 dB. The score is referred to as the SNR loss. SNR loss is a measure of how well a person with hearing loss will understand speech in noise relative to a person who hears normally in noise. SNR loss is defined as the dB increase in the signal-to-noise ratio required by a person with hearing impairment to understand speech in noise as well as a person with normal hearing. ST's SNR loss was 9 dB, which indicated a moderate SNR loss.

Additional Questions for the Reader

1. What do Sandra's additional test results suggest about her auditory system functioning?
2. Why should the audiologist be concerned about the functioning of the vestibular system in individuals with diabetes?
3. What is the role of the audiologist in managing a patient with diabetes?

Discussion of Additional Questions for the Reader

1. *What do Sandra's additional test results suggest about her auditory system functioning?* The reduced amplitudes of the DPOAEs could be the results of the normal aging process or may imply that cochlear function was impaired for the lower frequencies even though the pure tone thresholds were within normal limits. The results from the ABR suggested some retrocochlear damage. The QuickSIN results matched ST's description of having difficulty understanding speech in noisy situations. It was recommended that ST have annual hearing evaluations as well as be fitted with hearing aids. ST was not fitted with hearing aids at that time due to concerns about the costs of amplification. She and her family were provided with strategies for better communication as well as information on self-help groups for individuals with hearing loss. ST and her family had another chronic condition, hearing impairment, to cope with. She was going to have to self-manage behavioral changes associated with her hearing loss as well as her diabetes. She had some major challenges ahead of her.
2. *Why should the audiologist be concerned about the functioning of the vestibular system in individuals with diabetes?* Hyperglycemia can affect both small blood vessels (microangiopathy) and nerves throughout the body (neuropathy). In other words, diabetes can impact the cochlea, the vestibular system, and the VIII cranial nerve. Vestibular issues should be analyzed in conjunction with vision and foot care issues.
3. *What is the role of the audiologist in managing a patient with diabetes?* Audiologists should collect baseline audiological data, including pure tone thresholds, speech tests, immittance tests, OAEs, and ABRs (Dowd, 2019). For each individual patient audiologists should determine a schedule for monitoring a patient's hearing based on the case history of diabetes, other chronic diseases, medications, noise exposure, and any genetic issues. Audiologists should determine if a hearing aid, tinnitus, or cochlear implant evaluation is needed. Audiologists should also evaluate and treat balance problems. Audiologists can refer patients for diabetes education, vision and foot evaluation, and medication oversight.

Audiologists, therefore, should establish collaborative relationships with pharmacy for ototoxicity and vestibulotoxicity monitoring, podiatry for better foot and balance care, and optometry to lower risks of falls. Furthermore, audiologists should counsel patients to see the dentist several times a year because periodontal disease has been associated with poor glycemic control.

KEY POINTS

- Racial health disparities exist for developing diabetes in the United States. Type 2 diabetes is one of the biggest challenges facing African Americans in the United States because non-Hispanic African Americans are twice as likely as non-Hispanic Whites to develop type 2 diabetes.
- Audiologists need to be aware that there are several non-modifiable risk factors, which are often genetic, associated with the development of diabetes itself. These risk factors include race/ethnicity, parent or sibling with diabetes, and mother who had gestational diabetes.
- Diabetes ear disease involves the cochlea (hearing), the vestibular system (balance) and the VIII cranial nerve (central processing for both hearing and balance). Hearing impairment, both in high frequency and low/midfrequency ranges, is more common in people with diabetes than in those without, perhaps due to neuropathy and/or vascular disease.
- Audiological concerns for individuals with diabetes include ***hearing loss*** due to cochlear microangiopathy and neural degeneration, ***balance and fall risk*** due to foot neuropathy, vision problems, and vestibular system abnormalities, and ***diabetic pain and infection control medications*** that can lead to ototoxicity and vestibulotoxicity.
- Audiology and PPOD (Pharmacy, Podiatry, Optometry, Dentistry) need to adopt a team approach to diabetes care. All specialists need to be able to recognize signs of diabetes and systemic concerns resulting from diabetes. There is a PPOD Guide for diabetes management on the CDC (2016a) website. It is in the process of being modified to include audiology (Dowd, 2019).
- Diabetes and hearing impairment are both chronic conditions. Both require self-managed behavioral changes as well as interprofessional collaborative care.

ACKNOWLEDGMENT

The case described is not based on an actual patient but is a composite of several reports about patients with diabetes.

REFERENCES

Albu, J. B., Kovera, A. J., Allen, L., Wainwright, M., Berk, E., Raja-Khan, N., ... Gallagher, D. (2005). Independent association of insulin resistance with larger amounts of intermuscular adipose tissue and a greater acute insulin response to glucose in African American than in white nondiabetic women. *The American Journal of Clinical Nutrition*, *82*(6), 1210–1217. doi:10.1093/ajcn/82.6.1210 PubMed

American Diabetes Association. (2015). Cardiovascular disease and risk management. Sec. 8 in Standards of Medical Care in Diabetes—2015. *Diabetes Care*, *38*(Suppl. 1), S49–S57. doi:10.2337/dc15-S011

American Diabetes Association. (2017, October 4). Diabetes and hearing loss. Retrieved from http://www.diabetes.org/living-with-diabetes/treatment-and-care/seniors/diabetes-and-hearing-loss.html

American Diabetes Association. (2018, March 22). Statistics about diabetes. Retrieved from http://www.diabetes.org/diabetes-basics/statistics/

American Diabetes Association. (2019). Standards of Medical Care in Diabetes - 2019. *Diabetes Care, 42*(Suppl. 1), S34–S45. PubMed

Bainbridge, K. E., Hoffman, H. J., & Cowie, C. C. (2011). Risk factors for hearing impairment among U.S. adults with diabetes: National Health and Nutrition Examination Survey 1999-2004. *Diabetes Care, 34*(7), 1540–1545. doi:10.2337/dc10-2161 PubMed

Bainbridge, K. E., Hoffman, H. J., & Cowrie, C. C. (2008). Diabetes and hearing impairment in the United States: Audiometric evidence from the National Health and Nutrition Examination Survey, 1999 to 2004. *Annals of Internal Medicine, 149*(1), 1–10. doi:10.7326/0003-4819-149-1-200807010-00231 PubMed

Bancks, M. P., Kershaw, K., Carson, A. P., Gordon-Larsen, P., Schreiner, P. J., & Carnethon, M. R. (2017, December). Association of modifiable risk factors in young adulthood with racial disparity in incident Type 2 during middle adulthood. *Journal of the American Medical Association, 318*(24), 2457–2465. doi:10.1001/jama.2017.19546 PubMed

Blackwell, D.L., Lucas J.W., & Clarke T.C. (2014). Summary health statistics for U.S. adults: National Health Interview Survey, 2012. National Center for Health Statistics. Vital and Health Statistics, 10(260).

Centers for Disease Control and Prevention (CDC). (2016a, February 19). Working together to manage diabetes: A toolkit for pharmacy, podiatry, optometry, and dentistry (PPOD). Retrieved from https://www.cdc.gov/diabetes/ndep/toolkits/ppod.html

Centers for Disease Control and Prevention (CDC). (2016b). United States Diabetes Surveillance System. Retrieved from https://gis.cdc.gov/grasp/diabetes/DiabetesAtlas.html

Centers for Disease Control and Prevention (CDC). (2017). *National Diabetes Statistics Report, 2017.* Atlanta, GA: Centers for Disease Control and Prevention, US Department of Health and Human Services.

Centers for Disease Control and Prevention (CDC). (2018, April 10). Leading causes of death (LCOD) by race/ethnicity, all females-United States, 2015. Retrieved from https://www.cdc.gov/women/lcod/2015/race-ethnicity/index.htm

Chung, S. S. M., Ho, E. C. M., Lam, K. S. L., & Chung, S. K. (2003, August). Contribution of polyol pathway to diabetes-induced oxidative stress. *Journal of the American Society of Nephrology, 14*(8Suppl 3), S233–S236. doi:10.1097/01.ASN.0000077408.15865.06 PubMed

Dowd, K. (2019, May 28). Audiology in diabetes care: Merging into PPOD care interprofessional collaboration [Webinar]. Jointly provided by Postgraduate Institute for Medicine and The Audiology Project.

Etymotic Research. (2001). *QuickSIN test.* Elk Grove Village, IL: Etymotic Research.

Fukushima, H., Cureoglu, S., Schachern, P. A., Kusanoki, T., Oktay, M. F., Fukushima, N., ... Harada, T. (2005). Cochlear changes in patients with type 1 diabetes mellitus. *Otolaryngology - Head and Neck Surgery, 133*(1), 100–106. doi:10.1016/j.otohns.2005.02.004 PubMed

Fukushima, H., Cureoglu, S., Schachern, P. A., Paparella, M. M., Harada, T., & Oktay, M. F. (2006). Effects of type 2 diabetes mellitus on cochlear structure in humans. *Archives of Otolaryngology--Head & Neck Surgery, 132*(9), 934–938. doi:10.1001/archotol.132.9.934 PubMed

Golden, S. H., Brown, A., Cauley, J. A., Chin, M. H., Gary-Webb, T. L., Kim, C., ... Anton, B. (2012, September). Health disparities in endocrine disorders: Biological, clinical, and nonclinical factors—An Endocrine Society Scientific Statement. *The Journal of Clinical Endocrinology and Metabolism, 97*(9), E1579–E1639. doi:10.1210/jc.2012-2043 PubMed

Gupta, S., Bhat, J. S., & Kumar, K. (2015). Subcortical processing of speech in individuals with type 2 diabetes mellitus. *International Journal of Diabetes in Developing Countries, 35*(3), 327–331. doi:10.1007/s13410-015-0299-y

Haffner, S. M., D'Agostino, R., Saad, M. F., Rewers, M., Mykkänen, L., & Selby, J. (1996). Increased insulin resistance and insulin secretion in nondiabetic African-Americans and Hispanics compared with non-Hispanic whites. The Insulin Resistance Atherosclerosis Study. *Diabetes, 45*(6), 742–748. doi:10.2337/diab.45.6.742 PubMed

Hao, J., Fu, X., Zhang, C., Zhang, X., Zhao, S., & Li, X. (2017). Early detection of hearing impairment in patients with diabetes mellitus with otoacoustic emission. A systematic review and meta-analysis. *Acta Oto-Laryngologica, 137*(2), 179–185. doi:10.1080/00016489.2016.1223344 PubMed

Harris, M. I., Klein, R., Cowie, C. C., Rowland, M., & Byrd-Holt, D. D. (1998, August). Is the risk of diabetic retinopathy greater in non-Hispanic blacks and Mexican Americans than in non-Hispanic whites with type 2 diabetes? A U.S. population study. *Diabetes Care, 21*(8), 1230–1235. doi:10.2337/diacare.21.8.1230 PubMed

Hoffman, H. J., Dobie, R. A., Losonczy, K. G., Themann, C. L., & Flamme, G. A. (2017). Declining prevalence of hearing loss in US adults aged 20 to 69. *JAMA Otolaryngology-Head & Neck Surgery, 143*(3), 274–285. doi:10.1001/jamaoto.2016.3527 PubMed

Horikawa, C., Kodama, S., Tanaka, S., Fujihara, K., Hirasawa, R., Yachi, Y., ... Sone, H. (2013, January). Diabetes and risk of hearing impairment in adults: A meta-analysis. *The Journal of Clinical Endocrinology and Metabolism, 98*(1), 51–58. doi:10.1210/jc.2012-2119 PubMed

Kariya, S., Cureoglu, S., Fukushima, H., Morita, N., Boylan, M. Y., Maeda, Y., ... Paparella, M. M. (2010). Comparing the cochlear spiral modiolar artery in type-1 and type-2 diabetes mellitus: A human temporal bone study. *Acta Medica Okayama, 64*(6), 375–383. PubMed

Kim, M. B., Zhang, Y., Chang, Y., Ryu, S., Choi, Y., Kwon, M. J., ... Cho, J. (2017, April 1). Diabetes mellitus and the incidence of hearing loss: A cohort study. *International Journal of Epidemiology, 46*(2), 717–726. doi:10.1093/ije/dyw243 PubMed

Kirk, J. K., Bell, R. A., Bertoni, A. G., Arcury, T. A., Quandt, S. A., Goff, D. C. Jr, & Narayan, K. M. (2005). Ethnic disparities: Control of glycemia, blood pressure, and LDL cholesterol among US adults with type 2 diabetes. *The Annals of Pharmacotherapy, 39*(9), 1489–1501. doi:10.1345/aph.1E685 PubMed

Li, J., Zhang, Y., Fu, X., Bi, J., Li, Y., Liu, B., & Zhang, L. (2018). Alteration of auditory function in type 2 diabetic and pre-diabetic patients. *Acta Oto-Laryngologica, 138*(6), 542–547. doi:10.1080/00016489.2017.1422084 PubMed

Lin, F. R., & Ferruci, L. (2012). Hearing loss among older adults in the United States. *Archives of Internal Medicine, 172*(4), 369–371. doi:10.1001/archinternmed.2011.728 PubMed

Lisowska, G., Namysłowski, G., Morawski, K., & Strojek, K. (2001). Cochlear dysfunction and diabetic microangiopathy. *Scandinavian Audiology. Supplementum*, *52*(1), 199–203. doi:10.1080/010503901300007524 PubMed

Mener, D. J., Betz, J., Genther, D. J., Chen, D., & Lin, F. R. (2013). Hearing loss and depression in older adults. *Journal of the American Geriatrics Society*, *61*(9), 1627–1629. Available https://www.ncbi.nlm.nih.gov/pmc/articles/PMC3773611 doi:10.1111/jgs.12429 PubMed

National Institute on Deafness and Other Communication Disorders. (2015). Quick statistics. Retrieved from www.nidcd.nih.gov/health/statistics/Pages/quick.aspx

Office of Minority Health U.S. Department of Health and Human Sciences. (2016, July 13). Diabetes and African Americans. Retrieved from https://minorityhealth.hhs.gov/omh/browse.aspx?lvl=4&lvlid=18

Office of Minority Health U.S. Department of Health and Human Sciences. (2017, August 25) Obesity and African Americans. Retrieved from https://minorityhealth.hhs.gov/omh/browse.aspx?lvl=4&lvlID=25

Otoacoustics Emissions Portal. (2012, December 17). Concepts of DPOAEs. Retrieved from https://www.otoemissions.org/index.php/en/basics-of-oaes/dpoaes/14-concepts-of-dpoaes

The Audiology Project. (2019). Our vision – The Audiology Project story. Retrieved from https://www.theaudiologyproject.com/our-vision

The Hearing Review. (2012, January 30). More age-related hearing loss in female diabetics with poor glucose control. Retrieved from http://www.hearingreview.com/2012/01/more-age-related-hearing-loss-in-female-diabetics-with-poor-glucose-control/

World Health Organization (WHO). (2019). Diabetes programme: About diabetes. Retrieved from https://www.who.int/diabetes/action_online/basics/en/index3.html

KEY TERMS AND DEFINITIONS

Health Disparity: Is a difference in health status of people from different groups.
Hyperglycemia: Is high blood sugar.

Interprofessional Collaborative Practice: Occurs when multiple service providers from different professional backgrounds provide comprehensive healthcare, or educational services, by working with individuals and their families, caregivers, and communities to deliver the highest quality of care.

Microangiopathy: Is also known as microvascular disease, or small vessel disease. It is an angiopathy (i.e., disease of blood vessels) affecting small blood vessels in the body.

Neuropathy: Is a disease or dysfunction of one or more peripheral nerves, typically causing tinkling, numbness, or muscle weakness.

Oxidative Stress: Is an imbalance of free radicals (unstable atoms) and antioxidants (man-made or natural substances that may prevent or delay some types of cell damage caused by free radicals) in the body, which can lead to cell and tissue damage.

Prevalence: Is the proportion of a population who have a specific characteristic in a given time period.

Risk Factors: Is any attribute, characteristic or exposure of an individual that increases the likelihood of developing a disease or injury.

Chapter 15
Supervision:
The Other Side of Cultural Diversity

Katrina Evette Miller
North Carolina Central University, USA

EXECUTIVE SUMMARY

This chapter addresses the cultural diversity of supervisees encountered by supervisors. This case study addresses the cultural dynamics of a clinical fellow from Saudi Arabia who is completing her clinical fellowship in the United States. Aneshia is a clinical fellow who received her Bachelor of Science degree from King Saud University in Saudi Arabia and then earned her Master's degree from an American university. As a Muslim woman such topics as dress, religion, and culture are described and addressed as it relates to Aneshia and her interaction with patients, coworkers, and caregivers. Areas such as appropriate communication distance, appropriate greetings, and physical interactions (oral motor examination, etc.) are discussed along with strategies for addressing these challenges. Areas including documentation as it relates to Arabic syntax and morphology versus standard American English are described. Strategies for working with professionals from Middle Eastern and Arabic countries are also discussed.

INTRODUCTION

Why a case study on supervision as part of a book discussing cultural diversity?

The demographics of the United States dictate it. The shifting demographics of the U.S. are well documented through the United States Census Bureau (U. S. Census Bureau, 2012) and through the American Speech-Language-Hearing Association (ASHA). The U.S. Census Bureau projects that with the continued growth of minority populations, including Native Americans, African Americans, Asians, Pacific Islanders and Hispanics, the combined numbers of minorities will rise to over 60 percent of the population by the year 2060 versus 38 percent in 2017 (U.S. Census Bureau, 2012). This growth of minority residents in the United States also reflects a growth in cultural diversity including a growth in the variety of religions, foods and customs. This growth in minority inhabitants not only affects how speech-language pathologists (SLPs) serve clients from diverse populations, but how SLPs train culturally and linguistically diverse professionals.

DOI: 10.4018/978-1-7998-2261-5.ch015

Further supporting the need to understand cultural diversity, particularly in the field of communication disorders, is the fact that one out of five children in the United States is speaking a language other than English (U.S. Census Bureau, 2015). In addition, individuals who identify as European Americans have diverse histories, cultures and world views. These numbers make it imperative that practitioners have the knowledge and skills, along with the appropriate attitudes to adequately provide services in a culturally responsive manner to anyone from any racial or ethnic group.

ASHA first identified the need to address multicultural issues in the late 1960's. During that time the Black Caucus of ASHA was formed in an attempt to speak to the racial and social injustices of that time (Wiggins, 2014). Later in 1978, the National Black Association for Speech-Language-Hearing (NBASLH) was created and is still in existence today. These were the early attempts for the organizations to speak and provide research in the areas of communication differences versus communication disorders. Most of these original efforts were geared to African American children. From these initial efforts came the position statements that declared that dialects are variations on communication styles and not disorders (Wiggins, 2014).

Based on the increase in diversity as it relates to the populations being served by speech-language pathologists, as well as the increase in international students, one can see the need for communication sciences and disorders programs to vary teaching and training methodology. Over the past ten years the number of post-graduate international students admitted to universities in the United States has increased (Barta, et al., 2019). This increase in international students studying in American universities implies that professionals charged with educating international students are faced with a unique set of instructional challenges. These instructional challenges are exacerbated by the fact that speech-language pathology and audiology deal with human communication. In a field that must consider the content, form and use of language, understanding and being able to apply this standard to a variety of cultures is not only important in the treatment of communication disorders but in the training of those professionals.

Although the term globalization can be defined many ways depending on the theory being used (Hyter et al., 2017), the need for globalization competencies is imperative for speech-language pathologists and audiologists. This is supported by the increased degree of interdependence among nations and the increased opportunities to live and work with individuals and families from countries other than one's own.

Finally, thc disproportionate access to adequate health care by minority populations is well documented in the professional literature (ASHA, 2018). One strategy that has been implemented to increase the access of culturally and linguistically diverse (CALD) populations to health care, is to increase the number of CALD health care professionals. This includes persons in the allied health professions including speech-language pathologists (Attrill, Lincoln & McAllister, 2017). Along with the increase of CALD populations being served, comes the need to provide opportunities for practitioners serving these populations to develop adequate intercultural skills.

While supervision is a specialized area recognized by ASHA, it like other specialized areas requires training and experience to be as effective as possible. Often some of the first professionals students in the communication disorders field bond with are their clinical supervisors. Although young minority clinicians in the speech-language pathology field may not have clinical supervisors that look like them, having one that is culturally responsive can assist with any feelings of disconnection (Gauvin, 2016).

The Clinical Fellowship is viewed as a mentoring relationship since the professionals involved are actively working in the field of speech-language pathology. This case study discusses the mentorship of a Muslim woman as she completed her Clinical Fellowship in a state supported hospital setting. Topics that will be discussed include strategies to assist both the Clinical Fellowship mentor and the clinical fellow in becoming culturally competent and culturally responsive clinicians. In addition, issues faced by a Clinical Fellowship mentor will be discussed along with strategies that are affective within any supervisory relationship.

CASE STUDY

Background Information

Aneshia is a 28-year-old Muslim woman from Saudi Arabia. Aneshia received her Bachelor of Science degree in Speech and Hearing Science from King Saud University in Saudi Arabia. She recently completed a Master of Science degree in Communication Disorders from a small accredited university in the southeastern part of the United States.

Aneshia was a solid "B" student during her matriculation through graduate school but required an extra semester to complete her practicum hours requirement. Aneshia required additional assistance with transcription during her articulation course and when working with children with more severe articulation/motor speech disabilities. Her dialect affected her ability to provide appropriate clinical services. As a result, her advisor recommended that she participate in her University's accent modification program. This was a great resource for Aneshia, and it helped her with her practicum experiences. Aneshia worked well with her classmates during group projects but often challenged her professors as it related to topics she felt were "culturally irrelevant" to her.

Aneshia had six semesters of clinical practicum experiences that included pediatrics, school age children and a skilled nursing facility. She particularly enjoyed working with young children and found her "niche" with early intervention. Aneshia found that working in the skilled nursing facility was challenging. While she felt that she understood the disorders, she was not confident treating men and often felt uncomfortable when she had to treat or provide education to males.

Aneshia is a mother of a six-year-old son and a four-year-old daughter who are in the U.S. along with her husband. Her husband and her children traveled to the United States to be with Aneshia while she completed her studies. Although her husband has been generally supportive while Aneshia completed her studies, he has grown weary of the Western way of life and is threatening to take the children with him and return to Saudi Arabia. Aneshia just accepted a position at a local state supported hospital in order to complete her Clinical Fellowship. She will be working in the pediatric outpatient clinic. She is hoping her husband will give her one more year to complete her Clinical Fellowship. Besides, this was the plan when they left Saudi Arabia, so "why is he trying to change it now", Aneshia thinks at times.

Aneshia has had reasons to be grateful. Her parents were much more liberal Muslims than most of her friends and supported her desire and eagerness to continue her education including high school and college. She did very well with her studies in high school and had originally wanted to be a nurse. She learned about the field of speech-language pathology when she was volunteering at the local hospital in her city. She spent her weekends volunteering and developed a wonderful relationship with the speech-language pathologist that came to the local hospital several times a month. The speech-language pathologist helped her with her enrollment into King Saud University and even helped her with scholarship monies from the government.

She met and married her husband while she was at the university and was a little nervous that he might want her to end her studies when she got pregnant. Her husband was as liberal minded as her parents and he continued to support her efforts as a college student. When Aneshia received support from the Saudi government to continue her education in the United States, she was beyond thrilled. Not only was she going to be able to practice in a field that she loved, she would be able to earn her clinical certification and help train others who were also interested in the field.

Nevertheless, she was excited about her new job and about being a clinical fellow. She just needed to get through the next year and then she could go back to Saudi Arabia and make a difference in her country and within the field. Although it took her several months to secure a job with an employer that was willing to hire an international employee, she liked the team that interviewed her. She had gone through two interviews and felt like she would get along well with her colleagues and the administration. The program she was hired for would last one year. It was specifically designed for clinical fellows and would allow her to be mentored by several speech-language pathologists. Aneshia was particularly excited about specializing in pediatrics even though she would work mostly with the outpatient therapists.

Part of the discussion that follows includes strategies and techniques from a variety of professions that can assist supervisors in becoming culturally competent practitioners and supervisors/mentors. Mentorship can come in a variety of forms including formal relationships between a student and a professor or a less formal but beneficial one between a colleague and a colleague. One fact remains, that no matter what the area of expertise, a mentor or supervisor is generally someone who possesses more experience than the novice allied health professional or educator.

The Clinical Fellowship (CF) mentor and the clinical fellow is a relationship unique to the field of speech-language pathology. It is the CF mentor's charge to assist the CF mentee to bridge the gap from graduate student to novice professional and move on to a self-supervision level. While the clinical fellow and the Clinical Fellowship mentor relationship is not frequently addressed in the literature, there is evidence that this relationship may be one of the most influential of all mentoring relationships (Miller, 2018).

In the field of education, mentoring is seen as an essential component to the retention of special educators (D'Amato & Quinn, 2005). Based on the benefits of mentoring, the Council for Exceptional Children (CEC) and the National Council for the Accreditation of Teacher Education (NCATE) developed standards that require the completion of at least one year of mentorship for special educational professionals (CEC, 2019). The goals of these mentorship programs must include the following:

1. Facilitating the application of knowledge and skills learned
2. Conveying advanced knowledge and skills
3. Acclimation into the school's learning community
4. Reducing job stress and enhancing job satisfaction and
5. Supporting professional induction (CEC, 2019).

The mentoring programs instituted by the CEC are important to mention since most clinical fellows start their careers in the education arena. Incorporating these principles into a mentoring relationship can prove beneficial to a novice speech-language pathologist.

ASHA uses the term mentor to define the professional who assists the novice employee with the transition into an effective clinician following graduation. ASHA changed the term in 2007 from supervisor to mentor to reflect the shift in the way the clinical fellowship experience and the role of the professional overseeing this experience is perceived (McCarthy, 2008)

As the Communication Disorders field strives to meet the challenge of racial and cultural variations it is also important to recognize how these variables may and can affect the supervisor or supervisee relationship. For the discussion of this case study the terms supervisor and mentor will be used interchangeably.

Cultural Competence in Supervision

Schroeder, Andrews, and Hindes (2009) define a supervisor's multicultural competence as "the ability of supervisors to work with clients or trainees from other cultures and races" (p. 297). The concept of a multiculturally competent mentor supports the fact that, while a mentor can be competent from a professional or skills point of view, it is also possible for a professional to not be culturally competent as it relates to supervision or mentorship. Often professionals believe that cultural competence simply means treating everyone as an equal, but cultural competence addresses many more factors than respect alone.

Moore (2012) discusses a variety of research studies that addresses multicultural issues in supervision from several professions. Supervisors who are culturally competent are better able to discuss cultural differences than their counterparts. Supervisors must be able to dialogue about issues related to cultural differences (Moore, 2012) whether that cultural difference impacts colleagues or patients.

A supervisor's effectiveness as a culturally competent professional can be based on the type of feedback that was given to the mentee. This feedback can often include conflicting views on a patient's assessment and intervention strategies. Culturally competent supervisors did not hold stereotypical views of minorities and used cultural informants to better understand cultural/minority differences (Gardner, 2002). The ability to use cultural informants is a great way for supervisors to assist mentees in learning about other cultures and applying this knowledge.

Research further indicated that supervisees confidence improved with supervisors who were comfortable engaging in dialogue related to racial and cultural differences (Moore, 2012). Therefore, it is imperative that clinical mentors and supervisors spend time exploring their own biases and strive to assure that they are in a position to be as effective as possible. It is also important to note that supervisors who disregarded or ignored cultural concerns inevitably compromised patient care as alliances can be shattered and discontentment can occur (Burkard, Johnson, Madson, & Pruitt, 2006).

In a discussion of supervisory relationships, it is also important to mention the role that power has in these relationships. Supervisors and clinical fellowship mentors hold a substantial amount of power that can be perceived as positive or negative. Similarly, it is imperative that mentors are mindful of the historical events that have impacted racial and ethnic minorities in this country and how this dynamic can affect supervisory dyads (Moore, 2012).

Furthermore, Moore (2012) discusses the abuse of supervisory power when bilingual supervisees were given additional responsibilities including interpreting, translating documents and performing bilingual evaluations. These actions did not add to a positive working alliance since possessing these skills increased the workload of a supervisee.

Moore (2012) goes on to provide a discussion regarding the variety of mixed responses when supervisor and supervisee shared the same race as well as when they did not. One major item that was addressed is the importance of remembering that there are situations in which past experiences, specifically historical behaviors can impact the way in which individuals relate to each other.

Regardless, the overriding theme is that supervisors must be culturally competent and feel comfortable leading the discussion of issues as they relate to race and culture. In addition, if a mentor is not familiar with the norms of a culture, a culturally competent supervisor should feel free to utilize the expertise of supervisees and clients from diverse cultural groups. However, mentors should not assume all clinical fellows from CALD populations are culturally competent. They may need to receive training the same as anyone else.

Questions for the Reader

1. As a culturally competent and culturally responsive clinical fellowship mentor (supervisor) what matters should be discussed with Aneshia prior to her beginning her CF?
2. What challenges may arise related to the fact that Aneshia learned English as a second language? Should there be any concerns about the influence Arabic syntax and morphology on the provision of speech and language services in standard American English?
3. What are some of the assessment and intervention variables that need to be discussed with Aneshia as it relates to culturally responsive treatment?
4. What are some of the culture bound and power-distance variables that may impact the clinician-client relationship?
5. What are some of the communication style and child rearing variables that may impact speech and language treatment?
6. How may the Clinical Fellowship mentor and clinical fellow relationship impact Aneshia's ability to complete her Clinical Fellowship (CF) successfully?

Discussion of the Questions for the Reader

1. *As a culturally competent and culturally responsive clinical fellowship mentor (supervisor) what matters should be discussed with Aneshia prior to beginning her CF?* The supervisory process, observations, certification, licensure paperwork, and a general orientation should be discussed with Aneshia.

Supervisory Process

One area that is rarely addressed by supervisors, according to research by Miller (2018) is the supervisory model that the clinical mentor will follow. Most supervisors do not provide a guide as to the stages and final outcome a clinical fellow is striving to obtain. The supervisory model presented by McCrea and Brasseur (2020) is the Anderson Continuum of Supervision model. This model follows an evaluation-feedback, transitional and self-supervision emphasis which is not time-bound. The final stage of this model is the self-supervision level or a self-analysis stage (McCrea & Brasseur, 2020). At this level or stage the supervisee/clinical fellowship mentee and supervisor/clinical fellowship mentors are peers and strive to work together to achieve the targeted goal of self-supervision. Making sure that the CF mentee understands the standards in which she will be evaluated or expected to learn is important in establishing rapport and guidance.

Another supervisory model is the Dreyfus Model of Skills Acquisition. This model encompasses five stages of clinical knowledge including novice, advanced beginner, competent, proficient and expert (Dreyfus, 1981, Robke, 2016). It assesses the progression of acquired skills through formal instruction and practice.

The Hudson CORE Model of Supervision and Mentoring, which combines several concepts of supervision, is used by communication science and disorders professionals. The concepts of the Hudson model are collaboration, observation, reflection and evaluation. Each concept utilizes specific elements to assist the mentee in the progression through the model. The collaboration portion of the Hudson model emphasizes the importance of a trusting supervisory relationship. The observation component involves recording data, while the reflection component includes journaling. The self-evaluation portion of the model uses objective, systematic data and feedback in order to enhance the supervisee's performance (Robke, 2016).

While the models outlined previously provide a guide for supervisors and mentors in the field of speech-language pathology. There are four types of clinical supervision models that can be utilized across a variety of disciplines. These clinical supervision models can be described as: a psychotherapy-based model, a developmental-based model, a social-role model, and an eclectic model or an integrationist / supervisor's model of practice (Robke, 2016). These models can be used in a variety of fields including counseling and education and provide their users with a diverse approach to supervision.

While there are several other clinical models that can be identified and that are the basis for supervision and mentorship evaluation from an assortment of fields, it is important that mentees have an idea of the standards by which they will be evaluated and supervised. As with any model that is implemented, the goal is to move the novice professional through the beginning stages of learning to an independent level.

Observations, Certification and Licensure Paperwork

It is extremely important that the CF mentors review any local or state guidelines that would be important for the clinical fellow to follow especially as it relates to state licensure and documentation. Often CF mentors spend a great deal of time reviewing the clinical fellowship paperwork from ASHA and little time is spent reviewing local guidelines. It is imperative at this beginning stage that expectations and requirements are discussed and understood by the clinical fellow.

It is also important to discuss with the clinical fellow the observation format, review times and dates. While schedules in the speech-language pathology arena must be flexible, having a CF mentor on site adds to the ease and accessibility of observations of the clinical fellow. One of the challenges many clinical fellows identify, is the desire to have their mentors more accessible (Miller, 2018). Although most CF Mentors work for the same company as the clinical fellow, most are not in the same building as the clinical fellow. Therefore, the observations required by ASHA have to be scheduled in advance.

It is important that the clinical fellow is trained on any electronic record keeping and fully understands the documentation deadlines for the hospital, organization, city and state. These guidelines are extremely important for the clinical fellow to know when she is the only speech-language pathologist in the building or setting. Keeping abreast of the required paperwork is often a huge challenge for the novice allied health professional.

General Orientation

There is a general assumption that at this initial stage Aneshia should have participated in the hospital's new employee orientation. During this orientation basic information regarding employee expectations should be discussed. There may be a requirement that Aneshia complete a physical examination and obtain immunizations. Aneshia may also be required to complete a background check and educational modules that may have been developed by the hospital. Since Aneshia will be employed by a large state run institution she may also be eligible for benefits including health and life insurance. Finally, Aneshia should be given information regarding leave time including sick and vacation. She should also discuss with human resources any religious holidays she may observe that will require her to be absent from work. Procedures for requesting leave should also be discussed with human resources.

Aneshia and her CF mentor, or her immediate supervisor, if they are different persons, should also have a discussion regarding the hospitals procedures for requesting leave including sick time and vacation. The times when Aneshia is expected to start and stop each day should be reviewed along with uniform or dress expectations for the position. This topic regarding any dress restrictions Aneshia may have due to her religious beliefs should be handled at the human resources level in an effort to avoid any possible liability issues. Having these important topic discussions as soon as possible allows administration to prepare ahead and also helps to limit any stress that short notice may cause to other employees. In smaller organizations, the discussion of expectations may not be a priority, but it is important that the CF mentor make sure that expectations for the position and the Clinical Fellowship experience are reviewed and all parties involved understand the expectations of each other.

Aneshia should be part of a discussion regarding the environment and culture of the hospital. It is during this time that a culturally competent supervisor would emphasize any needs or expectations they may have. While it would be inappropriate to ask Aneshia about her fasting schedule etc., it would be appropriate to discuss her strategies for dealing with family members especially any male parents or caregivers. It may also be beneficial to discuss some of her previous challenges with family members and how she handled those. It is important at this point that Aneshia be honest about any level of insecurity as it relates to interactions with males. Muslim culture limits the interaction of women and men. Having this discussion early allows for both parties involved to completely understand expectations and be prepared for any challenges that may arise.

Having been reprimanded previously for not allowing adequate time regarding her need to be absent from a clinic site, Aneshia decided to provide a list of the religious holidays that she observed to not only human resources but to her CF Mentor, who was her immediate supervisor. This assisted with planning coverage for her absences. Aneshia also agreed to make up treatments after hours and on weekends if needed. She remembered it was unethical to leave her clients without treatment.

1. *What challenges may arise related to the fact that Aneshia learned English as a second language? Should there be any concerns about the influence of Arabic syntax and morphology on the provision of speech and language services in standard American English?* Aneshia is a non-native speaker of English; Arabic is her native language. Arab dialects are grouped into five geographic categories. The geographic categories are North African, Egyptian, Syrian, Arabian and Iraqi. In addition, written Arabic is different from spoken Arabic (Battle, 2012). Overall, Arabic spelling is phonetic and Arabic speakers produce English words. The consonants /p/, /v/, /n/ and /r/ do not have equivalents in Arabic. These patterns contribute to the phonological patterns of Aneshia.

While it is possible that none of these dialectical patterns may interfere with Aneshia's ability to treat clients, it is important that the CF mentor is fully aware of these dialectical patterns. Aneshia did have to participate in an accent modification program as a masters-level student.

Aneshia would naturally have to learn the record keeping system used by the hospital.

Aneshia's CF mentor should review record keeping programs utilized by the hospital. It would also be a good time for Aneshia and her CF mentor to talk about the diverse populations treated in the hospital. This would include the ethnic and racial make-up of the patients that are served by the state hospital. The CF mentor should review reports that Aneshia has written with her to assess any difficulties that may include grammatical variables.

It is important to note that a large percentage of communicatively impaired individuals of Arab descent live in metropolitan areas. This supports the fact that a shortage of speech-language pathologists and their skills must be viewed from a world-wide perspective (Battle, 2012).

2. *What are some of the assessment and intervention variables that may need to be discussed as it relates to culturally responsive treatment?* It is important, as a culturally competent clinician that Aneshia fully understand the difference between a communication difference and a communication disorder. This includes:
    a. recognizing cultural dimensions
    b. recognizing if a communication pattern is related to an individual's linguistic background
    c. understanding if communication differences are related to limited exposure to new cultural communication patterns
    d. understanding that a communication difference is a variation of a symbol system.

A CF mentor should make sure that Aneshia is aware that the use of standardized testing should not be the only method used for diagnostics. If a client is not reflected in the normalized group for standardization on a test, then the test scores are invalid.

It is accurate to state that Aneshia will more than likely encounter a variety of children with communication disorders from a variety of backgrounds, races and ethnicities. The CF mentor should also spend some time discussing with Aneshia that the definition of a communication disorder may vary among cultures. What is seen as a communication disorder by mainstream American standards, may not be seen as a problem in a child's diverse communities. It is important for the CF mentor to emphasize to Aneshia the importance of providing culturally appropriate education to parents and caregivers.

Since Aneshia will be providing early intervention services it is important that the CF Mentor helps Aneshia to realize the importance of incorporating her patients' culturally and linguistically diverse backgrounds into developing family-centered services. Family centered services include six key principles. These principles include viewing the client's family as the unit of attention, providing choices to the family, utilizing the family strength in intervention, building strong family professional relationships, focusing on the needs of the family and providing individual services (Peredo, 2016).

Aneshia should be made aware of the various forms of test bias, including linguistic bias, format bias, value bias and situational bias. Linguistic bias test items assess speech sounds and grammatical rules that do not exist in a client's native language or dialect. Format bias is the use of testing procedures, formats, items and vocabulary that are not familiar to the client due to differing cultural-linguistic experiences, exposure, and/or socialization influences. Value bias gives more credit to responses that are accepted in certain cultures-linguistic populations. Situational bias occurs when social/situational dynamics affects the responsiveness of clients (Battle, 2012).

Aneshia should be mindful that eye contact, seating arrangements and smiling are all factors that contribute to effective communication and whose appropriateness and use varies from culture to culture. Finally, it is important for Aneshia to participate in self-reflection, so that she is aware of her own value and belief system. She should also be aware that linguistic differences are affected by language differences (Roth & Worthington, 2021).

While these strategies can and should be utilized by practicing speech-language pathologists, it is important to remember that a CF mentor or supervisor should assist mentees with developing into a culturally competent professional. Helping a novice professional to reach a culturally competent level is an appropriate goal for a supervisor.

3. *What are some of the culture bound and power-distance variables that may impact the clinician-client relationship?* It is important that Aneshia understands that being a culturally competent clinician is ongoing and that being able to recognize sources that could potentially bring conflict to the clinic is an important skill to develop and maintain (Battle, 2012). Culture bound variables are vital because they help in the identification of the significance of the individual versus the group in any given culture.

ASHA reinforces the importance of a provider entering into the clinician-client relationship without making assumptions about the client based on their culture, ethnicity, language or life experiences (ASHA, 2005). In individualism, emphasis is placed on the freedom of an individual versus collectivism which considers the needs of an entire group (Battle, 2012). Individualism is seen with European countries and cultures while collectivism is part of Arab, African, Asian and Hispanic cultures.

Power-distance variables are variables that consider social relationships between people of different status. This can include the relationship with men and women, high power-distant relationships like superiors and lower power-distance cultures in which one does not necessarily accept a superior's orders.

Time orientation differs across cultures. When the culture is long-term and future oriented the establishment of long-term goals and priorities are highly valued. When the culture's focus is on the past the establishment of short-term goals are more attainable and preserving the present is more important. Western cultures are more oriented toward the future versus non-Western cultures that are more focused on the past. These variables can possibly have a major effect on client treatment and the clinician's interaction with family members.

Reviewing the impact that power and time has on culture and what is acceptable within a culture would greatly assist Aneshia as she works with patients and their families. As Aneshia is able to navigate across cultural time orientation, while developing long term goals and priorities versus short-term goals, she will be moving closer to a self-supervision level.

4. *What are some of the communication styles and child rearing variables that may impact speech and language treatment?* Nonverbal and verbal communication styles can possibly impact speech and language treatment. Language and communication styles are correlated to race, culture and ethnicity. Nonverbal communication includes communication distance, kinesics, (body language), eye contact, silence, loudness, inflection and stress. While verbal communications can include pragmatics or the way language is used in greetings and social distance. Non-Western cultures have

vertical communication patterns, flowing from those in higher prestige to those of lower prestige. Western cultures are more horizontal with communication partners.

Since Aneshia will be working with a pediatric population the clinical fellowship mentor should spend some time discussing child rearing practices and how these practices vary from culture to culture. Knowledge of these variables will assist with developing home programs and in educating family members. These child rearing variables include:

a. Asian cultures: children may be viewed as spoiled due to single-child policies. There are variations in bilingualism. Parents are seen as gratifying infants' every need.
b. American Indian cultures: child rearing activities may be left to family members other than parents (e.g., grandparents, aunts and uncles)
c. African American cultures: many households are headed by single adults, mainly females. Children are the future and need to know they are loved, and that they belong. Children must be disciplined and all responsible adults in *kinship* circles of influence play a role.
d. Anglo-European cultures: emphasis is placed on individuality, achievement, self-help and self-reliance. Typically, infants are placed in their own beds and have their own rooms early on. Children are involved in decision making. Mothers work outside of the home and children may be placed in day care.
e. Latino cultures: couples marry to have children; child relationship is more important than marital. Parents are nurturing and permissive. Focus on family member's dependence on family (Lynch & Hanson, 2011).

It is important to remember that these variables are generalizations and are not all encompassing.

5. How may the Clinical Fellowship mentor and clinical fellow relationship impact Aneshia's ability to complete her Clinical Fellowship (CF) successfully?

The Clinical Fellowship mentor and clinical fellow relationship can be one of the most important relationships in an early professional's career. For the most part the clinical fellowship experience is viewed as a positive one. Clinical Fellowship mentors not only assist an early career professional to transition from graduate student, they are often the person that orients the clinical fellow to a new position.

Having the skills needed to be an effective mentor is one of the greatest challenge a mentor can undertake. It is important that Aneshia and her CF mentor discuss methods by which Aneshia will receive feedback. The most consistent method that feedback is received has been identified as face-to-face, followed by phone then e-mail and finally text messaging (Miller, 2018). Clinical fellows felt that the face-to-face feedback along with the e-mail methods were effective. Often the method of feedback used had more to do with what was convenient for the CF mentor and the clinical fellow. While most clinical fellows do prefer face-to-face feedback, the greatest preference was that feedback was done as soon as possible. Clinical fellows felt that when a mentor was accessible the greatest amount of learning took place (Miller, 2018). As previously addressed, it did not matter how the feedback occurred, whether face-to-face or through phone calls or text messages. Clinical fellows that had the most positive CF experiences listed characteristics of their mentors. These characteristics included being knowledgeable, supportive, approachable, cultivating independence, and providing feedback and resources (Miller, 2018).

Other areas that may impact the success of Aneshia's experience includes generational differences. Research on generational differences as it relates to supervision has been documented. McCready (2007) discusses the four distinct generations that for the first time in history are working together. These generations, *Traditionalist (born 1900-1945)*, *Baby Boomers (born 1946-1964)*, *Generation X (born 1965-1980)* and *Millennials (born 1981-1999)*, represent distinct experiences, attitudes and images that affect everyday interactions, which in turn can and often have a greater impact on supervision and the mentoring process.

McCready (2011) implies that when dealing with persons from different generations one must try to avoid stereotyping and have an appreciation of the unique strengths each generations brings. This is an important concept for Aneshia and her CF Mentor to remember. This is also a concept that may impact her work environment and should be identified. An honest discussion of the variety of attitudes, as it relates to generational difference, that Aneshia may experience would be a unique way to begin dialog regarding strategies to address these differences. It would also be beneficial to identify that these differences may also impact working relationships.

Although gender differences may not play a major role, it is important for Aneshia's CF mentor to remember and recognize Aneshia's culture and her comfort with talking and/or interacting with male coworkers or family members. It would benefit both parties to discuss a strategic plan ahead of time when dealing with these issues.

OUTCOMES

Aneshia had challenges with documentation during her CF and required additional time and resources to assist in this area. Her mentor was particularly concerned with Aneshia's ability to teach her early intervention clients earlier-developing English speech sounds. Her mentor provided additional resources and recommendations.

Aneshia was not always receptive of these suggestions and as the time to complete her clinical fellowship was coming to an end, she realized that if she did not participate in additional remediation, she was in danger of not completing her fellowship successfully. While she had an excellent relationship with her mentor, she did not want to have to complete the additional work especially since she would be practicing in Saudi Arabia. Her mentor did explain to her that although she would be using her skills in another country, she must past the standards of ASHA in order to receive her certificate of clinical competence in speech-language pathology (CCC-SLP). Aneshia reconsidered and was able to complete her Clinical Fellowship successfully even though she required additional assistance and training.

KEY POINTS

- CF mentors or supervisors establish lines of effective communication between themselves and their clinical fellows or students early in the experience. They review and discuss the Supervisory Process with mentees.
- CF mentors or supervisors review the standards and/or the procedures that will be utilized for evaluations. This includes local, state and national standards if applicable.

- Culturally competent clinicians are aware of their own biases and provide reflective activities that will assist a clinical fellow or student in identifying their biases.
- Culturally competent clinicians discuss cultural issues that may arise with patients as soon as they occur and stay abreast of multicultural trends and issues through continuing education activities and experiences.
- CF mentors or supervisors seek additional professional resources when questions or concerns arise.

REFERENCES

American Speech-Language-Hearing Association (ASHA). (2015). *Cultural competence (Issues in Ethics).* Retrieved from http://www.asha.org/policy

American Speech-Language-Hearing Association (ASHA). (2017). *Issues in ethics: Cultural and linguistic competence.* Retrieved from www.asha.org/Practice/ethics/Cultural-and Linguistic-Competence/

American Speech-Language Hearing Association (ASHA). (2019). *Completing the Clinical Fellowship (CF) Experience.* Retrieved from: https://www.asha.org/Certification/Completing-the-Clinical-Fellowship-Experience/

Attrill, S., Lincoln, M., & McAllister, S. (2017). Culturally and linguistically diverse students' in speech-language pathology courses: A platform for culturally responsive services. *Journal for Speech-Language Pathology, 19*(3), 309–321. doi:10.1080/17549507.2017.1292548 PMID:28264593

Barta, P., Chen, T., Jou, D., McEnaney, C., & Fuller, A. (2019). *How international students are changing U.S. colleges.* Retrieved from: http://graphics.wsj.com/international-students/

Battle, D. E. (2012). *Communication disorders in multicultural populations and international populations* (4th ed.). Maryland Heights, MO: Elsevier Mosby.

Burkard, A., Johnson, A. J., Madson, M., Pruitt, N. T., Contreras-Tadych, D. A., Kozlowski, J. E. M., ... Knox, S. (2006, July). Supervisor cultural responsiveness and unresponsiveness in cross-cultural supervision. *Journal of Counseling Psychology, 53*(3), 288–301. doi:10.1037/0022-0167.53.3.288

Council for Exceptional Children (CEC). (2019). *CEC professional standards.* Retrieved from: https://www.cec.sped.org/Standards

D'Amato, B., & Quinn, R. (2005). The effects of mentoring on first-year teachers' perceptions of support received. *The Clearing House: A Journal of Educational Strategies, Issues and Ideas, 78*(3), 110–116. doi:10.3200/TCHS.78.3.110-117

Dreyfus, S. E. (1981). *Dreyfus Model of Skills Acquisition.* Retrieved from: http://www-personal.umich.edu/~mrother/KATA_Files/Dreyfus.pdf

Gardner, R. (2002). Cross cultural perspectives in supervision. *The Western Journal of Black Studies, 26*(2), 98–106.

Gauvin, G. M. (2016). *A study of cultural differences on the supervisory process in a graduate school program* (Doctoral dissertation). Retrieved from ProQuest Dissertations and Theses. (UMI 10127526)

Hyter, Y. D., Roman, T. R., Staley, B., & McPherson, B. (2017). Competence for effective global engagement: A proposal for communication sciences and disorders. *Perspectives on Global Issues in Communication Sciences and Disorders*, *2*, 9–20.

Hyter, Y. D., & Salas-Provance, M. B. (2019). *Culturally responsive practices in speech, language, and hearing sciences*. San Diego, CA: Plural Publishing.

Lynch, E. W., & Hanson, M. J. (2011). *Developing cross-cultural competence: A guide for working with children and their families* (4th ed.). Baltimore, MD: Paul H Brookes Publishing.

McCarthy, M. P., & Staub, K. J. (2008). Will you be my CF mentor? *Perspectives on Administration and Supervision*. Retrieved from: https://pubs.asha.org/doi/full/10.1044/aas18.3.82

McCrea, E., & Brasseur, J. (2020). *The supervisory process in speech-language pathology and audiology*. Thorafare, NJ: Slack, Incorporated.

McCready, V. (2011). Generational issues in supervision and administration. *The ASHA Leader, 16*, 12–15. doi:10:1044/leader FTR1.6052011.12

Miller, K. (2018) *Perceptions of speech-language pathologists in clinical fellowships* (Unpublished doctoral dissertation). Nova Southeastern University, Fort Lauderdale, FL.

Moore, R. (2012). Supervision and multicultural issues: Supervisors and supervisees. *Perspectives on Administration and Supervision*, *22*(1), 33–39. doi:10.1044/aas22.1.33

Peredo, T. N. (2016). Supporting culturally and linguistically diverse families in early intervention. *Perspectives of the ASHA Special Interest Groups SIG*, *1*(1), 154–167. doi:10.1044/persp1.SIG1.154

Qualls, C. D., & Munoz, M. L. (2005). Race-ethnicity, socioeconomic status, and cognitive communicative functioning in individuals with neurogenic communication disorders: Clinical implications and research directions. *ECHO: E-Journal for Black and Other Ethnic Group Research and Practices in Communication Sciences and Disorders*, *1*, 30–39.

Resendiz, M., Summers, C., Ruiz-Felter, R., Belasco, E., & Fox, K. (2017). Perceptions of mentoring SLPs and clinical fellows during the clinical fellowship. *Perspectives of ASHA Special Interest Groups, SIG 11, 2*, 25-41.

Robke, D. (2016). Foundational resources and terminology for supervision and mentorship. *Perspectives of ASHA Special Interest Group, SIG 11, 1,* 57-67. Retrieved from: https://pubs.asha.org/doi/10.1044/persp1.SIG11.57

Roth, F. P., & Worthington, C. K. (2021). *Treatment resources manual for speech-language pathology* (6th ed.). San Diego, CA: Plural Publishing.

Schroeder, M., Andrews, J. W., & Hines, Y. L. (2009). Cross-racial supervision: Critical issues in the supervisory relationship. *Canadian Journal of Counselling*, *43*(4), 295–310.

U.S. Census Bureau. (2018a, June 17). *American Community Survey (ACS): Comparing 2012 American Community Survey Data.* Retrieved from https://www.census.gov/programs surveys/acs/guidance/comparing-acs-data/2012.html

U.S. Census Bureau. (2018b, June 17). *American Community Survey (ACS): Comparing 2015 American Community Survey Data.* Retrieved from https://www.census.gov/programs-surveys/acs/guidance/comparing-acs-data/2015.html

Wiggins, E. (2014). *History of the National Black Association for Speech-Language and Hearing (NBASLH): The first twenty years.* Norfolk, VA: Poetica Publishing Company.

KEY TERMS AND DEFINITIONS

Clinical Fellow: First year SLP who is enrolled in a CF (ASHA, 2019).

Clinical Fellowship: A shift from graduate school student enrolled in a course of study to professional speech-language pathologist (SLP) (ASHA, 2019).

Clinical Fellowship Mentor: Is a certified SLP with a minimum of two years' experience assisting a clinical fellow through her or his CF (ASHA, 2019).

Cultural Responsiveness: The process of moving along a continuum to becoming a more effective in providing services across cultures (Hyter & Salas-Provance, 2019).

Culturally and Linguistically Diverse Populations: Children and families residing in the United States who come from homes that speak a language other than English and whose cultural identity differs from mainstream U.S. culture (Peredo, 2016).

Culturally Competent: A process of acceptance and respect for difference, continuing self-assessment regarding culture, and careful attention to the dynamics. At this stage, clinicians are able to effectively use their cultural knowledge during interviewing, assessment, and treatment (ASHA, 2019).

Self-Supervision: Is the stage in which a clinical fellow becomes independent and is responsible for his or her own professional growth. At this stage, the clinical fellow has the ability to accurately evaluate their clinical behavior and alter the behavior based on that evaluation (Miller, 2018).

Compilation of References

Abbeduto, L., Brady, N., & Kover, S. T. (2007). Language development and Fragile X Syndrome: Profiles, syndrome-specificity, and within-syndrome differences. *Mental Retardation and Developmental Disabilities Research Reviews*, *13*(1), 36–46. doi:10.1002/mrdd.20142 PMID:17326110

Abbeduto, L., Murphy, M. M., Cawthon, S. W., Richmond, E. K., Weissman, M. D., Karadottir, S., & O'Brien, A. (2003). Receptive language skills of adolescents and young adults with Down syndrome or Fragile X Syndrome. *American Journal of Mental Retardation*, *108*(3), 149–160. doi:10.1352/0895-8017(2003)108<0149:RLSOAA>2.0.CO;2 PMID:12691594

Abbeduto, L., Pavetto, M., Kesin, E., Weissman, M. D., Karadottir, S., O'Brien, A., & Cawthon, S. (2001). The linguistic and cognitive profile of Down syndrome: Evidence from a comparison with fragile x syndrome. *Down's Syndrome: Research and Practice*, *7*(1), 9–15. doi:10.3104/reports.109 PMID:11706811

Accredited Language Services. (2019). *The 10 most popular languages in the U.S.* Retrieved from https://www.accreditedlanguage.com/languages/the-10-most-popular-languages-in-the-us/

ACLU. (2019). *Family separation by the numbers*. Retrieved from https://www.aclu.org/issues/immigrants-rights/immigrants-rights-and-detention/family-separation

Adair, J. K. (2015). *The impact of discrimination on the early schooling experiences of children from immigrant families*. Migration Policy Institute. Available at http://www.migrationpolicy.org

Adamson, L. B., Bakeman, R., & Deckner, D. F. (2004). The development of symbol-infused joint engagement. *Child Development*, *75*(4), 1171–1187. doi:10.1111/j.1467-8624.2004.00732.x PMID:15260871

Albu, J. B., Kovera, A. J., Allen, L., Wainwright, M., Berk, E., Raja-Khan, N., ... Gallagher, D. (2005). Independent association of insulin resistance with larger amounts of intermuscular adipose tissue and a greater acute insulin response to glucose in African American than in white nondiabetic women. *The American Journal of Clinical Nutrition*, *82*(6), 1210–1217. doi:10.1093/ajcn/82.6.1210 PubMed

Ali, K., Dahra, D., Coelho, C., Jones, G., & Tredwin, C. (2017). Academic performance of undergraduate dental students with learning disabilities. *British Dental Journal*, *222*(3), 205–208. doi:10.1038j.bdj.2017.125 PMID:28184079

American Community Survey. (2008). *Selected population profile in the United States –Hispanic or Latino (1-year estimates)*. Washington, DC: U.S. Census Bureau.

American Diabetes Association. (2015). Cardiovascular disease and risk management. Sec. 8 in Standards of Medical Care in Diabetes—2015. *Diabetes Care*, *38*(Suppl. 1), S49–S57. doi:10.2337/dc15-S011

American Diabetes Association. (2017, October 4). Diabetes and hearing loss. Retrieved from http://www.diabetes.org/living-with-diabetes/treatment-and-care/seniors/diabetes-and-hearing-loss.html

American Diabetes Association. (2018, March 22). *Statistics about diabetes*. Retrieved from http://www.diabetes.org/diabetes-basics/statistics/

American Diabetes Association. (2019). Standards of Medical Care in Diabetes - 2019. *Diabetes Care*, *42*(Suppl. 1), S34–S45. PubMed

American Nutrition Association. (2019). USDA defines food deserts. *Nutrition Digest, 38*(2). Retrieved from http://americannutritionassociation.org/newsletter/usda-defines-food-deserts

American Psychiatric Association (APA). (2013). Diagnostic and statistical manual of mental disorders-5. Washington, DC: Author.

American Psychiatric Association. (2000). Diagnostic and statistical manual of mental disorders, text revision. (DSM-IV-TR). Washington, DC: American Psychiatric Association.

American Psychiatric Association. (2013). *Diagnostic and statistical manual of mental disorders* (5th ed.). Arlington, VA: American Psychiatric Publishing.

American Psychological Association. (2017). *Multicultural guidelines: An ecological approach to context, identity, and intersectionality*. Retrieved from http://www.apa.org/about/policy/multicultural-guidelines.pdf

American School Counselor Association. (2019). *ASCA School Counselor Professional Standards & Competencies*. Alexandria, VA: Author.

American Speech-Hearing-Language Association. (2013). *ASHA SLP health care survey*. Retrieved from https://www.asha.org/Research/memberdata/Healthcare-Survey/

American Speech-Hearing-Language Association. (2014). *Demographic profile of ASHA members providing bilingual services*. Retrieved from https://www.asha.org/uploadedFiles/Demographic-Profile-Bilingual-Spanish-Service-Members.pdf

American Speech-Hearing-Language Association. (2015). *Person centered focus on function: Aphasia*. Retrieved from https://www.asha.org/uploadedFiles/ICF-Aphasia.pdf

American Speech-Language Hearing Association (ASHA). (2019). *Completing the Clinical Fellowship (CF) Experience*. Retrieved from: https://www.asha.org/Certification/Completing-the-Clinical-Fellowship-Experience/

American Speech-Language-Hearing Association (2019a). *Cultural competence*. Retrieved from asha.org/Practice-Portal/Professional Issues/Cultural-Competence/.

American Speech-Language-Hearing Association (2019b). *Evidence-based practice*. Retrieved from asha.org/Research/EBP/Evidence-Based-Practice.

American Speech-Language-Hearing Association (ASHA). (2015). *Cultural competence (Issues in Ethics)*. Retrieved from http://www.asha.org/policy

American Speech-Language-Hearing Association (ASHA). (2017). *Issues in ethics: Cultural and linguistic competence*. Retrieved from www.asha.org/Practice/ethics/Cultural-and Linguistic-Competence/

American Speech-Language-Hearing Association (ASHA). (2019). *Practice portal: Speech sound disorders-articulation and phonology*. Retrieved from https://www.asha.org/PRPSpecificTopic.aspx?folderid=8589935321&section=Treatment

American Speech-Language-Hearing Association. (2004). *Knowledge and skills needed by speech-language pathologists and audiologists to provide culturally and linguistically appropriate services*. Retrieved from http://www.asha.org/docs/html/KS2004-00215.html

American Speech-Language-Hearing Association. (2008). *Service provision to children who are deaf and hard of hearing, birth to 36 months*. Joint Committee of the American Speech-Language-Hearing Association and Council on Education of the Deaf. Retrieved from http//www.asha.org/policy/ps2013-0339

American Speech-Language-Hearing Association. (2016). *2016 Schools Survey report: SLP workforce/work conditions*. Retrieved from https://www.asha.org/uploadedFiles/2018-Schools-Survey-Workforce-Report.pdf

American Speech-Language-Hearing Association. (2016). *Code of ethics*. Retrieved from www.asha.org/policy

American Speech-Language-Hearing Association. (2019a). *Autism*. Retrieved from https://www.asha.org/practice-portal/clinical-topics/autism/

American Speech-Language-Hearing Association. (2019b). *Cultural competence*. Retrieved from https://www.asha.org/PRPSpecificTopic.aspx?folderid=8589935230&section=Overview

American Speech-Language-Hearing Association. (2019c). *Evidence-Based Practice* Retrieved from https://www.asha.org/research/ebp/evidence-based-practice/

American Speech-Language-Hearing Association. (2019d). *Advantages of being bilingual*. Retrieved from https://www.asha.org/public/speech/development/The-Advantages-of-Being-Bilingual/

American Speech-Language-Hearing Association. (2019e). *Bilingual service delivery*. Retrieved from https://www.asha.org/practice-portal/professional-issues/bilingual-service-delivery/

American Speech-Language-Hearing Association. (2019f). *Family centered practices*. Retrieved from https://www.asha.org/Practice-Portal/Clinical-Topics/Autism/Family-Centered-Practice/

American Speech-Language-Hearing Association. (2019g). *Sample intervention goals based on core challenges in Autism Spectrum Disorder*. Retrieved from https://www.asha.org/uploadedFiles/ASHA/Practice_Portal/Clinical_Topics/Autism/Sample%20Intervention%20Goals.pdf

American Speech-Language-Hearing Association. (n.d.). *Adult Dysphagia*. Retrieved October 8, 2019 from http://www.asha.org/Practice-Portal/Clinical-Topics/Adult-Dysphagia/

American Stroke Association. (2019). *Stroke risk factors*. Retrieved from https://www.stroke.org/en/about-stroke/stroke-risk-factors

Antoniadou, N., & Kokkinos, C. (2013). A review of research on cyber-bullying in Greece. *International Journal of Adolescence and Youth*, *20*(2), 185–201. doi:10.1080/02673843.2013.778207

Anyon, Y. (2010). Reducing racial disparities and disproportionalities in the child welfare system: Policy perspectives about how to serve the best interests of African American youth. *Children and Youth Services Review*, *33*(2), 242–253. doi:10.1016/j.childyouth.2010.09.007

Apthorp, H. S. (2006). Effects of a supplemental vocabulary program in third-grade reading/language arts. *The Journal of Educational Research*, *100*(2), 67–79. doi:10.3200/JOER.100.2.67-79

Argeseanu, C. S., Ruben, J. D., & Narayan, K. M. (2008). Health of foreign-born people in the US: A review. *Health & Place*, *14*(4), 623–635. doi:10.1016/j.healthplace.2007.12.002 PMID:18242116

Arias, G., & Friberg, J. (2017). Bilingual language assessment: Contemporary versus recommended practice in American schools. *Language, Speech, and Hearing Services in Schools*, *48*(1), 1–15. doi:10.1044/2016_LSHSS-15-0090 PMID:27788525

Arioli, M., Crespi, C., & Canessa, N. (2018). Social cognition through the lens of cognitive and clinical neuroscience. *BioMed Research International*, *2018*, 4283427. doi:10.1155/2018/4283427 PMID:30302338

Arrastia, R. (2007). Ethnic differences in rehabilitation placement and outcome after TBI. *The Journal of Head Trauma Rehabilitation*, *22*(2), 113–121. doi:10.1097/01.HTR.0000265099.29436.56 PMID:17414313

Ascher, C. (1990). Assessing bilingual students for placement and instruction. *ERIC/CUE Digest No. 65*.

Attrill, S., Lincoln, M., & McAllister, S. (2017). Culturally and linguistically diverse students' in speech-language pathology courses: A platform for culturally responsive services. *Journal for Speech-Language Pathology*, *19*(3), 309–321. doi:10.1080/17549507.2017.1292548 PMID:28264593

Backhouse, G., & Morris, K. (2005). *Dyslexia?* London: Hodder Murray.

Bainbridge, K. E., Hoffman, H. J., & Cowie, C. C. (2011). Risk factors for hearing impairment among U.S. adults with diabetes: National Health and Nutrition Examination Survey 1999-2004. *Diabetes Care*, *34*(7), 1540–1545. doi:10.2337/dc10-2161 PMID:21593298

Bainbridge, K. E., Hoffman, H. J., & Cowrie, C. C. (2008). Diabetes and hearing impairment in the United States: Audiometric evidence from the National Health and Nutrition Examination Survey, 1999 to 2004. *Annals of Internal Medicine*, *149*(1), 1–10. doi:10.7326/0003-4819-149-1-200807010-00231 PubMed

Balestreri, M., Czosnyka, M., Chatfield, D. A., ... Pickard, D. (2004). Predictive value of Glasgow coma scale after brain trauma: Change in trend over the past ten years. *Journal of Neurology. Neurosurgery & Psychology*, *75*, 161–162. PMID:14707332

Bambara, L. M., Janney, R., & Snell, M. (2015). *Behavior support: Teachers' guides to inclusive practices* (3rd ed.). Baltimore, MD: Brookes.

Bambara, L. M., & Kern, L. (2005). *Individualized supports for students with problem behaviors: Designing positive behavior plans*. New York, NY: Guilford.

Banai, K., & Ahissar, M. (2006). Auditory processing deficits in dyslexia: Task or stimulus related? *Cerebral Cortex*, *16*(12), 1718–1728. doi:10.1093/cercor/bhj107 PMID:16407480

Bancks, M. P., Kershaw, K., Carson, A. P., Gordon-Larsen, P., Schreiner, P. J., & Carnethon, M. R. (2017, December). Association of modifiable risk factors in young adulthood with racial disparity in incident Type 2 during middle adulthood. *Journal of the American Medical Association*, *318*(24), 2457–2465. doi:10.1001/jama.2017.19546 PMID:29279935

Barragan, B., Castilla-Earls, A., Martinez-Nieto, M., Restrepo, A., & Gray, S. (2018). Performance of low-income dual language learners attending English-only schools on the Clinical Evaluation of Language Fundamentals-4th edition, Spanish. *Language, Speech, and Hearing Services in Schools*, *49*(2), 292–305. doi:10.1044/2017_LSHSS-17-0013 PMID:29330555

Barta, P., Chen, T., Jou, D., McEnaney, C., & Fuller, A. (2019). *How international students are changing U.S. colleges*. Retrieved from: http://graphics.wsj.com/international-students/

Barth, A. E., Stuebing, K. K., Anthony, J. L., Denton, C. A., Mathes, P. G., Fletcher, J. M., & Francis, D. J. (2008). Agreement among response to intervention criteria for identifying responder status. *Learning and Individual Differences*, *18*(3), 296–307. doi:10.1016/j.lindif.2008.04.004 PMID:19081758

Battle, D. (2002). Communication disorders in a multicultural and global society. In D. E. Battle (Ed.), *Communication disorders in multicultural populations* (3rd ed.; pp. 2–19). Boston: Butterworth-Heinemann.

Battle, D. E. (2012). *Communication disorders in multicultural populations and international populations* (4th ed.). Maryland Heights, MO: Elsevier Mosby.

Battle, D., & Anderson, N. (1998). Culturally diverse families and the development of language. In D. E. Battle (Ed.), *Communication disorders in multicultural populations* (pp. 213–245). Boston: Butterworth-Heinemann.

Bauman-Waengler, J. (2015). *Articulatory and phonological impairments: A clinical focus* (5th ed.). Boston, MA: Pearson, Allyn, & Bacon.

Bazarian, J., Pope, C., McClung, J., Cheng, Y., & Flesher, W. (2003). Ethnic and racial disparities in emergency department care for mild traumatic brain injury. *Academic Emergency Medicine*, *10*(11), 1209–1217. doi:10.1197/S1069-6563(03)00491-3 PMID:14597497

Beauvais, F. (1998). American Indians and alcohol. *Spotlight on Special Populations*, *22*(4), 253–259. PMID:15706751

Becker, D., Garcia, S., & Ellertson, C. (2004). Do Mexico City pharmacy workers screen women for health risks when they sell oral contraceptive pills over-the-counter? *Contraception*, *69*(4), 295–299. doi:10.1016/j.contraception.2003.11.014 PMID:15033404

Beck, I. L., McKeown, M. G., & Kucan, L. (2013). *Bringing words to life: Robust vocabulary instruction.* New York, NY: Guilford.

Beck, I. L., McKeown, M. G., Kucan, L., Hiebert, E. H., & Kamil, M. L. (2005). Choosing words to teach. In *Teaching and learning vocabulary: Bringing research to practice* (pp. 209–222). Mahwah, NJ: Lawrence Erlbaum Associates.

Bedore, L. M., & Peña, E. D. (2008). Assessment of bilingual children for identification of language impairment: Current findings and implications for practice. *International Journal of Bilingual Education and Bilingualism*, *11*(1), 1–29. doi:10.2167/beb392.0

Bedore, L. M., Pena, E. D., Joyner, D., & Macken, C. (2011). Parent and teacher rating of bilingual language proficiency and language development concerns. *International Journal of Bilingual Education and Bilingualism*, *14*(5), 489–511. doi:10.1080/13670050.2010.529102 PMID:29910668

Bedore, L., Pena, E., Anaya, J., Nieto, R., Lugo-Neris, M., & Baron, A. (2018). Production of English grammatical forms by English language learners. *Language, Speech, and Hearing Services in Schools*, *49*(2), 277–291. doi:10.1044/2017_LSHSS-17-0027 PMID:29621806

Belhassen, L., Pelle, G., Sediame, S., Bachir, D., Carville, C., Bucherer, C., ... Adnot, S. (2001). Endothelial dysfunction in patients with sickle cell disease is related to selective impairment of shear stress-mediated vasodilation. *Blood*, *97*(6), 1584–1589. doi:10.1182/blood.V97.6.1584 PMID:11238095

Benarous, X., Guile, J. M., Consoli, A., & Cohen, D. (2015). A systematic review of the evidence for impaired cognitive theory of mind in maltreated children. *Frontiers in Psychiatry*, *6*(108). doi:10.3389/fpsyt.2015.00108 PMID:26283975

Benavides, A., Kapantzoglou, M., & Murata, C. (2018). Two grammatical tasks for screening language abilities in Spanish-speaking children. *American Journal of Speech-Language Pathology*, *27*(2), 690–705. doi:10.1044/2017_AJSLP-17-0052 PMID:29554217

Beneria, L., Berik, G., & Floro, M. (2016). *Gender, development and globalization: Economics as if all people mattered* (2nd ed.). New York: Routledge.

Benkert, R., Hollie, B., Nordstron, C. K., Wickson, B., & Bins-Emerick, L. (2009). Trust, mistrust, racial identity and patient satisfaction in urban African American primary care patients of nurse practitioners. *Journal of Nursing Scholarship*, *41*(2), 211–219. doi:10.1111/j.1547-5069.2009.01273.x PMID:19538706

Bergstrom, S., Carr, H., Petersson, G., Stephansson, O., Bonamy, A. K., Dahlstrom, A., ... Johansson, S. (2016). Trends in congenital heart defects in infants with Down syndrome. *Pediatrics*, *138*(1), e20160123. doi:10.1542/peds.2016-0123 PMID:27252035

Berjis, N., Moeinimehr, M., & Nasiri, S. (2016). Endothelial dysfunction in patients with sudden sensorineural hearing loss. *Advanced Biomedical Research*, *5*, 1–4. PMID:26955626

Beveridge, M. E., & Bak, T. H. (2011). The languages of aphasia research: Bias and diversity. *Aphasiology*, *25*(12), 1451–1468. doi:10.1080/02687038.2011.624165

Bhattacharyya, N. (2014). The prevalence of dysphagia among adults in the United States. *Otolaryngology - Head and Neck Surgery*, *151*(5), 765–769. doi:10.1177/0194599814549156 PMID:25193514

Binford, W. (2019, June 21). A firsthand report of 'inhumane conditions' at a migrant children's detention center. *Interview on PBS News Hour*. Retrieved from https://www.pbs.org/newshour/show/a-firsthand-report-of-inhumane-conditions-at-a-migrant-childrens-detention-facility

Bishop, D. V. M. (2006). *The Children's Communication Checklist* (2nd ed.). San Antonio, TX: Psychological Corporation.

Blackmer, S. C., & Marshall, J. (1999). A comparison of traumatic brain injury in the Saskatchewan native North American and non-native north American populations. *Brain Injury: [BI]*, *13*(8), 627–635. doi:10.1080/026990599121359 PMID:10901690

Black-Pond, C., & Henry, J. (2008). A trauma-informed Child Welfare System practice: The essential elements. *The Michigan Child Welfare Law Journal*, *11*(2), 11–23.

Blackwell, D.L., Lucas J.W., & Clarke T.C. (2014). Summary health statistics for U.S. adults: National Health Interview Survey, 2012. National Center for Health Statistics. Vital and Health Statistics, 10(260).

Bland-Stewart, L. M. (2003). Phonetic inventories and phonological patterns of African American two-year-olds: A preliminary investigation. *Communication Disorders Quarterly*, *24*(3), 109–120. doi:10.1177/15257401030240030201

Bledsoe, B. (2009). Understand folk medicine's role in prehospital care of many Mexican Americans. *Journal of Emergency Medical Services*, *12*(34). Retrieved from https://www.jems.com/2009/11/30/understand-folk-medicines-role/

Bopp, K. D., Brown, K. E., & Mirenda, P. (2004). Speech-language pathologists' roles in the delivery of positive behavior support for individuals with developmental disabilities. *American Journal of Speech-Language Pathology*, *13*(1), 5–19. doi:10.1044/1058-0360(2004/003) PMID:15101810

Borella, E., Carretti, B., Cornoldi, C., & De Beni, R. (2020). Working memory training from an individual differences perspective: Efficacy in older adults. In J. M. Novick, M. F. Bunting, M. R. Dougherty, & R. W. Engle (Eds.), *Cognitive and working memory training: Perspectives from Psychology, Neuroscience, and Human Development* (pp. 14–39). New York, NY: Oxford University Press.

Borg, E. (1973). On the neuronal organization of the acoustic middle ear reflex. A physiological and anatomical study. *Brain Research*, *49*(1), 101–123. doi:10.1016/0006-8993(73)90404-6 PMID:4349006

Bowman, B., Comer, J., & Johns, D. (2018). Addressing the African-American achievement gap: Three leading educators issue a call to action. *Young Children*, *73*(2). Retrieved from https://www.naeyc.org/resources/pubs/yc/may2018/achievement-gap

Bracken, B. A., & McCallum, R. S. (2016). Universal Nonverbal Intelligence Test – Second Edition (UNIT-2). Austin, TX: Pro-Ed.

Brice, A. (2002). *The Hispanic child: Speech, language culture, and education.* Boston, MA: Pearson Education.

Brittian, A. S., & Gray, D. L. (2014). African American students' perceptions of differential treatment in learning environments: Examining the moderating role of peer support, connection to heritage, and discrimination efficacy. *Journal of Education, 194*(1), 1–9. doi:10.1177/002205741419400103

Bronfernbrenner, U. (1994). Ecological models of human development. In International Encyclopedia of Education (2nd ed.; vol. 3). Oxford, UK: Elsevier.

Brown Waesche, J. S., Schatschneider, C., Maner, J. K., Ahmed, Y., & Wagner, R. K. (2011). Examining agreement and longitudinal stability among traditional and RTI-based definitions of reading disability using the affected-status agreement statistic. *Journal of Learning Disabilities, 44*(3), 296–307. doi:10.1177/0022219410392048 PMID:21252372

Brown, R. (1973). *A first language: The early stages.* London: George Allen & Unwin. doi:10.4159/harvard.9780674732469

Brussel, S. A., & González-Fernandez, M. (2011). Racial disparities in the development of dysphagia after stroke: Further evidence from the Medicare database. *Archives of Physical Medicine and Rehabilitation, 92*(5), 737–742. doi:10.1016/j.apmr.2010.12.005 PMID:21457943

Burgos, V. (2007, November 14). Mexico-Guatemala: The other border. *Upside Down World.* Retrieved from http://upsidedownworld.org/archives/mexico/mexico-guatemala-the-other-border/

Burkard, A., Johnson, A. J., Madson, M., Pruitt, N. T., Contreras-Tadych, D. A., Kozlowski, J. E. M., ... Knox, S. (2006, July). Supervisor cultural responsiveness and unresponsiveness in cross-cultural supervision. *Journal of Counseling Psychology, 53*(3), 288–301. doi:10.1037/0022-0167.53.3.288

Burke-Harris, N. (2018). *The deepest well: Healing the long-term effects of childhood adversity.* New York: Houghton Mifflin Harcourt.

Burnett, D. M., Kolakowsky-Hayner, S. A., Slater, D., Stringer, A., Bushnik, T., Zafonte, R., & Cifu, D. X. (2003). Ethonographic analysis of traumatic brain injury patients in the national model systems database. *Archives of Physical Medicine and Rehabilitation, 84*(2), 263–267. doi:10.1053/apmr.2003.50091 PMID:12601659

Camarata, S. (2010). Naturalistic intervention for speech intelligibility and speech accuracy. In A. L. Williams, S. McLeod, & R. McCauley (Eds.), *Interventions for speech sound disorders in children* (pp. 381–406). Baltimore, MD: Brookes.

Campbell, T., Dollaghan, C., Needleman, H., & Janosky, J. (1997). Reducing bias in language assessment: Processing-dependent measures. *Journal of Speech, Language, and Hearing Research: JSLHR, 40*(3), 519–526. doi:10.1044/jslhr.4003.519 PMID:9210111

Cannon, J. E., Guardino, C., & Gallimore, E. (2016). A new kind of heterogeneity: What we can learn from d/Deaf and hard of hearing multilingual learners. *American Annals of the Deaf, 161*(1), 8–16. doi:10.1353/aad.2016.0015 PMID:27156914

Carrow-Woolfolk, E. (2011). *Oral and Written Language Scales* (2nd ed.). Torrance, CA: Western Publishing Services.

Casale, M., Mangiacapra, F., Bressi, E., Pace, A., Sabatino, L., Moffa, A., ... Salvinelli, F. (2016). Idiopathic sensorineural hearing loss is associated with endothelial dysfunction. *International Journal of Cardiology Heart & Vasculature, 12,* 32–33. doi:10.1016/j.ijcha.2016.05.001 PMID:28616539

Casalis, S., Colé, P., & Sopo, D. (2004). Morphological awareness in developmental dyslexia. *Annals of Dyslexia, 54*(1), 114–138. doi:10.100711881-004-0006-z PMID:15765006

Cavallo, M. M., & Saucedo, C. (1995). TBI in families from culturally diverse populations. *The Journal of Head Trauma Rehabilitation, 10*(2), 66–77. doi:10.1097/00001199-199504000-00008

Centeno, J. G. (2015). Assessing services with communicatively impaired bilingual adults in culturally and linguistically diverse neurorehabilitation programs. *Journal of Communication Disorders*, *58*, 58–73. doi:10.1016/j.jcomdis.2015.10.005 PMID:26513217

Centeno, J. G., & Ansaldo, A. (2013). Aphasia in multilingual populations. In I. Papathanasious, P. Coppens, & C. Potagas (Eds.), *Aphasia and related neurogenic communication disorders* (pp. 275–294). Boston: Jones and Bartlett.

Centers for Disease Control & Prevention. (2016). *Summary of 2016 national CDC EHDI data*. Retrieved from https://www.cdc.gov/ncbddd/hearingloss/2016-data/01-2016-HSFS-Data-Summary-h.pdf

Centers for Disease Control and Prevention (CDC). (2000a). *Weight-for-age percentiles: Girls, 2 to 20 years*. CDC Growth Charts: United States. Retrieved from https://www.cdc.gov/growthcharts/data/set2/chart-08.pdf

Centers for Disease Control and Prevention (CDC). (2000b). *Stature-for-age percentiles: Girls, 2 to 20 years*. CDC Growth Charts: United States. Retrieved from https://www.cdc.gov/growthcharts/data/set2/chart-08.pdf

Centers for Disease Control and Prevention (CDC). (2016a, February 19). Working together to manage diabetes: A toolkit for pharmacy, podiatry, optometry, and dentistry (PPOD). Retrieved from https://www.cdc.gov/diabetes/ndep/toolkits/ppod.html

Centers for Disease Control and Prevention (CDC). (2016b). United States Diabetes Surveillance System. Retrieved from https://gis.cdc.gov/grasp/diabetes/DiabetesAtlas.html

Centers for Disease Control and Prevention (CDC). (2017). *National Diabetes Statistics Report, 2017*. Atlanta, GA: Centers for Disease Control and Prevention, US Department of Health and Human Services.

Centers for Disease Control and Prevention (CDC). (2018, April 10). Leading causes of death (LCOD) by race/ethnicity, all females-United States, 2015. Retrieved from https://www.cdc.gov/women/lcod/2015/race-ethnicity/index.htm

Centers for Disease Control and Prevention (CDC). (2019). *Adverse childhood experiences*. Retrieved from https://www.cdc.gov/violenceprevention/childabuseandneglect/acestudy/index.html

Centers for Disease Control and Prevention (CDC). (2019). *Data & statistics on Autism Spectrum Disorders*. Retrieved from https://www.cdc.gov/ncbddd/autism/data.html

Centers for Disease Control and Prevention. (2002). Access to healthcare and preventive services among Hispanics and non-Hispanics. *Morbidity and Mortality Weekly Report*, *53*(40), 937–941.

Centers for Disease Control and Prevention. (2008). Work-related injury deaths among Hispanics—United States, 1992–2006. *Morbidity and Mortality Weekly Report*, *57*(22), 597–600. PMID:18528315

Centers for Disease Control and Prevention. (2017). *FastStats: Health of Hispanic or Latino Population*. National Center for Health Statistics.

Centers for Disease Control and Prevention. (2019, June 12). *Complications and treatments of sickle cell disease*. Retrieved from https://www.cdc.gov/ncbddd/sicklecell/treatments.html

Chapman, R. S. (2006). Language learning in Down Syndrome: The speech and language profile compared to adolescents with cognitive impairment of unknown origin. *Down's Syndrome: Research and Practice*, *10*(2), 61–66. doi:10.3104/reports.306 PMID:16869363

Chase, S., Ratcliff, G., Vernich, L., Al-Sukhni, E., Yasseen, B., & Colantonio, A. (2012). Preventive health practices and behavioral risk factors in women surviving traumatic brain injury. *Health Care for Women International*, *33*(7), 631–645. doi:10.1080/07399332.2012.673652 PMID:22681747

Child Welfare Information Gateway. (2016). *Racial disproportionality and disparity in child welfare*. Retrieved from https://www.childwelfare.gov/pubpdfs/racial_disproportionality.pdf

Chung, S. S. M., Ho, E. C. M., Lam, K. S. L., & Chung, S. K. (2003, August). Contribution of polyol pathway to diabetes-induced oxidative stress. *Journal of the American Society of Nephrology*, *14*(8Suppl 3), S233–S236. doi:10.1097/01.ASN.0000077408.15865.06 PubMed

Cicchetti, D., Rogosch, F. A., Maughan, A., Toth, S. L., & Bruce, J. (2003). False belief understanding in maltreated children. *Development and Psychopathology*, *15*(4), 1067–1091. doi:10.1017/S0954579403000440 PMID:14984138

Cichero, J. A. Y., Lam, P., Steele, C. M., Hanson, B., Chen, J., Dantas, R., ... Stanschus, S. (2017). Development of international terminology and definitions for texture-modified foods and thickened fluids used in dysphagia management: The IDDSI framework. *Dysphagia*, *32*(2), 293–314. doi:10.100700455-016-9758-y PMID:27913916

Ciolino, C. (2018). *Language profiles of children who have experienced complex trauma and fetal alcohol spectrum disorders* (Unpublished master's thesis). Western Michigan University, Kalamazoo, MI.

Cobo-Lewis, A. B., Oller, D. K., Lynch, M. P., & Levine, S. L. (1996). Relations of motor and vocal milestones in typically developing infants and infants with Down syndrome. *American Journal of Mental Retardation: AJMR*, *100*(5), 456–467. PMID:8852298

Cohen, J. A., Deblinger, E., Mannarino, A. P., & Steer, R. (2004). A multi-site, randomized controlled trial for children with abuse-related PTSD symptoms. *Journal of the American Academy of Child and Adolescent Psychiatry*, *43*(4), 393–402. doi:10.1097/00004583-200404000-00005 PMID:15187799

Collier, C. (2016). Acculturation Quick Screen-Third Edition (AQS-III). Administration Manual and Scoring Form. Cross Cultural Developmental Education Services.

Collier, C., Brice, A. E., & Oades-Sese, G. V. (2007). Assessment of acculturation. In G. B. Esquivel, E. C. Lopez, & S. Nahari (Eds.), *Handbook of multicultural school psychology: An interdisciplinary perspective* (pp. 353–380). Mahwah, NJ: Lawrence Erlbaum Associates.

Comos-Diaz, L. (2012). *Multicultural care: A clinician's guide to cultural competence*. Washington, DC: American Psychological Association. doi:10.1037/13491-000

Cook, A., Blaustein, M., Spinazzola, J., & Van Der Kolk, B. (2003). *Complex trauma in children and adolescents*. National Child Traumatic Stress Network. Retrieved from http://www.NCTSNet.org

Cook-Benjamin, L. (2001). Portfolio assessment: Benefits, issues of implementation, and reflections on its use. *Assessment Update*, *13*(4), 6–7.

Cortiella, C. (2011). *The state of learning disabilities*. New York, NY: National Center for Learning Disabilities.

Costley, K. C. (2012). *Learners on the move: Responsive teachers fill in the gap for highly mobile students*. Retrieved from http://eric.ed.gov/?id=ED533514

Council for Exceptional Children (CEC). (2019). *CEC professional standards*. Retrieved from: https://www.cec.sped.org/Standards

Counts, J., Katsiyannis, A., & Whitford, D. K. (2018). Culturally and linguistically diverse learners in special education: English Learners. *NASSP Bulletin*, *102*(1), 5–21. doi:10.1177/0192636518755945

Crawford, M. R., Gould, H. J., Smith, W. R., Beckford, N., Gibson, W. R., & Bobo, L. (1991). Prevalence of hearing loss in adults with sickle cell disease. *Ear and Hearing*, *12*(5), 349–351. doi:10.1097/00003446-199110000-00007 PMID:1783238

Creaghead, N. & Marguilies, C. (1982). Evaluating pragmatic skills of verbal and nonverbal children. *Communicative Disorders: A Journal for Continuing Education*, *7*, 73-86.

Culp, R. E., Watkins, R. V., Lawrence, H., Letts, D., Kelly, D. J., & Rice, M. L. (1991). Maltreated children's language and speech development: Abused, neglected, and abused and neglected. *First Language*, *11*(33), 377–389. doi:10.1177/014272379101103305

Curenton, S. (2015). African American preschooler' emotion explanations can provide evidence of their pragmatic skills. *Topics in Language Disorders*, *35*(1), 46–60. doi:10.1097/TLD.0000000000000045

Cuskelly, M., Povey, J., & Jobling, A. (2016). Trajectories of development of receptive vocabulary in individuals with Down syndrome. *Journal of Policy and Practice in Intellectual Disabilities*, *13*(2), 111–119. doi:10.1111/jppi.12151

D'Amato, B., & Quinn, R. (2005). The effects of mentoring on first-year teachers' perceptions of support received. *The Clearing House: A Journal of Educational Strategies, Issues and Ideas*, *78*(3), 110–116. doi:10.3200/TCHS.78.3.110-117

Daggett, A., Logemann, J., Rademaker, A., & Pauloski, B. (2006). Laryngeal penetration during deglutition in normal subjects of various ages. *Dysphagia*, *21*(4), 270–274. doi:10.100700455-006-9051-6 PMID:17216388

Damico, J. S. (1991). Descriptive assessment of communicative ability in limited English proficient students. In E. V. Hamayan & J. S. Damico (Eds.), *Limiting bias in the assessment of bilingual students* (pp. 157–217). Austin, TX: PRO-ED.

Damico, J. S., & Damico, S. K. (1993). Clinical forum: Language and social skills in the school-age population. *Language, Speech, and Hearing Services in Schools*, *24*, 236–243. doi:10.1044/0161-1461.2404.236

Darling, S. M., & Gallagher, P. A. (2004). Needs of and supports for African American and European American caregivers of young children with special needs in urban and rural settings. *Topics in Early Childhood Special Education*, *24*(2), 98–109. doi:10.1177/02711214040240020501

Dar, M., Anwaar, H., Vihman, M., & Keren-Portnoy, T. (2015). Developing an Urdu CDI for early language acquisition in Pakistan. *Journal of Child Speech and Language Studies*, *16*, 12–27.

Daugherty, J. C., Puente, A. E., Fasfous, A. F., Hidalgo-Ruzzante, N., & Pérez-Garcia, M. (2017). Diagnostic mistakes of culturally diverse individuals when using North American neuropsychological tests. *Applied Neuropsychology. Adult*, *24*(1), 16–22. doi:10.1080/23279095.2015.1036992 PMID:27485042

DaVanzo, J. E., Dobson, A., El-Gamil, A., Li, J. W., & Manolov, N. (2014). *Assessment of patient outcomes of rehabilitative care provided in inpatient rehabilitation facilities and after discharge*. Presentation to ARA Research Institute. Retrieved from https://amrpa.org/Portals/0/ARA%20Research%20Institute%20Final%20Dobson%20Da Vanzo%20 Senate%20Briefing%207%2010%2014.pdf

Davis-McFarland, E. (2008). Family and cultural issues in a school swallowing and feeding program. *Language, Speech, and Hearing Services in Schools*, *39*(2), 199–213. doi:10.1044/0161-1461(2008/020) PMID:18420523

De Haan, R., Horn, J., Limburg, M., van der Meulen, J., & Bossuyt, P. (1993). A comparison of 5 stroke scales with measures of disability, handicap, and quality-of-life. *Stroke*, *24*(8), 1178–1181. doi:10.1161/01.STR.24.8.1178 PMID:8342193

De Houwer, A., Bornstein, M. H., & Putnick, D. L. (2014). A bilingual-monolingual comparison of young children's vocabulary size: Evidence from comprehension and production. *Applied Psycholinguistics*, *35*(6), 1189–1211. doi:10.1017/S0142716412000744 PMID:29527076

De Jong, E. J. (2011). *Foundations of multilingualism in education: From principles to practice*. Philadelphia, PA: Caslon Publishing.

De Jong, E. J., & Freeman, R. (2010). Bilingual approaches. In C. Leung & A. Creese (Eds.), *English as an additional language. A reader for teachers working with linguistic minority pupils* (pp. 108–122). UK: Sage publications.

De Jong, E. J., & Harper, C. A. (2011). Accommodating diversity: Pre-service teachers' views on effective practices for English language learners. In T. Lucas (Ed.), *Teacher preparation for linguistically diverse classrooms. A resource for teacher educators*. New York: Routledge.

De Jong, E. J., Harper, C. A., & Coady, M. (2013). Enhanced knowledge and skills for elementary mainstream teachers of English Language Learners. *Theory into Practice*, *52*(2), 89–97. doi:10.1080/00405841.2013.770326

De Lamo White, C., & Jin, L. (2011). Evaluation of speech and language assessment approaches with bilingual children. *International Journal of Language & Communication Disorders*, *46*(6), 613–627. doi:10.1111/j.1460-6984.2011.00049.x PMID:22026564

de Lange, C. (2011, May 5). How sickle-cell carriers fend off malaria. *New Scientist*. Retrieved from https://www.newscientist.com/article/dn20450-how-sickle-cell-carriers-fend-off-malaria/#ixzz68ag80o2F

DeBellis, M. D. (2001). Developmental traumatology: The psychobiological development of maltreated children and its implications for research, treatment and policy. *Development and Psychopathology*, *13*, 537–561. PMID:11523847

DeBellis, M. D., Woolley, D. P., & Hooper, S. R. (2013). Neuropsychological findings in pediatric maltreatment: Relationship of PTSD, dissociative symptoms, and abuse/neglect indices to neurocognitive outcomes. *Child Maltreatment*, *18*(3), 171–183. doi:10.1177/1077559513497420 PMID:23886642

DeBellis, M. D., & Zisk, A. (2014). The biological effects of trauma. *Child and Adolescent Psychiatric Clinics of North America*, *23*(2), 185–222. doi:10.1016/j.chc.2014.01.002 PMID:24656576

Decker, K. B., Vallotton, C. D., & Johnson, H. A. (2012). Parents' communication decision for children with hearing loss: Sources of information and influence. *American Annals of the Deaf*, *157*(4), 326–339. doi:10.1353/aad.2012.1631 PMID:23259352

Demaerschalk, B. M., Kleindorfer, D. O., Adeoye, O. M., Demchuk, A. M., Fugate, J. E., Grotta, J. C., ... Smith, E. E. (2016). Scientific rationale for the inclusion and exclusion criteria for intravenous alteplase in acute ischemic stroke: A statement for healthcare professionals from the American Heart Association/American Stroke Association. *Stroke*, *47*(2), 581–641. doi:10.1161/STR.0000000000000086 PMID:26696642

Dennis, M. S., Lewis, S. C., & Warlow, C. (2005). FOOD trial collaboration. Effect of timing and method of enteral tube feeding for dysphagic stroke patients (FOOD): A multicentre randomised controlled trial. *Lancet*, *365*(9461), 764–772. doi:10.1016/S0140-6736(05)17983-5 PMID:15733717

DeThorne, L. S., & Schaefer, B. A. (2004). A guide to child nonverbal IQ measures. *American Journal of Speech-Language Pathology*, *13*(4), 275–290. doi:10.1044/1058-0360(2004/029) PMID:15719895

Dhingra, L., Ahmed, E., Shin, J., Scharaga, E., & Magun, M. (2015). Cognitive effects and sedation. *Pain Medicine*, *16*(1suppl 1), 37–43. doi:10.1111/pme.12912 PMID:26461075

Di Sante, M., Sylvestre, A., Bouchard, C., & Leblond, J. (2019). The pragmatic language skills of severely neglected 420month old children: Results of the ELLAN study. *Child Maltreatment*, *24*(3), 244–253. doi:10.1177/1077559519828838 PMID:30782015

DiMatteo, M. R. (1994). Enhancing patient adherence to medical recommendations. *Journal of the American Medical Association*, *271*(1), 79–83. doi:10.1001/jama.271.1.79 PMID:8258895

Dispaldro, M., Leonard, L. B., & Deevy, P. (2013). Real-word and nonword repetition in Italian-speaking children with specific language impairment: A study of diagnostic accuracy. *Journal of Speech, Language, and Hearing Research: JSLHR*, *56*(1), 232–336. doi:10.1044/1092-4388(2012/11-0304) PMID:22761319

Dodd, B., & Thompson, L. (2001). Speech disorder in children with Down syndrome. *Journal of Intellectual Disability Research*, *45*(4), 308–316. doi:10.1046/j.1365-2788.2001.00327.x PMID:11489052

Dollaghan, C., & Campbell, T. (1998). Nonword repetition and child language impairment. *Journal of Speech, Language, and Hearing Research: JSLHR*, *41*(5), 1136–1146. doi:10.1044/jslhr.4105.1136 PMID:9771635

Dowd, K. (2019, May 28). Audiology in diabetes care: Merging into PPOD care interprofessional collaboration [Webinar]. Jointly provided by Postgraduate Institute for Medicine and The Audiology Project.

Downs, C. R., Stuart, A., & Holbert, D. (2000). Distortion product otoacoustic emissions in normal-hearing African-American children with homozygous sickle cell disease. *Journal of Communication Disorders*, *33*(2), 111–129. doi:10.1016/S0021-9924(99)00027-1 PMID:10834829

Dreyfus, S. E. (1981). *Dreyfus Model of Skills Acquisition*. Retrieved from: http://www-personal.umich.edu/~mrother/KATA_Files/Dreyfus.pdf

Dunn, D. M. (2018). Peabody Picture Vocabulary Test – Fifth Edition (PPVT-5). Minneapolis, MN: Pearson Education.

Dunn, L. M., & Dunn, D. M. (2007). *Peabody Picture Vocabulary Test-4*. Minneapolis, MN: Pearson.

Dunn, L. M., & Dunn, L. M. (1981). *Peabody Picture Vocabulary Test- Revised*. Circle Pines, MN: American Guidance Service.

Dunn, L. M., & Dunn, L. M. (1997). *Peabody Picture Vocabulary Test-III* (3rd ed.). Circle Pines, MN: American Guidance Service.

Dunn, W. (2014). *Sensory Profile-2*. New York: Pearson.

Dunst, C., & Trivette, C. (2009). Capacity building family systems intervention practices. *Journal of Family Social Work*, *12*(2), 119–143. doi:10.1080/10522150802713322

Earland, J., Gilchrist, M., McFarland, L., & Harrison, K. (2011). Dietetics students' perceptions and experiences of interprofessional education. *Journal of Human Nutrition and Dietetics*, *24*(2), 135–143. doi:10.1111/j.1365-277X.2010.01141.x PMID:21332834

Ebert, K., & Pham, G. (2017). Synthesizing information from language samples and standardized tests in school-age bilingual assessment. *Language, Speech, and Hearing Services in Schools*, *48*(1), 42–65. doi:10.1044/2016_LSHSS-16-0007 PMID:28055056

Edutopia. (2019). *Response to intervention*. Retrieved from https://www.edutopia.org/topic/response-to-intervention

Edwards, A. (2019). Hispanic poverty rate hit an all-time low. Rate dropped to 18.3 percent, down 1.1. points from 2016. *U.S. Census Bureau*. Retrieved at https://www.census.gov/library/stories/2019/02/hispanic-poverty-rate-hit-an-all-time-low-in-2017.html

Elliot, C. D. (2007). *Differential abilities scales* (2nd ed.). San Antonio, TX: The Psychological Corporation.

Ellis Weismer, S., Tomblin, B., Zhang, X., Buckwalter, P., Chynoweth, J., & Jones, M. (2000). Nonword repetition performance in school-age children with and without language impairment. *Journal of Speech, Language, and Hearing Research: JSLHR*, *43*(4), 865–878. doi:10.1044/jslhr.4304.865 PMID:11386474

English, L. H., Wisener, M., & Bailey, H. N. (2018). Childhood emotional maltreatment, anxiety, attachment and mindfulness: Associations with facial emotion recognition. *Child Abuse & Neglect*, *80*, 146–160. doi:10.1016/j.chiabu.2018.02.006 PMID:29605464

Erber, N. (1982). *Auditory training*. Washington, DC: Alexander Graham Bell Association for the Deaf.

Escobar, N. (2018, August 14). Family separation isn't new: U. S. Immigration policy has traumatized migrant children and parents for nearly a century. *The Atlantic*. Retrieved from https://www.theatlantic.com/family/archive/2018/08/us-immigration-policy-has-traumatized-children-for-nearly-100-years/567479/

Etymotic Research. (2001). *QuickSIN test*. Elk Grove Village, IL: Etymotic Research.

Fabbro, F. (2001). The bilingual brain: Bilingual aphasia. *Brain and Language*, *79*(2), 201–210. doi:10.1006/brln.2001.2480 PMID:11712844

Faigle, R., Bahouth, R., Urrutia, V. C., & Gottesman, R. F. (2016). Racial and socioeconomic disparities in gastrostomy tube placement after intracerebral hemorrhage in the United States. *Stroke*, *47*(4), 31–36. doi:10.1161/STROKEAHA.115.011712 PMID:26892281

Fannin, D. (2016). The intersection of culture and ICF-CY personal and environmental factors for alternative and augmentative communication. *Perspectives of the ASHA Special Interest Groups, SIG 12, 1*(3), 63-82.

Farmer, P. (2004). An anthropology of structural violence. *Current Anthropology*, *45*(3), 305–325. doi:10.1086/382250

Farmer, P. (2005). *Pathologies of power. Health, human rights, and the new war on the poor*. Berkeley, CA: University of California Press.

Farrell, A. N., Landry, A. M., Yee, M. E., Leu, R. M., & Goudy, S. L. (2019). Sensorineural hearing loss in children with sickle cell disease. *International Journal of Pediatric Otorhinolaryngology*, *118*, 110114. doi:10.1016/j.ijporl.2018.12.002 PMID:30599285

Fasfous, A. F., Hidalgo-Russante, N., Vilar-López, R., Catena-Martinez, A., & Pérez-Garcia, M. (2013). Cultural differences in neuropsychological abilities related to perform intelligence tasks. *Archives of Clinical Neuropsychology*, *28*(8), 784–790. doi:10.1093/arclin/act074 PMID:24055883

Feder, K. P., Michaud, M., McNamee, J., Fitzpatrick, E., Ramage-Morin, P., & Beauregard, Y. (2017). Prevalence of hearing loss among a representative sample of Canadian children and adolescents, 3 to 19 years of age. *Ear and Hearing*, *38*(1), 7–20. doi:10.1097/AUD.0000000000000345 PMID:27556530

Feldman, P.H., McDonald, M.V., Eimicke, J., & Teresi. (2019). Racial and ethnic health disparities a vulnerable post-stroke home care population. *Journal of Racial and Ethnic Health Disparities, 6*(3), 525-535. https://doi-org.libproxy.uncg.edu/10.1007/s40615-018-00551-y

Feliciano, C. (2018). How family, immigrant group, and school contexts shape ethnic educational disparities. *Ethnic and Racial Studies*, *41*(2), 189–209. doi:10.1080/01419870.2017.1355974

Felitti, V. J., Nordenberg, A. R. F., Williamson, D. F., Spitz, A. M., Edwards, B., Kross, M. P., & Marks, J. S. (1998). Relationship of childhood abuse and household dysfunction to many of the leading causes of death in adults. The Adverse Childhood Experiences (ACE) Study. *American Journal of Preventive Medicine*, *14*(4), 245–258. doi:10.1016/S0749-3797(98)00017-8 PMID:9635069

Fenson, L., Marchman, V. A., Thal, D. J., Dale, P. S., Reznick, J. S., & Bates, E. (2007). *MacArthur-Bates Communicative Development Inventories: User's guide and technical manual* (2nd ed.). Baltimore, MD: Brookes.

Fiestas, C. E., & Pena, E. D. (2004). Narrative discourse in bilingual children: Language and task effects. *Language, Speech, and Hearing Services in Schools, 35*(2), 155–168. doi:10.1044/0161-1461(2004/016)

Figueroa, R. A. (1989). Psychological testing of linguistic-minority students: Knowledge gaps and regulations. *Exceptional Children, 56*(2), 145–153. doi:10.1177/001440298905600206 PMID:2792161

Filho, J. O. (2018). Neuroimaging of acute ischemic stroke. *UpToDate.* Retrieved from https://www.uptodate.com/contents/neuroimaging-of-acute-ischemic-stroke

Fletcher, J. M., Lyon, G. R., Fuchs, L. S., & Barnes, M. A. (2019). *Learning disabilities: From identification to intervention* (2nd ed.). New York, NY: Guilford Press.

Fletcher, J. M., & Miciak, J. (2017). Comprehensive cognitive assessments are not necessary for the identification and treatment of learning disabilities. *Archives of Clinical Neuropsychology, 32*, 2–7.

Fletcher, J. M., Stuebing, K. K., Barth, A. E., Denton, C. A., Cirino, P. T., Francis, D. J., & Vaughn, S. (2011). Cognitive correlates of inadequate response to reading intervention. *School Psychology Review, 40*(1), 3–22. PMID:23125475

Fletcher, J. M., Stuebing, K. K., Morris, R. D., & Lyon, G. R. (2013). Classification and definition of learning disabilities: A hybrid model. In H. L. Swanson, K. R. Harris, & S. Graham (Eds.), *Handbook of learning disabilities*. New York, NY: The Guilford Press.

Flores, A. (2017). How the US Hispanic population is changing. *Pew Research Center*. Retrieved from https://www.pewresearch.org/fact-tank/2017/09/18/how-the-u-s-hispanic-population-is-changing/

Ford, D. Y. (2012). Culturally different students in special education: Looking backward to move forward. *Exceptional Children, 78*(4), 391–405. doi:10.1177/001440291207800401

Fouriea, I., & van Niekerk, D. (2001). Follow-up on the use of portfolio assessment for a module in research information skills: An analysis of its value. *Education for Information, 19*(2), 107–126. doi:10.3233/EFI-2001-19202

Fraser, K., MacKenzie, D., & Versnel, J. (2017). Complex trauma in children and youth: A scoping review of sensory-based interventions. *Occupational Therapy in Mental Health, 33*(3), 199–216. doi:10.1080/0164212X.2016.1265475

Friedman, E. M., Luban, N. L. C., Herer, G. R., & Williams, I. (1980). Sickle cell anemia and hearing. *The Annals of Otology, Rhinology, and Laryngology, 89*(4), 342–349. doi:10.1177/000348948008900409 PMID:7416684

Fudala, J. B., & Stegall, S. (2017). *Arizona Articulation and Phonology Scale* (4th ed.). Torrance, CA: Western Psychological Services.

Fukushima, H., Cureoglu, S., Schachern, P. A., Kusanoki, T., Oktay, M. F., Fukushima, N., ... Harada, T. (2005). Cochlear changes in patients with type 1 diabetes mellitus. *Otolaryngology - Head and Neck Surgery, 133*(1), 100–106. doi:10.1016/j.otohns.2005.02.004 PubMed

Fukushima, H., Cureoglu, S., Schachern, P. A., Paparella, M. M., Harada, T., & Oktay, M. F. (2006). Effects of type 2 diabetes mellitus on cochlear structure in humans. *Archives of Otolaryngology--Head & Neck Surgery, 132*(9), 934–938. doi:10.1001/archotol.132.9.934 PubMed

Gaffney, M., Green, D. R., & Gaffney, C. (2010). Newborn hearing screening and follow-up: Are children receiving recommended services? *Public Health Reports, 125*(2), 199–207. doi:10.1177/003335491012500208 PMID:20297746

Gallaudet Research Institute. (2010). *Annual survey of deaf and hard of hearing children & youth.* Retrieved from https://www.gallaudet.edu/research-support-and-international-affairs/research-support/research-resources/demographics

Gallaudet Research Institute. (2013). *Regional and National Summary Report of Data from the 2011-12 Annual survey of deaf and hard of hearing children and youth.* Washington, DC: GRI, Gallaudet University.

Gallaudet University Laurent Clerc National Deaf Education Center and California School for the Deaf-Riverside. (2018). *The College and Career Readiness for ASL: K-12 Standards.* Washington, DC: Clerc Center, Gallaudet University.

Galtung, J. (1969). Violence, peace, and peace research. *Journal of Peace Research*, *6*(3), 167–191. doi:10.1177/002234336900600301

Gao, S., Kumar, R. G., Wisniewski, S. R., & Fabio, A. (2018). Disparities in health care utilization of adults with TBI are related to insurance, race, and ethnicity: A systematic review. *The Journal of Head Trauma Rehabilitation*, *33*(3), E40–E50. doi:10.1097/HTR.0000000000000338 PMID:28926481

Garcia-Coll, C., Lamberty, C., Jenkins, R., MacAdoo, H., Crnic, K., Wasik, B., & Vasquesz, G. (1996). An Integrative Model for the study of developmental competencies in minority children. *Child Development*, *67*(5), 1891–1914. doi:10.2307/1131600 PMID:9022222

Garcia, H. H., Gonzales, A. E., Tsang, V. C., & Gilman, R. H. (2006). Neurocysticercosis: Some of the essentials. *Practical Neurology*, *6*(5), 288–297. doi:10.1136/jnnp.2006.101253

Garcia, J. M., Chambers, E. T. IV, & Molander, M. (2005). Thickened liquids: Practice patterns of speech-language pathologists. *American Journal of Speech-Language Pathology*, *14*(1), 4–13. doi:10.1044/1058-0360(2005/003) PMID:15962843

Gardner, R. (2002). Cross cultural perspectives in supervision. *The Western Journal of Black Studies*, *26*(2), 98–106.

Gary, K. W., Arango-Lasprilla, J. C., & Stevens, L. F. (2009). Do racial/ethnic differences exist in post-injury outcomes after TBI? A comprehensive review of the literature. *Brain Injury: [BI]*, *23*(10), 775–789. doi:10.1080/02699050903200563 PMID:19697166

Gathercole, S. E., & Alloway, T. P. (2006). Practitioner review: Short-term and working memory impairments in neurodevelopmental disorders: Diagnosis and remedial support. *Journal of Child Psychology and Psychiatry, and Allied Disciplines*, *47*(1), 4–15. doi:10.1111/j.1469-7610.2005.01446.x PMID:16405635

Gauvin, G. M. (2016). *A study of cultural differences on the supervisory process in a graduate school program* (Doctoral dissertation). Retrieved from ProQuest Dissertations and Theses. (UMI 10127526)

Geary, D. C., & Hoard, M. K. (2001). Numerical and arithmetical deficits in learning-disabled children: Relation to dyscalculia and dyslexia. *Aphasiology*, *15*(7), 635–647. doi:10.1080/02687040143000113

Genesee, F. (2016). *At-risk learners and bilingualism: Is it a good idea?* Retrieved from http://www.colorincolorado.org/article/at-risk-learners-and-bilingualism-is-it-a-good

GeneseeF.idea.

Genesee, F., Lindholm-Leary, K., Saunders, W., & Christian, D. (2005). English language learn-ers in U.S. schools: An overview of research findings. *Journal of Education for Students Placed at Risk*, *10*(4), 363–385. doi:10.120715327671espr1004_2

Gerrish, K., Chau, R., Sobowale, A., & Birks, E. (2004). Bridging the language barrier: The use of interpreters in primary care nursing. *Health & Social Care in the Community*, *12*(5), 407–413. doi:10.1111/j.1365-2524.2004.00510.x PMID:15373819

Gillam, R. B., & Pearson, N. (2017). Test of Narrative Language, Second Edition (TNL-2). Austin, TX: Pro-Ed.

Gillam, S., & Justice, L. (2010). Progress monitoring tools for SLPs in response to intervention (RTI): Primary grades. *The ASHA Leader, 9*(21).

Gillam, S., Gillam, R. B., Fargo, J., Olszewski, A., & Segura, H. (2016). Monitoring Indicators of Scholarly Language (MISL): A progress-monitoring instrument for measuring narrative discourse skills. *Communicative Disorders and Deaf Education Faculty Publications. Paper 494*. Retrieved from https://digitalcommons.usu.edu/comd_facpub/494

Gilliam, J. (2006). Gilliam Autism Rating Scale Second Edition GARS-2. Austin, TX: Pro-Ed.

Gillman, A., Winkler, R., & Taylor, N. F. (2017). Implementing the free water protocol does not result in aspiration pneumonia in carefully selected patients with dysphagia: A systematic review. *Dysphagia, 32*(3), 345–361. doi:10.100700455-016-9761-3 PMID:27878598

Ginieri-Coccossis, M., Rotsika, V., Skevington, S., Papaevangelou, S., Malliori, M., Tomaras, V., & Kokkevi, A. (2013). Quality of life in newly diagnosed children with specific learning disabilities (SpLD) and differences from typically developing children: A study of child and parent reports. *Child: Care, Health and Development, 39*(4), 581–591. doi:10.1111/j.1365-2214.2012.01369.x PMID:22372869

Gioia, G. A., Isquith, P. K., Guy, S. C., & Kenworthy, L. (2003). *Behavior Rating Inventory of Executive Function (BRIEF)*. Lutz, FL: PAR, Inc.

Glymour, M., Berkman, L., Ertel, K., Fay, M., Glass, T., & Furie, K. (2007). Lesion characteristics, NIH Stroke Scale, and functional recovery after stroke. *American Journal of Physical Medicine & Rehabilitation, 86*(9), 725–733. doi:10.1097/PHM.0b013e31813e0a32 PMID:17709996

Goh, S. K. Y., & Ng, C. W. (2015). Hard truths about Chinese language policy and planning in Singapore. *Global Chinese, 1*, 267–279.

Goh, S. K. Y., Tham, E. K. H., Magiati, I., Sim, L., Sanmugam, S., Aiu, A., ... Rifkin-Graboi, A. (2017). Analysis of item-level bias in the Bayley-III Language Subscales: The validity and utility of standardized language assessment in a multilingual setting. *Journal of Speech, Language, and Hearing Research: JSLHR, 60*(9), 2663–2671. doi:10.1044/2017_JSLHR-L-16-0196 PMID:28813555

Golden, S. H., Brown, A., Cauley, J. A., Chin, M. H., Gary-Webb, T. L., Kim, C., ... Anton, B. (2012, September). Health disparities in endocrine disorders: Biological, clinical, and nonclinical factors—An Endocrine Society Scientific Statement. *The Journal of Clinical Endocrinology and Metabolism, 97*(9), E1579–E1639. doi:10.1210/jc.2012-2043 PubMed

Goldman, R., & Fristoe, M. (2000). *Goldman-Fristoe Test of Articulation-2*. Circle Pines, MN: American Guidance Service, Inc.

Goldman, R., & Fristoe, M. (2015). *Goldman Fristoe Test of Articulation* (3rd ed.). Bloomington, MN: PsychCorp.

Goldman, R., & Fristoe, M. (2015). *Goldman-Fristoe Test of Articulation* (3rd ed.). Bloomington, MN: NCS Pearson, Inc.

Goldstein, G., & Bebko, J. M. (2003). The profile of multiple language proficiencies: A measure for evaluation language samples of deaf children. *Journal of Deaf Studies and Deaf Education, 4*(8), 452–463. doi:10.1093/deafed/eng027 PMID:15448075

Goldstein, L. B., Bertels, C., & Davis, J. N. (1989). Interrater Reliability of the NIH Stroke Scale. *Archives of Neurology, 46*(6), 660–662. doi:10.1001/archneur.1989.00520420080026 PMID:2730378

Gonzales, R. (2018, June 20). Trumps' executive order on family separation: What it does and doesn't do. *NPR News*. Retrieve from https://www.npr.org/2018/06/20/622095441/trump-executive-order-on-family-separation-what-it-does-and-doesnt-do

González-Frenández, M., Kuhlemeirer, K. V., & Palmer, J. B. (2008). Racial disparities in the development of dysphagia after stroke: Analysis of the California (MIRCal) and New York (SPARCS) inpatient databases. *Archives of Physical Medicine and Rehabilitation, 89*, 1258–1359. PMID:18586139

Gonzalez, L., Stein, G., Kiang, L., & Cupito, A. (2014). The impact of discrimination and support on developmental competencies in Latino adolescents. *Journal of Latina/o Psychology, 2*(2), 79–91. doi:10.1037/lat0000014

Goral, M., & Conner, P. S. (2013). Language disorders in multilingual and multicultural populations. *Annual Review of Applied Linguistics, 33*, 128–161. doi:10.1017/S026719051300010X PMID:26257455

Gould, H. J., Crawford, M. R., Smith, W. R., Beckford, N., Gibson, W. R., Pettie, L., & Bobo, L. (1991). Hearing disorders in sickle cell disease: Cochlear and retrocochlear findings. *Ear and Hearing, 12*(5), 352–354. doi:10.1097/00003446-199110000-00008 PMID:1783239

Gray, C. (2010). *The new social story book.* Arlington, TX: Future Horizons.

Grimes, B. F. (1996). *Ethnologue: Languages of the world.* Dallas, TX: Summer Institute of Linguistics, Inc.

Grosjean, F. (1994). Individual bilingualism. In *The Encyclopedia of Language and Linguistics.* Oxford, UK: Pergamon Press.

Grosjean, F. (2010). *Bilingual life and reality.* Cambridge, MA: Harvard University Press. doi:10.4159/9780674056459

Gross, M., Buac, M., & Kaushanskaya, M. (2014). Conceptual scoring of receptive and expressive vocabulary measures in simultaneous and sequential bilingual children. *American Journal of Speech-Language Pathology, 23*(4), 574–586. doi:10.1044/2014_AJSLP-13-0026 PMID:24811415

Guiberson, M. M., & Rodriguez, B. L. (2013). Classification accuracy of nonword repetition when used with preschool-age Spanish-speaking children. *Language, Speech, and Hearing Services in Schools, 44*(2), 121–132. doi:10.1044/0161-1461(2012/12-0009) PMID:23188260

Guiberson, M. M., Rodriguez, B. L., & Dale, P. S. (2011). Classification accuracy of brief parent report measures of language development in Spanish-speaking toddlers. *Language, Speech, and Hearing Services in Schools, 42*(4), 536–549. doi:10.1044/0161-1461(2011/10-0076) PMID:21844403

Guiberson, M., & Ferris, K. P. (2019). Early language interventions for young dual language learners: A scoping review. *American Journal of Speech-Language Pathology, 28*(3), 945–963. doi:10.1044/2019_AJSLP-IDLL-18-0251 PMID:31398304

Gundykunst, W. B. (1998). *Bridging differences: Effective intergroup communication.* Newbury Park, CA: Sage.

Gupta, S., Bhat, J. S., & Kumar, K. (2015). Subcortical processing of speech in individuals with type 2 diabetes mellitus. *International Journal of Diabetes in Developing Countries, 35*(3), 327–331. doi:10.1007/s13410-015-0299-y

Gutierrez-Clellen, C., & Kreiter, J. (2003). Understanding child bilingual acquisition using parent and teacher reports. *Applied Psycholinguistics, 24*(2), 267–288. doi:10.1017/S0142716403000158

Haas, J. S., & Goldman, L. (1994). Acutely injured patients with trauma in Massachusetts: Differences in care and mortality, by insurance status. *American Journal of Public Health, 84*(10), 1605–1608. doi:10.2105/AJPH.84.10.1605 PMID:7943478

Haffner, S. M., D'Agostino, R., Saad, M. F., Rewers, M., Mykkänen, L., & Selby, J. (1996). Increased insulin resistance and insulin secretion in nondiabetic African-Americans and Hispanics compared with non-Hispanic whites. The Insulin Resistance Atherosclerosis Study. *Diabetes, 45*(6), 742–748. doi:10.2337/diab.45.6.742 PubMed

Haft, S., Duong, P. H., Hp, T., Hendren, R., & Hoeft, F. (2018). Anxiety and attentional bias in children with specific learning disorders. *Journal of Abnormal Child Psychology*. Retrieved from https://link.springer.com/article/10.1007/s10802-018-0458-y

Haider, A. H., Chang, D. C., Efron, D. T., Haut, E. R., Crandall, M., & Cornwell, E. E. (2008). Race and insurance status as risk factors for trauma mortality. *Archives of Surgery*, *143*(10), 945–949. doi:10.1001/archsurg.143.10.945 PMID:18936372

Hallowell, B. (2017). *Aphasia and other acquired neurogenic language disorders: A guide for clinical excellence*. San Diego, CA: Plural Publishing.

Hammer, C., Komaroff, E., Rodriguez, B., Lopez, L., Scarpino, S., & Goldstein, B. (2012). Predicting Spanish-English bilingual children's language abilities. *Journal of Speech, Language, and Hearing Research: JSLHR*, *55*(5), 1251–1264. doi:10.1044/1092-4388(2012/11-0016) PMID:22337497

Hammer, C., Lawrence, F., & Micco, A. (2008). Exposure to English before and after entry into Head Start: Bilingual children's receptive language growth in Spanish and English. *Journal of Bilingual Education and Bilingualism*, *11*(1), 30–56. doi:10.2167/beb376.0 PMID:26430382

Hammer, C., & Rodriguez, B. (2012). Bilingual language acquisition and the child socialization process. In B. Goldstein (Ed.), *Bilingual language development and disorders in Spanish-English speakers* (2nd ed.; pp. 31–46). Baltimore, MD: Paul H. Brookes.

Hammer, C., Rodriguez, B., Davidson, M., Lawrence, F., & Miccio, A. (2011). Changes in language usage of Puerto Rican mothers and their children. Do gender and timing of exposure to English matter? *Applied Psycholinguistics*, *32*(2), 275–297. doi:10.1017/S014271641000041X PMID:23258946

Hanson, M. F., & Gilkerson, D. (1999). Portfolio assessment: More than ABCs and 123s. *Early Childhood Education Journal*, *27*(2), 81–86. doi:10.1023/A:1026044126583

Hao, J., Fu, X., Zhang, C., Zhang, X., Zhao, S., & Li, X. (2017). Early detection of hearing impairment in patients with diabetes mellitus with otoacoustic emission. A systematic review and meta-analysis. *Acta Oto-Laryngologica*, *137*(2), 179–185. doi:10.1080/00016489.2016.1223344 PubMed

Happé, F. (1994). An advanced test of theory of mind: Understanding of story characters' thoughts and feelings by able autistic, mentally handicapped, and normal children and adults. *Journal of Autism and Developmental Disorders*, *24*(2), 129–154. doi:10.1007/BF02172093 PMID:8040158

Harris, J., & Fleming, V. (2009). Toward model-driven interventions for African-Americans with cognitive-communicative disorders. *Seminars in Speech and Language*, *30*(3), 207–216. doi:10.1055-0029-1225957 PMID:19711238

Harris, M. I., Klein, R., Cowie, C. C., Rowland, M., & Byrd-Holt, D. D. (1998, August). Is the risk of diabetic retinopathy greater in non-Hispanic blacks and Mexican Americans than in non-Hispanic whites with type 2 diabetes? A U.S. population study. *Diabetes Care*, *21*(8), 1230–1235. doi:10.2337/diacare.21.8.1230 PubMed

Harrison, P. L., & Oakland, T. (2015). *Adaptive Behavior Assessment System* (3rd ed.). Torrance, CA: Western Psychological Services.

Hays, P. A. (2001). Sorting things out: Culturally responsive assessment. In *Addressing cultural complexities in practice: A framework for clinicians and counselors* (pp. 89–109). Washington, DC: American Psychological Association; doi:10.1037/10411-006

Hays, P. A. (2016). Conducting a culturally responsive assessment. In *Addressing cultural complexities in practice: Assessment, diagnosis, and therapy* (3rd ed.; pp. 127–160). Washington, DC: American Psychological Association; doi:10.1037/14801-007

Hedge, M. N., & Pomaville, F. (2008). *Assessment of communication disorders in children.* San Diego, CA: Plural Publishing.

Heffernan, D. S., Vera, R. M., Monaghan, S. F., Thakkar, R. K., Kolzloff, M. S., Connolly, M. D., ... Cioffi, W. G. (2011). Impact of socioethnic factors on outcomes following traumatic brain injury. *The Journal of Trauma Injury Infection and Critical Care*, *70*(3), 527–534. doi:10.1097/TA.0b013e31820d0ed7 PMID:21610339

Heilmann, J., Miller, J. F., & Dunaway, C. (2010). Properties of the Narrative Scoring Scheme using narrative retells in young school-age children. *American Journal of Speech-Language Pathology*, *19*(2), 154–166. doi:10.1044/1058-0360(2009/08-0024) PMID:20008470

Henderson, D. E., & Restrepo, M. A. (2016, November). *Navajo student's performance on the CELF – 4.* Paper presented at the American Speech-Language-Hearing Association Convention, Philadelphia, PA.

Henderson, D. E., Restrepo, M. A., & Aiken, L. S. (2018). Dynamic assessment of narratives among Navajo preschoolers. *Journal of Speech, Language, and Hearing Research: JSLHR*, *61*(10), 2547–2560. doi:10.1044/2018_JSLHR-L-17-0313 PMID:30304364

Henry, J. (2016). The CTAC in Action. In W. Steele, & C. Malchiodi (Eds.), Trauma-informed practices with children and adolescents (pp. 36 – 40). New York: Routledge.

Henry, J., Richardson, M., Black-Pond, C., Sloane, M., Atchison, B., & Hyter, Y. D. (2011). A grassroots prototype for trauma-informed child welfare system change. *Child Welfare*, *90*(6), 169–186. PMID:22533048

Henry, J., Sloane, M., & Black-Pond, C. (2007). Neurobiology and neurodevelopment of childhood traumatic stress and alcohol exposure. *Language. Speech and Hearing in Schools*, *38*, 99–108. doi:10.1044/0161-1461(2007/010) PMID:17428956

Hernandez, A. E., Dapretto, M., Mazziotta, J., & Bookheimer, S. (2001). Language switching and language representation in Spanish-English bilinguals: An fMRI study. *Neuroimaging*, *14*(2), 510–520. doi:10.1006/nimg.2001.0810 PMID:11467923

Hoepfl, M. (1993). Portfolio assessment. *Technology Teacher*, *53*(2), 28–29.

Hoff, E., Core, C., Place, S., Rumiche, R., Señor, M., & Parra, M. (2012). Dual language exposure and early bilingual development. *Journal of Child Language*, *39*(1), 1–27. doi:10.1017/S0305000910000759 PMID:21418730

Hoffman, H. J., Dobie, R. A., Losonczy, K. G., Themann, C. L., & Flamme, G. A. (2017). Declining prevalence of hearing loss in US adults aged 20 to 69. *JAMA Otolaryngology-Head & Neck Surgery*, *143*(3), 274–285. doi:10.1001/jamaoto.2016.3527 PubMed

Ho, K. (2007). Structural violence as a human rights violation. *Essex Human Rights Review*, *4*(2), 1–17.

Hollebrandse, B., van Hout, A., & Hendriks, P. (2014). Children's first and second-order false belief reasoning in a verbal and a low-verbal task. *Synthese*, *191*(3), 321–333. doi:10.100711229-012-0169-9

Horikawa, C., Kodama, S., Tanaka, S., Fujihara, K., Hirasawa, R., Yachi, Y., ... Sone, H. (2013, January). Diabetes and risk of hearing impairment in adults: A meta-analysis. *The Journal of Clinical Endocrinology and Metabolism*, *98*(1), 51–58. doi:10.1210/jc.2012-2119 PubMed

Horton-Ikard, R., Munoz, M. L., Thomas-Tate, S., & Keller-Bell, Y. (2009). Establishing a pedagogical framework for the multicultural course in communication sciences and disorders. *American Journal of Speech-Language Pathology, 18*(2), 192–206. doi:10.1044/1058-0360(2008/07-0086) PMID:19106206

Hough, R. L., Landsverk, J. A., Karno, M., Burnam, M. A., Timbers, D. M., Escobar, J. I., & Regier, D. A. (1987). Utilization of health and mental health services by Los Angeles Mexican Americans and non-Hispanic whites. *Archives of General Psychiatry, 44*(8), 702–709. doi:10.1001/archpsyc.1987.01800200028005 PMID:3632245

Hudson, B. (2010). *Evaluating and enhancing children's phonological systems: Research and theory to practice.* Wichita, KS: PhonoComp.

Huerta, M., Bishop, S., Duncan, A., Hus, V., & Lord, C. (2012). Application of DSM-5 criteria for autism spectrum disorder to three samples of children with DSM-IV diagnoses of pervasive developmental disorders. *The American Journal of Psychiatry, 169*(10), 1056–1064. doi:10.1176/appi.ajp.2012.12020276 PMID:23032385

Human Rights Watch. (2019, July 11). *US: Family separation harming children, families*. Retrieved from https://www.hrw.org/news/2019/07/11/us-family-separation-harming-children-families

Humbert, I. A., & Robbins, J. (2008). Dysphagia in the elderly. *Physical Medicine and Rehabilitation Clinics of North America, 19*(4), 853–866. doi:10.1016/j.pmr.2008.06.002 PMID:18940645

Hunter, M. (2016). Colorism in the classroom: How skin tone stratifies African American and Latina/o Students. *Theory into Practice, 55*(1), 54–61. doi:10.1080/00405841.2016.1119019

Hwang, W. (2006). The psychotherapy adaptation and modification framework: Application to Asian Americans. *The American Psychologist, 61*(7), 702–715. doi:10.1037/0003-066X.61.7.702 PMID:17032070

Hyter, Y. D. (2010 April). Prenatal alcohol exposure, complex trauma and language outcomes. Seminar presented at the annual conference of the National Black Association of Speech-Language and Hearing, Tampa, FL.

Hyter, Y. D., & Ciolino, C. (2017, November). *Providing SLP services through a trauma informed lens.* Seminar presented at the annual convention of the American Speech-Language-Hearing Association, Los Angeles, CA.

Hyter, Y. D., Henry, J., Sloane, M., Suarez, M., & Ciolino, C. (2018). *The effects of complex trauma and alcohol exposure: The brain, language and skills for daily living*. Short course presented at the Annual Convention of the Michigan Speech-Language-Hearing Association, Kalamazoo, MI.

Hyter, Y.D. (2012). Complex trauma and prenatal alcohol exposure: Clinical implications. *ASHA Perspectives on School-Based Issues, 13*(2), 32 – 42. doi/ doi:10.1044bi13.2.32

Hyter, Y.D., Roman, T.R., Staley, B., & McPherson, B. (2017). Competencies for effective global engagement: A proposal for communication sciences and disorders. *Perspectives of the ASHA Special Interest Groups, SIG 17, 2*(1), 9 – 20.

Hyter, Y. D. (2003). Language intervention for children with emotional and behavioral disorders. *Behavioral Disorders, 29*(1), 65–76. doi:10.1177/019874290302900104

Hyter, Y. D. (2008, January 22). Considering conceptual frameworks in communication sciences and disorders. *ASHA Leader, 13*(1), 30–31. doi:10.1044/leader.FMP.13012008.30

Hyter, Y. D. (2014). Conceptual framework for responsive global engagement in communication sciences and disorders. *Topics in Language Disorders, 34*(2), 103–120. doi:10.1097/TLD.0000000000000015

Hyter, Y. D. (2017). Pragmatic assessment and intervention in children. In L. Cummings (Ed.), *Research in clinical pragmatics* (pp. 493–526). New York: Springer International Publishing. doi:10.1007/978-3-319-47489-2_19

Hyter, Y. D., & Applegate, E. B. (2012). *Assessment of Pragmatic Language and Social Communication (APLSC). Unpublished research version*. Kalamazoo: Western Michigan University.

Hyter, Y. D., & Black-Pond, C. (2005). *Juan and Maria Cell Phone Task: Second order belief attribution script. Unpublished assessment protocol*. Kalamazoo: Western Michigan University.

Hyter, Y. D., Henry, J., Atchison, B., Sloane, M., Black-Pond, C., & Shangraw, K. (2003). Children affected by trauma and alcohol exposure. *ASHA Leader*, *8*(21), 6–14. doi:10.1044/leader.FTR2.08212003.6

Hyter, Y. D., & Jackson, J. J. (2010). *Hyter Pragmatic Protocol Revised: 9 – 15-years old. Unpublished assessment protocol*. Kalamazoo: Western Michigan University.

Hyter, Y. D., Rogers-Adkinson, D. L., Self, T. L., Friederich Simmons, B., & Jantz, J. (2011). Pragmatic language intervention for children with language and emotional/behavioral disorders. *Communication Disorders Quarterly*, *23*(1), 4–16. doi:10.1177/152574010102300103

Hyter, Y. D., Roman, T. R., Staley, B., & McPherson, B. (2017). Competence for effective global engagement: A proposal for communication sciences and disorders. *Perspectives on Global Issues in Communication Sciences and Disorders*, *2*, 9–20.

Hyter, Y. D., & Salace-Provance, M. (2019). *Culturally responsive practices in speech, language, and hearing sciences*. San Diego, CA: Plural Publishing.

Hyter, Y. D., & Salas-Provance, M. B. (2019). *Culturally responsive practices in speech, language and hearing sciences*. San Diego, CA: Plural Publishing.

Hyter, Y., & Salas-Provance, M. (2019). Definitions. In Y. D. Hyter & M. B. Salas-Provance (Eds.), *Culturally responsive practices in speech, language, and hearing sciences* (pp. 15–38). San Diego, CA: Plural Publishing.

IDEA-2004, Individuals with Disabilities Education Act, 20 U.S.C. § 1400 (2004).

Iglesias, A., & Rojas, R. (2012). Bilingual language development of English language learners: Modeling the growth of two languages. In B. Goldstein (Ed.), *Bilingual language development and disorders in Spanish-English speakers* (2nd ed.; pp. 31–46). Baltimore, MD: Paul H. Brookes.

Iluz-Cohen, P., & Walters, J. (2012). Telling stories in two languages: Narratives of preschool children with typical and impaired language. *Bilingualism: Language and Cognition*, *15*(1), 58–74. doi:10.1017/S1366728911000538

Individuals with Disabilities Education Act, 20 u.S.C. § 1400 (2004).

Individuals with Disabilities Education Improvement Act of 2004 (IDEA). (2004). *Public Law 108-446, 108th Congress*. Retrieved from https://sites.ed.gov/idea/

Isaac, K. (2002). *Speech pathology and cultural and linguistic diversity*. London: Whurr.

Ivanova, M. V., & Hallowell, B. (2013). A tutorial on aphasia test development in any langauage: Key substantive and psychometric considerations. *Aphasiology*, *27*(8), 891–920. doi:10.1080/02687038.2013.805728 PMID:23976813

Ivins, B. J., Schwab, K., Warden, D., Harvey, S., Hoilien, M., Powell, C. O., ... Salazar, A. M. (2003). Traumatic brain injury in US army paratroopers: Prevalence and character. *The Journal of Trauma Injury Infection and Critical Care*, *55*(4), 617–621. doi:10.1097/01.TA.0000052368.97573.D4 PMID:14566111

Jalomo, R. Jr. (2000). Assessing minority student performance. *New Directions for Community Colleges*, *112*(112), 7–18. doi:10.1002/cc.11201

Jarger, T. E., Weiss, H. B., Cohen, J. H., & Pepe, P. E. (2000). Traumatic brain injuries evaluated in US emergency departments, 1992-1994. *Academic Emergency Medicine*, *7*(2), 134–140. doi:10.1111/j.1553-2712.2000.tb00515.x PMID:10691071

Johnson, J. K., Miller, S. H., & Horowitz, S. D. (2008). Systems-Based Practice: Improving the safety and quality of patient care by recognizing and improving the systems in which we work. In *Advances in patient safety: New directions and alternative approaches (Vol. 2: Culture and Redesign).* Rockville, MD: Agency for Healthcare Research and Quality (US). Available from https://www.ncbi.nlm.nih.gov/books/NBK43731

Joint Committee on Infant Hearing. (2007). Year 2007 position statement: Principles and guidelines for early hearing detection and intervention programs. *American Academy of Pediatrics*, *120*(4), 898–921. PMID:17908777

Joint Committee on Infant Hearing. (2013). Supplement to the JCIH 2007 position statement: Principles and guidelines for intervention after confirmation that a child is deaf or hard of hearing. *American Academy of Pediatrics*, *131*, 1324–1349. PMID:23530178

Jones, S. (2019, February 4). Trump administration: Reuniting some separated migrant families might be too hard. *Intelligencer*. Retrieved from http://nymag.com/intelligencer/2019/02/hhs-reuniting-separated-migrant-families-hard.html

Jonson Reid, M., Drake, B., Kim, J., Porterfield, S., & Han, L. (2004). A prospective analysis of the relationship between reported child maltreatment and special education eligibility among poor children. *Child Maltreatment*, *9*(4), 382–394. doi:10.1177/1077559504269192 PMID:15538037

Jordan, K. A. (n.d.). *Sensory strategies for classroom sensory avoiders*. Retrieved from https://www.iidc.indiana.edu/styles/iidc/defiles/IRCA/SensoryAvoiders.pdf

Jorge, R. E., Robinson, R. G., Starkstein, S. E., & Arndt, S. (1994). Influence of major depression on 1 year outcome in patients with traumatic brain injury. *Journal of Neurosurgery*, *81*(5), 726–733. doi:10.3171/jns.1994.81.5.0726 PMID:7931619

Kapantzoglou, M., Restrepo, M. A., Gray, S., & Thompson, H. (2015). Language ability groups in bilingual children: A latent profile analysis. *Journal of Speech, Language, and Hearing Research: JSLHR*, *58*(5), 1549–1562. doi:10.1044/2015_JSLHR-L-14-0290 PMID:26200211

Kapantzoglou, M., Restrepo, M. A., & Thompson, M. S. (2012). Dynamic assessment of word learning skills: Identifying language impairment in bilingual children. *Language, Speech, and Hearing Services in Schools*, *43*(1), 81–96. doi:10.1044/0161-1461(2011/10-0095) PMID:22052970

Karanth, P. (2000). Multilingual/multiliterate/multicultural studies of aphasia – the Rosetta Stone of neurolinguistics in the new millennium. *Brain and Language, 71*(1), 113-115.

Karanth, P., Roseberry-McKibbin, C., & James, P. (2017). *Intervention for preschoolers with communication delays: Practical strategies*. San Diego, CA: Plural Publishing, Inc.

Kariya, S., Cureoglu, S., Fukushima, H., Morita, N., Boylan, M. Y., Maeda, Y., ... Paparella, M. M. (2010). Comparing the cochlear spiral modiolar artery in type-1 and type-2 diabetes mellitus: A human temporal bone study. *Acta Medica Okayama*, *64*(6), 375–383. PubMed

Kayle, M., Docherty, S. L., Sloane, R., Tanabe, P., Maslow, G., Pan, W., & Shah, W. N. (2019). Transition to adult care in sickle cell disease: A longitudinal study of clinical characteristics and disease severity. *Pediatric Blood & Cancer*, *66*(1), e27463. doi:10.1002/pbc.27463 PMID:30251318

Kayser, H. (2012). Hispanic and Latino cultures in the United States and Latin America. In D. Battle (Ed.), *Communication disorders in multicultural and international populations* (4th ed.; pp. 102–118). St Louis, MO: Elsevier. doi:10.1016/B978-0-323-06699-0.00015-7

Keller-Bell, Y., & Short, M. (2019). Positive behavioral interventions and supports in schools: A tutorial. *Language, Speech, and Hearing Services in Schools*, *50*(1), 1–15. doi:10.1044/2018_LSHSS-17-0037 PMID:30950772

Kemp, C., & Rasbridge, L. A. (2004). Mexico. In *Refugee and immigrant health: A handbook for health professionals*. Cambridge, UK: Cambridge University Press.

Kenny, B. (2015). Food culture, preferences, and ethics in dysphagia management. *Bioethics*, *29*(9), 646–652. doi:10.1111/bioe.12189 PMID:26481206

Kent, R. D., & Vorperian, H. K. (2013). Speech impairment in Down syndrome: A review. *Journal of Speech, Language, and Hearing Research: JSLHR*, *56*(1), 178–210. doi:10.1044/1092-4388(2012/12-0148) PMID:23275397

Kids Count Data Center (KCDC). (2018). *The number of bilingual kids in America continues to rise*. Retrieved from https://datacenter.kidscount.org/updates/show/184-the-number-of-bilingual-kids-in-america-continues-to-rise?utm_source=eblast&utm_medium=email&utm_campaign=KIDS-COUNT

Kids Count Data Center (KCDC). (2019). *Children who speak a language other than English at home in the United States.* Retrieved on Sep 28th, 2019 online from https://datacenter.kidscount.org/data/tables/81-children-who-speak-a-language-other-than-english-at-home#detailed/1/any/false/871,870,573,869,36,868,867,133,38,35/any/396,397

Kim, M. B., Zhang, Y., Chang, Y., Ryu, S., Choi, Y., Kwon, M. J., ... Cho, J. (2017, April 1). Diabetes mellitus and the incidence of hearing loss: A cohort study. *International Journal of Epidemiology*, *46*(2), 717–726. doi:10.1093/ije/dyw243 PubMed

Kim, M., Pae, S., & Bak, C. (2007). *Assessment of phonology and articulation for children (APAC)*. Inchon, South Korea: Human Brain Research and Consulting Company.

King, D. E., & Bushwick, B. (1994). Beliefs and attitudes of hospital inpatients about faith healing and prayer. *The Journal of Family Practice*, *39*(4), 349–352. PMID:7931113

Kirk, J. K., Bell, R. A., Bertoni, A. G., Arcury, T. A., Quandt, S. A., Goff, D. C. Jr, & Narayan, K. M. (2005). Ethnic disparities: Control of glycemia, blood pressure, and LDL cholesterol among US adults with type 2 diabetes. *The Annals of Pharmacotherapy*, *39*(9), 1489–1501. doi:10.1345/aph.1E685 PubMed

Kirsch, T. (2017). *IPE/IPP in academic and clinical curriculum*. Retrieved from https://caa.asha.org/news/ipeipp-in-academic-and-clinical-curriculum/

Kisser, J., Waldstein, S. R., Evans, M. K., & Zonderman, A. B. (2017). Lifetime prevalence of TBI in a demographically diverse community sample. *Brain Injury: [BI]*, *31*(5), 620–623. doi:10.1080/02699052.2017.1283057 PMID:28326858

Kleinman, A., Eisenberg, L., & Good, B. (1978). Culture, illness, and care: Clinical lessons from anthropologic and cross-cultural research. *Annals of Internal Medicine*, *88*(2), 251–258. doi:10.7326/0003-4819-88-2-251 PMID:626456

Klingner, J. K., & Edwards, P. A. (2006). Cultural considerations with response to intervention models. *Reading Research Quarterly*, *41*(1), 108–117. doi:10.1598/RRQ.41.1.6

Knoors, H., & Marschark, M. (2014). *Teaching deaf learners; psychological and developmental foundations*. New York, NY: Oxford University Press. doi:10.1093/acprof:oso/9780199792023.001.0001

Kohnert, K. (2013). *Language disorders in bilingual children and adults* (2nd ed.). San Diego, CA: Plural Publishing.

Kohnert, K., & Bates, E. (2002). Balancing bilinguals II: Lexical comprehension and cognitive processing in children learning Spanish and English. *Journal of Speech, Language, and Hearing Research: JSLHR*, *45*(2), 347–359. doi:10.1044/1092-4388(2002/027) PMID:12003516

Koidou, I., Kollias, N., Sdravou, K., & Grouios, G. (2013). Dysphagia: A short review of the current state. *Educational Gerontology*, *39*(11), 812–827. doi:10.1080/03601277.2013.766518

Koussi, A., Zafeiriou, D. I., Kontzoglou, G., Tsatra, I., Noussios, G., & Athanassiou, M. (2001). Hearing loss in children with sickle cell disease. *Acta Oto-Rhino-Laryngologica Belgica*, *55*, 235–239. PMID:11685961

Kraemer, R., & Fabiano-Smith, L. (2017). Language assessment of Latino English learning children: A records abstraction study. *Journal of Latinos and Education*, *16*(4), 349–358. doi:10.1080/15348431.2016.1257429

Kraus, J., & McArthur, D. (1996). Epidemiologic Aspects of Brain Injury. *Neuroepidemiology*, *14*(2), 435–450. PMID:8827181

Kreicher, K. L., Weir, F. W., Nguyen, S. A., & Meyer, T. A. (2018). Characteristics and progression of hearing loss in children with Down syndrome. *The Journal of Pediatrics*, *193*, 27–33. doi:10.1016/j.jpeds.2017.09.053 PMID:29174076

Kreutzer, J. S., Marwitz, J. H., Walker, W., Sander, A., Sherer, M., Bogner, J., ... Bushnik, T. (2003). Moderating factors in return to work and job stability after traumatic brain injury. *The Journal of Head Trauma Rehabilitation*, *18*(2), 128–138. doi:10.1097/00001199-200303000-00004 PMID:12802222

Krogstad, J., & Noe-Bustamente. (2019). *7 facts for National Hispanic Heritage Month.* Retrieved from https://www.pewresearch.org/fact-tank/2019/10/14/facts-for-national-hispanic-heritage-month/

Kucik, J. E., Shin, M., Siffel, C., Marengo, L., & Correa, A. (2013). Trends in survival among children with Down syndrome in 10 regions of the United States. *Pediatrics*, *131*(1), e27–e36. doi:10.1542/peds.2012-1616 PMID:23248222

Kumin, L. (2001). Speech intelligibility in individuals with Down syndrome: A framework for targeting specific factors for assessment and treatment. *Down Syndrome Quarterly*, *6*(3), 1-8.

Kummerer, S. E. (2012). Promising strategies for collaborating with Hispanic parents during family-centered speech-language intervention. *Communication Disorders Quarterly*, *33*(2), 84–95. doi:10.1177/1525740109358453

Laing, S., & Kamhi, A. (2003). Alternative assessment of language and literacy in culturally and linguistically diverse populations. *Language, Speech, and Hearing Services in Schools*, *34*(1), 44–55. doi:10.1044/0161-1461(2003/005) PMID:27764486

Langdon, H. (2008). *Assessment and intervention for communication disorders in culturally and linguistically diverse populations*. Clifton Park, NY: Thomson Delmar.

Langdon, H. W. (2015). For parents raising their children bilingually with important messages for those who have children with special needs. *Health Psychology Review*, *3*(2), 1–9.

Langlois, J., Rutland-Brown, W., & Thomas, K. (2004). Traumatic brain injury in the United States, emergency department visits, hospitalizations, and deaths. *Centers for Disease Control and Prevention*. Retrieved from https://www.cdc.gov/traumaticbraininjury/tbi_ed.html

Langmore, S. E., Terpenning, M. S., Schork, A., Chen, Y., Murray, J. T., Lopatin, D., & Loesche, W. (1998). Predictors of aspiration pneumonia: How important is dysphagia? *Dysphagia*, *13*(2), 69–81. doi:10.1007/PL00009559 PMID:9513300

Lazewnik, R., Creaghead, N. A., Smith, A. B., Prendeville, J., Raisor-Becker, L., & Silbert, N. (2019). Identifiers of language impairment for Spanish-English dual learners. *Language, Speech, and Hearing Services in Schools*, *50*(1), 126–137. doi:10.1044/2018_LSHSS-17-0046 PMID:30521665

Leap, W. L. (1993). *American Indian English*. Salt Lake City, UT: University of Utah Press.

Lederberg, A. R., Schick, B., & Spencer, P. E. (2013). Language and literacy development of deaf and hard-of-hearing children: Successes and challenges. *Developmental Psychology*, *49*(1), 15–30. doi:10.1037/a0029558 PMID:22845829

Ledger, S. D. (2002). Reflections on communicating with non-English speaking patients. *British Journal of Nursing (Mark Allen Publishing)*, *11*(11), 773–780. doi:10.12968/bjon.2002.11.11.773 PMID:12070380

Leigh, G., & Crowe, K. (2015). Responding to cultural and linguistic diversity among deaf and hard-of-hearing learnings. In H. Knoors & M. Marschark (Eds.), *Educating deaf learners: Creating a global evidence base* (pp. 68–91). New York, NY: Oxford University Press. doi:10.1093/acprof:oso/9780190215194.003.0004

Leiter, A. E., & Windsor, J. (1996). Compliance of geriatric dysphagic patients with safe swallowing instructions. *Journal of Medical Speech-Language Pathology*, *4*, 289–299.

Lequerica, A., & Krch, D. (2014). Issues of cultural diversity in acquired brain injury (ABI) rehabilitation. *Journal of Neurologic Rehabilitation*, *34*, 645–653. PMID:24796439

Leslie, P., & Coyle, J. (2010). Complex decisions involving gastrostomy feeding tubes: When you're never right or wrong. *Perspectives on Gerontology*, *5*(2), 42–47. doi:10.1044/gero15.2.42

Le, T. H., & Gean, A. D. (2009). Neuroimaging of traumatic brain injury. *The Mount Sinai Journal of Medicine, New York*, *76*(2), 145–162. doi:10.1002/msj.20102 PMID:19306377

Levey, S., Cheng, L.L., & Langdon, H.W. (2013). The relationship between ethical principles and clinical practice in working with culturally and linguistically diverse (CLD) populations: A tutorial. *Speech and Hearing Review: A bilingual Annual, 11*, 77-104.

Li, J., Zhang, Y., Fu, X., Bi, J., Li, Y., Liu, B., & Zhang, L. (2018). Alteration of auditory function in type 2 diabetic and pre-diabetic patients. *Acta Oto-Laryngologica*, *138*(6), 542–547. doi:10.1080/00016489.2017.1422084 PubMed

Linan-Thompson, S., Cirino, P. T., & Vaughn, S. (2007). Determining English Language Learners' Response to Intervention: Questions and some answers. *Learning Disability Quarterly*, *30*(3), 185–195. doi:10.2307/30035563

Lind, D. (2019, June 25). *The horrifying conditions facing kids in the border detention, explained*. Retrieved from https://www.vox.com/policy-and-politics/2019/6/25/18715725/children-border-detention-kids-cages-immigration

Linden, M., & Redpath, S. (2011). A comparative study of nursing attitudes towards young male survivors of brain injury: A questionnaire survey. *International Journal of Nursing Studies*, *48*(1), 62–69. doi:10.1016/j.ijnurstu.2010.05.011 PMID:20965077

Lin, F. R., & Ferruci, L. (2012). Hearing loss among older adults in the United States. *Archives of Internal Medicine*, *172*(4), 369–371. doi:10.1001/archinternmed.2011.728 PubMed

Lisowska, G., Namysłowski, G., Morawski, K., & Strojek, K. (2001). Cochlear dysfunction and diabetic microangiopathy. *Scandinavian Audiology. Supplementum*, *52*(1), 199–203. doi:10.1080/010503901300007524 PubMed

Livingston, G., Minushkin, S., & Cohn, D. (2008). Hispanics and healthcare in the US: Access, information, and knowledge. *Pew Research Center*. Retrieved from https://www.pewhispanic.org/2008/08/13/hispanics-and-health-care-in-the-united-states-access-information-and-knowledge/

Livingston, G., & Kahn, J. R. (2002). An American dream unfulfilled: The limited mobility of Mexican Americans. *Social Science Quarterly*, *83*(4), 1003–1012. doi:10.1111/1540-6237.00129

Lo, L., & Hiatt-Michael, D. (2014). *Promising practices to empower culturally and linguistically diverse families of children with disabilities*. Charlotte, NC: Information Age Publishing.

Lorenzen, B., & Murray, L. (2008). Bilingual aphasia: A theoretical and clinical review. *American Journal of Speech-Language Pathology*, *17*(3), 299–317. doi:10.1044/1058-0360(2008/026) PMID:18663112

Losen, D., Hodson, C., Ee, J., & Martinez, T. (2014). Disturbing inequities: Exploring the relationship between racial disparities in special education identification and discipline. *The Journal of Applied Research on Children*, *5*(2). Retrieved from https://digitalcommons.library.tmc.edu/childrenatrisk/vol5/iss2/15/

Loveall, S. J., Channell, M. M., Phillips, B. A., Abbeduto, L., & Conners, F. A. (2016). Receptive vocabulary analysis in Down syndrome. *Research in Developmental Disabilities*, *55*, 161–172. doi:10.1016/j.ridd.2016.03.018 PMID:27084992

Lovelace, S., & Stewart, S. R. (2009). Effects of robust vocabulary instruction and multicultural text on the development of word knowledge among African American children. *American Journal of Speech-Language Pathology*, *18*(2), 168–179. doi:10.1044/1058-0360(2008/08-0023) PMID:19106209

Lovelace, T. S., Tamayo, S., & Robertson, R. E. (2018). Experiences of African American mothers of sons with autism spectrum disorder: Lessons for improving service delivery. *Education and Training in Autism and Developmental Disabilities*, *53*(1), 3–16.

Low, J., Wyles, C., Wilkinson, T., & Sainsbury, R. (2001). The effect of compliance outcomes for patients with dysphagia on videofluoroscopy. *Dysphagia*, *12*(2), 123–127. doi:10.1007004550011002 PMID:11305222

Luckner, J. L., & Bowen, S. (2006). Assessment practices of professionals serving students who are deaf or hard of hearing: An initial investigation. *American Annals of the Deaf*, *151*(4), 410–417. doi:10.1353/aad.2006.0046 PMID:17225635

Ludwig, D., & Kerins, M (2019). Interprofessional education: Application of interprofessional education collaborative core competencies to school settings. *Perspectives of the ASHA Special Interest Groups, SIG 2, 1*(3), 1-6.

Lujan, J. (2010). Meeting religious needs of Hispanic clients to provide culturally competent care. *The Internet Journal of Allied Health Sciences and Practice*, *8*(2), 4.

Luke, N., & Banerjee, R. (2013). Differential associations between childhood maltreatment experiences and social understanding: A meta-analysis and systemic review. *Developmental Review*, *33*(1), 1–28. doi:10.1016/j.dr.2012.10.001

Lynch, E. W., & Hanson, M. J. (2011). *Developing cross-cultural competence: A guide for working with children and their families* (4th ed.). Baltimore, MD: Paul H Brookes Publishing.

Lynch, E. W., & Hanson, M. J. (2011). *Developing cross-cultural competence: A guide for working with young children and their families* (4th ed.). Baltimore, MD: Paul H. Brookes.

MacDonald, C. B., Bauer, P. W., Cox, L. C., & McMahon, L. (1999). Otologic findings in pediatric cohort with sickle cell disease. *International Journal of Pediatric Otorhinolaryngology*, *47*(1), 23–28. doi:10.1016/S0165-5876(98)90152-5 PMID:10206391

Ma, E., Threats, T., & Worrall, L. (2008). An introduction to the International Classification of Functioning, Disability, and Health for speech-language pathology. *International Journal of Speech-Language Pathology*, *10*(1-2), 2–8. doi:10.1080/14417040701772612

Maguire-Jack, K., Lanier, P., & Lombardi, B. (2019). Investigating racial differences in clusters of adverse childhood experiences. *The American Journal of Orthopsychiatry*; Advance online publication. doi:10.1037/ort0000405 PMID:30816722

Maki, K. E., & Adams, S. R. (2018). A current landscape of specific learning disability identification: Training, practices, and implications. *Psychology in the Schools*, *56*(1), 18–31. doi:10.1002/pits.22179

Maki, K. E., Floyd, R. G., & Roberson, T. (2015). State learning disability eligibility criteria: A comprehensive review. *School Psychology Quarterly*, *30*(4), 457–469. doi:10.1037pq0000109 PMID:25581001

Malchiodi, C. A. (2005). Expressive therapies: History, theory, and practice. In C. A. Malchiodi (Ed.), *Expressive therapies* (pp. 1–15). New York: Guilford Publications.

Maloney, J., & Walsh, M. (2019). Managing and supporting quality-of-life in dysphagia: A survey of clinical practice patterns and perspectives in the UK, Ireland, and South Africa. *International Journal of Communication Disorders*, *54*(1), 41–49. doi:10.1111/1460-6984.12429 PMID:30362200

Manarino, A. P., Cohen, J. A., Deblinger, E., Runyon, M. K., & Steer, R. A. (2012). Trauma focused cognitive-behavioral therapy for children: Sustained impact of treatment 6 and 12 months later. *Child Maltreatment*, *17*(3), 231–241. doi:10.1177/1077559512451787 PMID:22763575

Mann, W., Pena, E. D., & Morgan, G. (2014). Exploring the use of dynamic language assessment with deaf children, who use American Sign Language: Two case studies. *Journal of Communication Disorders*, *52*, 16–30. doi:10.1016/j.jcomdis.2014.05.002 PMID:24908340

Marik, P. E., & Kaplan, D. (2003). Aspiration pneumonia and dysphagia in the elderly. *Chest*, *124*(1), 328–336. doi:10.1378/chest.124.1.328 PMID:12853541

Marks, A., & Garcia-Coll, C. (2018, December). (201). Education and developmental competencies of ethnic minority children: Recent theoretical and methodological advances. *Developmental Review*, *50*, 90–98. doi:10.1016/j.dr.2018.05.004

Marquardt, T. P., & Gillam, R. B. (1999). Assessment in communication disorders: Some observations on current issues. *Language Testing*, *16*(3), 249–269. doi:10.1177/026553229901600302

Martinez, O., Wu, E., Sandfort, T., Dodge, B., Carballo-Dieguez, A., Pinto, R., ... Chavez-Baray, S. (2015). Evaluating the impact of immigration policies on health status among undocumented immigrants: A systematic review. *Journal of Immigrant and Minority Health*, *17*(3), 947–970. doi:10.100710903-013-9968-4 PMID:24375382

Martin, N., & Brownell, R. (2011). *Expressive One Word Picture Vocabulary Test* (4th ed.). Novato, CA: Academic Therapy Publications.

Masten, A. S. (2012). Risk and resilience in the educational success of homeless and highly mobile children: Introduction to the special section. *Educational Researcher*, *41*(9), 363–365. doi:10.3102/0013189X12467366

Masten, A. S., Cutuli, J. J., Herbers, J. E., Hinz, E., Obradovic, J., & Wenzel, A. J. (2014). Academic risk and resilience in the context of homelessness. *Child Development Perspectives*, *8*(4), 201–206. doi:10.1111/cdep.12088 PMID:29623104

Masten, A. S., Fiat, A. E., Labella, M. H., & Strack, R. A. (2015). Educating homeless and highly mobile students: Implications of research on risk and resilience. *School Psychology Review*, *44*(3), 315–330. doi:10.17105pr-15-0068.1

Matthew, D. B., Rodrigue, E., & Reeves, R. V. (2016). *Time for justice: Tackling race inequalities in health and housing. Report.* Washington, DC: Brookings. Retrieved from https://www.brookings.edu/research/time-for-justice-tackling-race-inequalities-in-health-and-housing/

McCarthy, M. P., & Staub, K. J. (2008). Will you be my CF mentor? *Perspectives on Administration and Supervision*. Retrieved from: https://pubs.asha.org/doi/full/10.1044/aas18.3.82

McCloskey, G., Perkins, L. A., & Van Diner, B. (2009). *Assessment and intervention for executive function difficulties*. New York: Routledge.

McCready, V. (2011). Generational issues in supervision and administration. *The ASHA Leader, 16*, 12–15. doi:10:1044/leader FTR1.6052011.12

McCrea, E., & Brasseur, J. (2020). *The supervisory process in speech-language pathology and audiology*. Thorafare, NJ: Slack, Incorporated.

McFarland, J. (2016, February 18). *Diversity in home languages: Examining English learners in public schools*. Retrieved from https://nces.ed.gov/blogs/nces/post/diversity-in-home-languages-examining-english-learners-in-u-s-public-schools

McNeiley, L. (2018). Using the International Classification of Functioning, Disability, and Health framework to achieve interprofessional functional outcomes for young children: A speech-language pathology perspective. *Pediatric Clinics of North America, 65*(1), 125–134. doi:10.1016/j.pcl.2017.08.025 PMID:29173712

Meadow-Orlans, K. P., Sass-Lehrer, M., & Mertens, D. M. (2003). *Parents and their deaf children: The early years*. Washington, DC: Gallaudet University Press.

Meagher, A. D., Beadles, C. A., Doorey, J., & Charles, A. G. (2015). Racial and ethnic disparities in discharge to rehabilitation following traumatic brain injury. *Journal of Neurosurgery, 122*(3), 595–601. doi:10.3171/2014.10.JNS14187 PMID:25415069

Meinzen-Derr, J., Wiley, S., Creighton, J., & Choo, D. (2007). Auditory skills checklist: Clinical tool for monitoring functional auditory skill development in young children with cochlear implants. *The Annals of Otology, Rhinology, and Laryngology, 116*(11), 812–818. doi:10.1177/000348940711601104 PMID:18074665

Mener, D. J., Betz, J., Genther, D. J., Chen, D., & Lin, F. R. (2013). Hearing loss and depression in older adults. *Journal of the American Geriatrics Society, 61*(9), 1627–1629. Available https://www.ncbi.nlm.nih.gov/pmc/articles/PMC3773611 doi:10.1111/jgs.12429 PubMed

Migration Policy Institute. (2016). *ELL information center*. Retrieved from http://www.migrationpolicy.org/programs/ell-information-center

Miller, K. (2018) *Perceptions of speech-language pathologists in clinical fellowships* (Unpublished doctoral dissertation). Nova Southeastern University, Fort Lauderdale, FL.

Miller, J. F., Andriacchi, K., & Nockerts, A. (2012). *Assessing Language Production Using SALT Software: A Clinician's Guide to Language Sample Analysis*. Middleton, WI: Salt Software, LLC.

Miller, J. M., & Dengerink, H. (1988, November-December). Control of inner ear blood flow. *American Journal of Otolaryngology, 9*(6), 302–316. doi:10.1016/S0196-0709(88)80038-3 PMID:3067593

Minke, K. M., Sheridan, S. M., Kim, E. M., Ryoo, J. H., & Koziol, N. A. (2014). Congruence in parent-teacher relationships. *The Elementary School Journal, 114*(4), 527–546. doi:10.1086/675637

Mitchell, R. E., & Karchmer, M. A. (2004). Chasing the mythical ten percent: Parental hearing status of deaf and hard of hearing students in the United States. *Sign Language Studies, 4*(2), 138–163. doi:10.1353ls.2004.0005

Moeller, M. P., Carr, G., Seaver, L., Stredler-Brown, A., & Holzinger, D. (2013). Best practices in family-centered early intervention for children who are deaf or hard of hearing: An international consensus statement. *Journal of Deaf Studies and Deaf Education*, *18*(4), 429–445. doi:10.1093/deafed/ent034 PMID:24030911

Montes-Jovellar, L., Carrillo, A., Muriel, A., Barbera, R., Sanchez, F., & Cobeta, I. (2019). Translation and validation of the MD Anderson Dysphagia Inventory (MDADI) for Spanish-speaking patients. *Head & Neck*, *41*, 122–129. doi:10.1002/hed.25478 PMID:30549341

Moore, B., & Montgomery, J. K. (2018). *Making a difference for America's children: Speech-language pathologists in public schools* (3rd ed.). Austin, TX: Pro-Ed.

Moore, R. (2012). Supervision and multicultural issues: Supervisors and supervisees. *Perspectives on Administration and Supervision*, *22*(1), 33–39. doi:10.1044/aas22.1.33

Moreno, J. M., Garcia-Baamonde, M. E., & Blazquez, M. (2010). Desarrollo linguistico y adaptacion escolar en ninos en acogimiento residencial [Linguistic development and adaptation in children in residential care]. *Anales de Psicología*, *26*, 189–196.

Moreno-Manso, J. M., Garcia-Baamonde, M. E., Blazquez-Alonso, M., Pozueco-Romero, J. M., & Godoy-Merino, M. J. (2016). Social communication disorders and social cognitive attitudes in victims of child abuse. *Journal of Child and Family Studies*, *25*(1), 241–250. doi:10.100710826-015-0192-9

Morgan, P. L., Farkas, G., Hillemeier, M. M., Mattison, R., Maczuga, S., Li, H., & Cook, M. (2015). Minorities are disproportionately underrepresented in special education: Longitudinal across five disability conditions. *Educational Researcher*, *44*(5), 278–292. doi:10.3102/0013189X15591157 PMID:27445414

Morgan, P. L., Hammer, C. S., Farkas, G., Hillemeier, M. M., Maczuga, S., Cook, M., & Morano, S. (2016). Who receives speech/language services by 5 years of age in the United States? *American Journal of Speech-Language Pathology*, *25*(2), 183–199. doi:10.1044/2015_AJSLP-14-0201 PMID:26579989

Morganstein, K. M., & Manace, E. D. (1969). Temporal bone histopathology in sickle cell disease. *Laryngoscope*, *79*(12), 2172–2180. doi:10.1288/00005537-196912000-00013 PMID:5362685

Mothes, L., Kristensen, C. H., Grassi-Oliveira, R., Fonseca, R. P., de Lima Argimon, I. I., & Irigaray, T. Q. (2015). Childhood maltreatment and executive functions in adolescents. *Child and Adolescent Mental Health*, *20*(1), 56–62. doi:10.1111/camh.12068

Muir, K. W., Weir, C. J., Murray, G. D., Povey, C., & Lees, K. R. (1996). Comparison of neurological scales and scoring systems for acute stroke prognosis. *Stroke*, *27*(10), 1817–1820. doi:10.1161/01.STR.27.10.1817 PMID:8841337

Mulkey, P., Lacock, M., & Scott, K. (2004). *Guidelines for Healthcare Providers Interacting with American Indian Patients and Their Families*. Chicago, IL: Metropolitan Chicago Healthcare Council.

Murphy, J., & Busch, Z. (2015, August 5). *CAFTA-DR Notches 10-year record of success*. Retrieved from https://www.uschamber.com/issue-brief/cafta-dr-notches-10-year-record-success

Myer, M. (1969). *Frog, where are you?* New York: Dial Press.

Myers, P., & Hammill, D. (1976). *Methods for learning disorders*. New York, N.Y.: Wiley.

Naniwadekar, K. (2018). Stress and anxiety among parents of children with communication disorders. In *Handbook of research on psychosocial perspectives of human communication disorders* (pp. 141–156). Hershey, PA: Information Science Publishing/IGI Global. doi:10.4018/978-1-5225-4955-0.ch008

National Alliance for Hispanic Health. (2004). *Delivering preventive health care to Hispanics: A manual for providers.* US Department of Health and Human Services, Health Resources and Services Administration.

National Association of Social Workers. (2012). *NASW Standards for School Social Work Services.* Available at https://www.socialworkers.org/LinkClick.aspx?fileticket=1Ze4-9Os7E%3D&portalid=0

National Center for Education Statistics. (2018). *Table 204.30. Children 3-21 years old served under Individuals with Disabilities Education Act, Part B, by type of disability: Selected years, 1976-77 through 2011-12.* Retrieved from https://nces.ed.gov/programs/digest/d13/tables/dt13_204.30.asp

National Center for Education Statistics. (2019). *English language learners in public schools.* Retrieved from https://nces.ed.gov/programs/coe/indicator_cgf.asp

National Center for Education Statistics. (2019, May). *English language learners in public schools.* Retrieved from https://nces.ed.gov/programs/coe/indicator_cgf.asp

National Center for Health Statistics. (2008). *Trends in the health of Americans.* Department of Health and Human Services, National Center for Health Statistics. Retrieved from https://www.cdc.gov/nchs/data/hus/hus08.pdf

National Center for Homeless Education at SERVE. (2015). *Navigating the intersections of the Mckinney-Vento Act and Individuals with Disabilities Education Act: Coordination to help homeless children and youth with disabilities. Best practices in homeless education brief series.* Retrieved from http://www.nclive.org/cgi-bin/nclsm?url=http://search.ebscohost.com/login.aspx?direct=true&db=eric&AN=ED574610&site=ehost-live

National Center for Homelessness. (2019). *Federal data summary: School years 2014-15 to 2016-17.* Retrieved from https://nche.ed.gov/wp-content/uploads/2019/02/Federal-Data-Summary-SY-14.15-to-16.17-Final-Published-2.12.19.pdf

National Child Traumatic Stress Network (NCTSN). (2016). *Complex trauma.* Retrieved from http://www.nctsn.org/trauma-types/complex-trauma

National Child Traumatic Stress Network (NTCSN). (n.d.). *Complex trauma.* Retrieved from https://www.nctsn.org/what-is-child-trauma/trauma-types/complex-trauma

National Heart, Lung, and Blood Institute. (2019). *Sickle cell disease.* Retrieved from https://www.nhlbi.nih.gov/health-topics/sickle-cell-disease

National Institute on Deafness and Other Communication Disorders. (2015). Quick statistics. Retrieved from www.nidcd.nih.gov/health/statistics/Pages/quick.aspx

National Institute on Deafness and Other Communication Disorders. (2019). *Aphasia.* Retrieved from https://www.nidcd.nih.gov/health/aphasia

National Scientific Council on the Developing Child. (2012). *The science of neglect: The persistent absence of responsive care disrupts the developing brain: Working paper 12.* Retrieved from https://developingchild.harvard.edu/resources/the-science-of-neglect-the-persistent-absence-of-responsive-care-disrupts-the-developing-brain/

Nguyen, H. T., Evans, M., & Zonderman, A. B. (2004). Poverty and self-reported mental disorders: Findings from the healthy aging in neighborhoods of diversity across the life span study (HANDLS). *Annals of Epidemiology*, *17*(9), 736. doi:10.1016/j.annepidem.2007.07.042

Nichols, H. (2019, July 4). *The top 10 leading causes of death in the United States.* Retrieved from https://www.medicalnewstoday.com/articles/282929.php

Niemeier, J., & Carlos Arango-Lasprilla, J. (2007). Toward improved rehabilitation services for ethnically diverse survivors of traumatic brain injury. *The Journal of Head Trauma Rehabilitation*, *22*(2), 75–84. doi:10.1097/01.HTR.0000265095.06565.7b PMID:17414309

Nightengale, E., Yoon, P., Wolter-Warmerdam, K., Daniels, D., & Hickey, F. (2017). Understanding hearing and hearing loss in children with Down syndrome. *American Journal of Audiology*, *26*(3), 301–308. doi:10.1044/2017_AJA-17-0010 PMID:28854301

Noe-Bustamente, L. (2019). *Key facts about U.S. Hispanics and their diverse heritage*. Retrieved from https://www.pewresearch.org/fact-tank/2019/09/16/key-facts-about-u-s-hispanics/

Norman, M. A., Moore, D. J., Taylor, M., Franklin Jr, D., Cysique, L., & Ake, C. (2011). Demographically corrected norms for African Americans and Caucasians on the Hopkins Verbal Learning Test–Revised, brief visuospatial memory test–revised, stroop color and word test, and Wisconsin card sorting test 64-card version. *Journal of Clinical and Experimental Neuropsychology, 33*(7), 793-804.

Office of Minority Health U.S. Department of Health and Human Sciences. (2016, July 13). Diabetes and African Americans. Retrieved from https://minorityhealth.hhs.gov/omh/browse.aspx?lvl=4&lvlid=18

Office of Minority Health U.S. Department of Health and Human Sciences. (2017, August 25) Obesity and African Americans. Retrieved from https://minorityhealth.hhs.gov/omh/browse.aspx?lvl=4&lvlID=25

Office of the U.S. Trade Representative. (2004, February). *Putting CAFTA into perspective: Fact sheet on agriculture*. Retrieved from https://ustr.gov/about-us/policy-offices/press-office/fact-sheets/archives/2004/february/putting-cafta-perspective-fact-sheet-agricu

Ogura, T., Watamaki, T., & Inaba, T. (2016). *The Japanese MacArthur-Bates Communicative Development Inventories*. Kyoto: Nakanishiya Co.

Olivos, E. M., Gallagher, R. J., & Aguilar, J. (2010). Fostering collaboration with culturally and linguistically diverse families of children with moderate to severe disabilities. *Journal of Educational & Psychological Consultation*, *20*(1), 28–40. doi:10.1080/10474410903535372

Oller, D., & Eilers, R. (2002). *Language and literacy in bilingual children*. Tonawanda, NY: Multilingual Matters. doi:10.21832/9781853595721

Oller, J. W. Jr. (1979). *Language tests at school*. Longman Group UK Limited.

Oller, J. W. Jr. (1997). Monoglottosis: What's wrong with the idea of the IQ meritocracy and its racy cousins? *Applied Linguistics*, *18*(4), 467–507. doi:10.1093/applin/18.4.467

Oller, J. W. Jr, Kim, K., & Choe, Y. (2000). Testing verbal (language) and non-verbal abilities in language minorities: A socio-educational problem in historical perspective. *Language Testing*, *17*(3), 341–360. doi:10.1177/026553220001700304

Oller, J. W. Jr, Kim, K., Choe, Y., & Jarvis, L. H. (2001). Testing relations between language (verbal) and nonverbal abilities in children and adults acquiring a nonprimary language. *Language Testing*, *18*(1), 33–54. doi:10.1177/026553220101800102

Olswang, L. B., Coggins, T. E., & Timler, G. R. (2001). Outcome measures for school-age children with social communication problems. *Topics in Language Disorders*, *21*(4), 50–73. doi:10.1097/00011363-200111000-00006

Olusanya, B. O., Luxon, L. M., & Wirz, S. L. (2004). Benefits and challenges of newborn hearing screening for developing countries. *International Journal of Pediatric Otorhinolaryngology*, *68*(3), 287–305. doi:10.1016/j.ijporl.2003.10.015 PMID:15129939

Olver, J. H., Ponsford, J. L., & Curran, C. (1996). Outcome following traumatic brain injury: A comparison between 2 and 5 years after injury. *Brain Injury: [BI]*, *10*(11), 841–848. doi:10.1080/026990596123945 PMID:8905161

Ong, S., Talan, D. A., Moran, G. J., Mower, W., Newdew, M., Tsang, V. C. W., & Pinner, R. W. (2002). Neurcysticercosis in radiography imaged seizure patients in US emergency departments. *Emerging Infectious Diseases*, *8*(6), 608–612. doi:10.3201/eid0806.010377 PMID:12023918

Ooi, C. C.-W., & Wong, A. M.-Y. (2012). Assessing bilingual Chinese – English young children in Malaysia using language sample measures. *International Journal of Speech-Language Pathology*, *14*(6), 499–508. doi:10.3109/17549507.2012.712159 PMID:23039126

Oommen, K. J. (2004). *Neurological history and physical examination*. Retrieved from https://emedicine.medscape.com/article/1147993-overview

Ortega, D. M., Graybill, L., & Lasch, C. N. (2015). Enacting and sustaining trauma and violence through policy enforcement: Family immigration detention. *Journal of Women and Social Work*, *30*(3), 281–285. doi:10.1177/0886109915595190

Orttman, J. M., Velkoff, V. A., & Howard, H. (2014). An Aging Nation: The Older Population in the United States Population Estimates and Projections Current Population Reports. *United States Census Bureau*. Retrieved from https://www.census.gov/prod/2014pubs/p25-1140.pdf

Otoacoustics Emissions Portal. (2012, December 17). Concepts of DPOAEs. Retrieved from https://www.otoemissions.org/index.php/en/basics-of-oaes/dpoaes/14-concepts-of-dpoaes

Ovando, C. (2008). Acculturation. In J. M. Gonzalez (Ed.), *Encyclopedia of bilingual education* (pp. 9–10). Thousand Oaks, CA: Sage.

Owens, R. E. (2020). *Language development: An introduction* (10th ed.). New York: Pearson Education.

Owens, R. E. Jr, Meta, D. E., & Haas, A. (2002). *Communication disorders: A life span perspective*. New York, NY: Pearson Education.

Padilla, A. H., Palmer, P. M., & Rodriguez, B. L. (2019). The relationship between culture, quality of life and stigma in Hispanic New Mexicans with dysphagia: A preliminary investigation using quantitative and qualitative analysis. *American Journal of Speech-Language Pathology*, *28*(2), 1–16. doi:10.1044/2018_AJSLP-18-0061 PMID:31136241

Pae, S., & Kwak, K. C. (2011). *Korean MacArthur-Bates Communicative Development Inventories (K M-B CDI)*. Seoul: Mindpress.

Palafox, P. L. (2017). The unique speech needs of children in poverty. *ASHA Leader*, *22*(3), 30–31. doi:10.1044/leader.SCM.22032017.30

Palardy, J. M. (1994). Theoretical underpinning of portfolio assessment. *Journal of Instructional Psychology*, *21*(1), 90–93.

Palisano, R. J., Walter, S. D., Russell, D. J., Rosenbaum, P. L., Gemus, M., Galuppi, B. E., & Cunningham, L. (2001). Gross motor function of children with Down syndrome: Creation of motor growth curves. *Archives of Physical Medicine and Rehabilitation*, *82*(4), 494–500. doi:10.1053/apmr.2001.21956 PMID:11295010

Paniagua, F. A., & Yamada, A. M. (Eds.). (2013). *Handbook of multicultural mental health: Assessment and treatment of diverse populations*. Cambridge, UK: Academic Press.

Panther, K. (2005). The Frazier free water protocol. *Perspectives on Swallowing and Swallowing Disorders (Dysphagia)*, *14*(1), 4–9. doi:10.1044asd14.1.4

Paradis, J. (2016). The development of English as a second language with and without specific language impairment: Clinical implications. *Journal of Speech, Language, and Hearing Research: JSLHR*, *59*(1), 171–182. doi:10.1044/2015_JSLHR-L-15-0008 PMID:26501845

Paradis, J., Emmerzael, K., & Duncan, T. (2010). Assessment of English learners: Using parent reports on first language development. *Journal of Communication Disorders*, *43*(6), 474–497. doi:10.1016/j.jcomdis.2010.01.002 PMID:20304411

Paradis, J., Genesee, R., & Crago, M. (2011). *Dual language development & disorders* (2nd ed.). Baltimore, MD: Brookes Publishing.

Paradis, J., Schneider, P., & Duncan, T. S. (2013). Discriminating children with language impairment among English-language learners from diverse first language backgrounds. *Journal of Speech, Language, and Hearing Research: JSLHR*, *56*(3), 971–981. doi:10.1044/1092-4388(2012/12-0050) PMID:23275391

Paradis, M., & Libben, G. (2014). *The assessment of bilingual aphasia*. New York: Psychology Press. doi:10.4324/9781315802138

Parangimalil, G. J. (2001). Latino health in the new millennium: The need for a culture-centered approach. *Sociological Spectrum*, *21*(3), 423–429. doi:10.1080/027321701300202064

Parker, S. E., Fau, M. C., Canfield, M. A., Fau, C. M., Rickard, R., Fau, R. R., . . . Correa, A. (2010). *Updated national birth prevalence estimates for selected birth defects in the United States, 2004-2006*. (1542-0760 (Electronic)).

Passel, J. S., & Cohn, D. V. (2009). *A portrait of unauthorized immigrants in the United States. Pew Hispanic Center Report*. Washington, DC: Pew Research Center.

Paterakis, K., Karantanas, A. H., Komnos, A., & Volikas, Z. (2000). Outcome of patients with diffuse axonal injury: The significance and prognostic value of MRI in the acute phase. *The Journal of Trauma Injury Infection and Critical Care*, *49*(6), 1071–1075. doi:10.1097/00005373-200012000-00016 PMID:11130491

Paul, R., & Norbury, C. (2012). *Language disorders from infancy through Adolescence* (5th ed.). St. Louis, MO: Elsevier Mosby.

Paul, R., & Norbury, C. (2012). *Language disorders from infancy through adolescence: Listening, speaking, reading, writing, and communicating* (4th ed.). St. Louis, MO: Elsevier.

Payne, J. C. (2014). *Adult neurogenic language disorders: Assessment and treatment. A comprehensive ethnobiological approach*. San Diego, CA: Plural Publishing.

Pearson, B., Velleman, S., Bryant, T., & Charko, T. (2008). Phonological milestones for African American English-speaking children learning Mainstream American English as a second dialect. *Language, Speech, and Hearing Services in Schools*, *40*(3), 229–244. doi:10.1044/0161-1461(2008/08-0064) PMID:18952815

Peña, E. D., Gillam, R. B., & Bedore, L. M. (2014). Dynamic assessment of narrative ability in English accurately identifies language impairment in English language learners. *Journal of Speech, Language, and Hearing Research: JSLHR*, *57*(6), 2208–2220. doi:10.1044/2014_JSLHR-L-13-0151 PMID:25075793

Peña, E. D., Gutiérrez-Clellen, V. F., Iglesias, A., Goldstein, B., & Bedore, L. M. (2018). *Bilingual English Spanish Assessment (BESA)*. Baltimore, MD: Brookes.

Penn, C., & Armstrong, E. (2017). Intercultural aphasia: New models of understanding for Indigenous populations. *Aphasiology*, *31*(5), 563–594.

Peredo, T. N. (2016). Supporting culturally and linguistically diverse families in early intervention. *Perspectives of the ASHA Special Interest Groups SIG, 1*(1), 154–167. doi:10.1044/persp1.SIG1.154

Perez Foster, R. (2001). When immigration is trauma: Guidelines for the individual and family clinician. *The American Journal of Orthopsychiatry, 71*(2), 153–170. doi:10.1037/0002-9432.71.2.153 PMID:11347358

Perez-Brena, N., Rivas-Drake, D., Toomey, R., & Umana-Taylor, A. (2018). Contributions of the integrative model for the study of developmental competencies in minority children: What have we learned about adaptive culture. *The American Psychologist, 73*(6), 713–726. doi:10.1037/amp0000292 PMID:30188161

Perez-Rocha, M., & Paley, J. (2014, November 21). What "Free Trade" has done to Central America. *Foreign Policy in Focus*. Retrieved from https://fpif.org/free-trade-done-central-america/

Perla, H. (2016 March 1). *The impact of CAFTA: Drugs, gangs and immigration.* Retrieved from https://www.telesurenglish.net/opinion/The-Impact-of-CAFTA-Drugs-Gangs-and-Immigration-20160301-0008.html

Perner, J. (1988). Higher-order beliefs and intentions in children's understanding of social interaction. In J. W. Astington, P. L. Harris, & D. R. Olson (Eds.), *Developing theories of mind* (pp. 271–294). Cambridge, UK: Cambridge University Press.

Perner, J., & Wimmer, H. (1985). "John thinks that Mary thinks that. . .": Attribution of second order beliefs by 5- to 10-year-old children. *Journal of Experimental Child Psychology, 39*(3), 437–471. doi:10.1016/0022-0965(85)90051-7

Perry, B. D. (2006). The neurosequential model of therapeutics: Applying principles of neuroscience to clinical work with traumatized and maltreated children. In N. Boyd Webb (Ed.), *Working with traumatized youth in child welfare* (pp. 27–52). New York: Guilford Press.

Perry, B. D. (2009). Examining child maltreatment through a neurodevelopmental lens: Clinical applications of the neurosequential model of therapeutics. *Journal of Loss and Trauma, 14*(4), 240–255. doi:10.1080/15325020903004350

Petersen, D. B., & Spencer, T. D. (2014). *The Predictive Early Assessment of Reading and Language (PEARL): Screener.* Available from www.LanguageDynamicsGroup.com

Peterson, C., & Slaughter, V. (2003). Opening windows into the mind: Mothers' preferences for explanations and children's theory of mind. *Cognitive Development, 18*(3), 399–429. doi:10.1016/S0885-2014(03)00041-8

Pew Hispanic Center. (2010). *Country of origin profiles- Hispanics in the United States.* Retrieved from http://pewhispanic.org/data/origins/

Pew Research Center. (2019). *Key findings about U.S. immigrants.* Retrieved from https://www.pewresearch.org/fact-tank/2019/06/03/key-findings-about-u-s-immigrants/

Pewewardy, C., & Fitzpatrick, M. (2009). Working with American Indian students and families: Disabilities, issues, and interventions. *Intervention in School and Clinic, 45*(2), 91–98. doi:10.1177/1053451209340223

Pham, G., Ebert, K., & Kohnert, K. (2015). Bilingual children with primary language impairment: Three months after treatment. *Journal of Language and Communication Disorders, 50*(1), 94–105. doi:10.1111/1460-6984.12123 PMID:25134887

Phelan, E., Pal, R., Henderson, L., Green, K. M. J., & Bruce, I. A. (2016). The management of children with Down syndrome and profound hearing loss. *Cochlear Implants International, 17*(1), 52–57. doi:10.1179/1754762815Y.0000000019 PMID:26252564

Plowman, E., Hentz, B., & Ellis, C. (2012). Post-stroke aphasia prognosis: A review of patient related and stroke-related factors. *Journal of Evaluating Clinical Practices, 18*(3), 689–694. doi:10.1111/j.1365-2753.2011.01650.x PMID:21395923

Pollan, M. (2009). *Food rules: An eater's manual*. New York, NY: Penguin.

Portes, A., & Rumbaut, R. (2001). *Legacies: The story of the immigrant second generation*. Berkeley, CA: University of California.

Prezas, R. F., & Hodson, B. W. (2010). The Cycles Phonological Remediation approach. In A. L. Williams, S. McLeod, & R. McCauley (Eds.), *Interventions for speech sound disorders in children* (pp. 137–158). Baltimore, MD: Brookes.

Price-Wise, G. (2008). Language, culture, and medical tragedy: The case of Willie Ramirez. *Health Affairs Blog*. Retrieved from https://www.healthaffairs.org/do/10.1377/hblog20081119.000463/full/

Proctor, A., Yairi, E., Duff, M. C., & Zhang, J. (2008). Prevalence of stuttering in African American preschoolers. *Journal of Speech, Language, and Hearing Research: JSLHR*, *51*(6), 1465–1479. doi:10.1044/1092-4388(2008/07-0057) PMID:18664698

Pua, E. P. K., Lee, M. L. C., & Liow, S. J. R. (2017). Screening bilingual preschoolers for language difficulties: Utility of teacher and parent reports. *Journal of Speech, Language, and Hearing Research: JSLHR*, *60*(4), 950–968. doi:10.1044/2016_JSLHR-L-16-0122 PMID:28297001

Puente, A. E., Perez-Garcia, M., Lopez, R. V., Hidalgo-Ruzzante, N. A., & Fasfous, A. F. (2013). Neuropsychological assessment of culturally and educationally dissimilar individuals. In *Handbook of Multicultural Mental Health* (pp. 225–241). Cambridge, UK: Academic Press. doi:10.1016/B978-0-12-394420-7.00012-6

Qualls, C. D., & Munoz, M. L. (2005). Race-ethnicity, socioeconomic status, and cognitive communicative functioning in individuals with neurogenic communication disorders: Clinical implications and research directions. *ECHO: E-Journal for Black and Other Ethnic Group Research and Practices in Communication Sciences and Disorders*, *1*, 30–39.

Quaranta, N., De Ceglie, V., & D'Elia, A. (2016). Endothelial dysfunction in idiopathic sudden sensorineural hearing loss: A review. *Audiology Research*, *6*(1), 17–21. doi:10.4081/audiores.2016.151 PMID:27588164

Quinn, C. T., Rogers, Z. R., McCavit, T. L., & Buchanan, G. R. (2010). Improved survival of children and adolescents with sickle cell disease. *Blood*, *115*(17), 3447–3452. doi:10.1182/blood-2009-07-233700 PMID:20194891

Quintana, S. M., & Mahgoub, L. (2016). Ethnic and racial disparities in education: Psychology's role in understanding and reducing disparities. *Theory into Practice*, *55*(2), 94–103. doi:10.1080/00405841.2016.1148985

Ramirez, R. R. (2004). *We the people: Hispanics in the US. (Census 2000 special reports)*. Washington, DC: Bureau of the Census, US Department of Commerce.

Rancho Los Amigos National Rehabilitation Center. (2011). *The rancho levels of cognitive functioning*. Retrieved from: https://web.archive.org/web/20110514024558/http://rancho.org/Research_RanchoLevels.aspx

Redpath, S., & Linden, M. (2004). Attitudes towards behavioral versus organic acquisition of brain injury. *Brain Injury: [BI]*, *18*(9), 861–869. doi:10.1080/02699050410001671838 PMID:15223739

Resendiz, M., Summers, C., Ruiz-Felter, R., Belasco, E., & Fox, K. (2017). Perceptions of mentoring SLPs and clinical fellows during the clinical fellowship. *Perspectives of ASHA Special Interest Groups, SIG 11, 2*, 25-41.

Reuterskiold-Wagner, C., Sahlen, B., & Nyman, A. (2005). Non-word repetition and non-word discrimination in Swedish preschool children. *Clinical Linguistics & Phonetics*, *19*(8), 681–699. doi:10.1080/02699200400000343 PMID:16147409

Rezzonico, S., Goldberg, A., Mak, K. K., Yap, S., Milburn, T., Belletti, A., & Girolametto, L. (2016). Narratives in two languages: Storytelling of Bilingual Cantonese-English Preschoolers. *Journal of Speech, Language, and Hearing Research: JSLHR*, *59*(3), 521–532. doi:10.1044/2015_JSLHR-L-15-0052 PMID:27253078

Rice, M. L., Smolik, F., Perpich, D., Thompson, T., Rytting, N., & Blossom, M. (2010). Mean length of utterance levels in 6-month intervals for children 3 to 9 years with and without language impairments. *Journal of Speech, Language, and Hearing Research: JSLHR*, *53*(2), 333–349. doi:10.1044/1092-4388(2009/08-0183) PMID:20360460

Richardson, M., Black-Pond, C., Sloane, M., Atchison, B., Hyter, Y. D., & Henry, J. (2015). Neurodevelopmental impact of child maltreatment. *Mental Health Issues in Childhood Maltreatment*. Retrieved from https://wmich.edu/sites/default/files/attachments/u354/2016/Neurodevelopmental%20Impact%20of%20Child%20Trauma%20Chaper-1.pdf

Riquelme, L. (2004). Cultural Competence in Dysphagia. *ASHA Leader*, *9*(7), 8–22. doi:10.1044/leader.FTR5.09072004.8

Riquelme, L. (2013). SIGnatures: Evolving Expressions of Culture. *ASHA Leader*, *18*(11), 52–55. doi:10.1044/leader.SIGN.18112013.52

Rivera, M., Ortíz, M., Lawson, M. E., & Verma, K. M. (2002). Evaluation of the use of complementary and alternative medicine in the largest Southwest United States Mexico border city. *Pharmacotherapy*, *22*(2), 256–264. doi:10.1592/phco.22.3.256.33543 PMID:11837563

Rizzo, S. (2018, June 19). The facts about Trump's policy of separating families at the border. *The Washington Post*. Retrieved from https://www.washingtonpost.com/news/fact-checker/wp/2018/06/19/the-facts-about-trumps-policy-of-separating-families-at-the-border/?noredirect=on

Robbins, J., Gensler, G., Hind, J., Logemann, J. A., Lindblad, A. S., Brandt, D., ... Miller Gardner, P. J. (2008). Comparison of 2 interventions for liquid aspiration on pneumonia incidence. *Annals of Internal Medicine*, *148*(7), 509–518. doi:10.7326/0003-4819-148-7-200804010-00007 PMID:18378947

Roberts, J. E., Price, J., & Malkin, C. (2007). Language and communication development in Down Syndrome. *Mental Retardation and Developmental Disabilities Research Reviews*, *13*(1), 26–35. doi:10.1002/mrdd.20136 PMID:17326116

Roberts, J., Price, J., Barnes, E., Nelson, L., Burchinal, M., Hennon, E. A., ... Hooper, S. R. (2007). Receptive vocabulary, expressive vocabulary, and speech production of boys with Fragile X Syndrome in comparison to boys with Down Syndrome. *American Journal of Mental Retardation*, *112*(3), 177–193. doi:10.1352/0895-8017(2007)112[177:RVEVAS]2.0.CO;2 PMID:17542655

Robke, D. (2016). Foundational resources and terminology for supervision and mentorship. *Perspectives of ASHA Special Interest Group, SIG 11, 1,* 57-67. Retrieved from: https://pubs.asha.org/doi/10.1044/persp1.SIG11.57

Rodekohr, R. K., & Haynes, W. O. (2001). Differentiating dialect from disorder: A comparison of two processing tasks and a standardized language test. *Journal of Communication Disorders*, *34*(3), 255–272. doi:10.1016/S0021-9924(01)00050-8 PMID:11409607

Rodriguez, B., & Olswang, L. (2003). Mexican-American and Anglo-American mothers' beliefs and values about child rearing, education, and language impairment. *American Journal of Speech-Language Pathology*, *12*(4), 452–462. doi:10.1044/1058-0360(2003/091) PMID:14658997

Roger, P., & Code, C. (2011). Lost in translation? Issues of content validity in interpreter mediated aphasia assessments. *International Journal of Speech-Language Pathology*, *13*(1), 61–73. doi:10.3109/17549507.2011.549241 PMID:21329412

Roger, P., Code, C., & Sheard, C. (2000). Assessment and management of aphasia in a linguistically diverse society. *Asia Pacific Journal of Speech, Language and Hearing*, *5*(1), 21–34. doi:10.1179/136132800807547573

Romero, J. M. (2012). Pragmatic communicative intervention strategies for victims of child abuse. *Children and Youth Services Review*, *34*(9), 1729–1734. doi:10.1016/j.childyouth.2012.05.003

Romero, V., Robertson, R., & Warner, A. (2018). *Building resilience in students impacted by adverse childhood experiences: A whole staff approach*. London, UK: Sage Publications.

Roseberry-McKibbin, C. (2008). *Increasing language skills of students from low income backgrounds*. San Diego, CA: Plural Publishing.

Roseberry-McKibbin, C. (2018). *Multicultural students with special language needs: Practical strategies for assessment and intervention* (5th ed.). Oceanside, CA: Academic Communication Associates.

Roseberry-McKibbin, C., Hegde, M. N., & Tellis, G. E. (2019). *An advanced review of speech-language pathology: Preparation for the Praxis SLP and comprehensive examination* (5th ed.). Austin, TX: Pro-Ed. Inc.

Rosenbek, J., Robbins, J., Roecker, E., Coyle, J., & Woods, J. (1996). A penetration-aspiration scale. *Dysphagia*, *11*(2), 93–98. doi:10.1007/BF00417897 PMID:8721066

Rosenbloom, S. R., & Way, N. (2004). Experiences of discrimination among African American, Asian American, and Latino adolescents in an urban high school. *Youth & Society*, *35*(4), 420–451. doi:10.1177/0044118X03261479

Rossetti, L. (2006). *The Rossetti infant toddler language scale*. East Moline, IL: Linguisystems.

Rossignol, L. N., & Paasche-Orlow, M. K. (2013). Empowering patients who have specific learning disabilities. *Journal of the American Medical Association*, *310*(14), 1445. doi:10.1001/jama.2013.278068 PMID:24052008

Roth, F. P., Dixon, D. A., Paul, D. R., & Bellini, P. I. (2013). RtI grades 3-5 in action: Oral and written language activities for the Common Core State Standards. Rockville, MD: American Speech and Hearing Association.

Roth, F. P., & Worthington, C. K. (2021). *Treatment resources manual for speech-language pathology* (6th ed.). San Diego, CA: Plural Publishing.

Rumbaut, R. G., & Massey, D. S. (2013). Immigration & language diversity in the United States. *Daedalus*, *142*(3), 141–154. doi:10.1162/DAED_a_00224 PMID:25018562

Ruppar, A., Allcock, H., & Gonsier-Gerdin, J. (2017). Ecological factors affecting access to general education content and contexts for students with significant disabilities. *Remedial and Special Education*, *38*(1), 53–63. doi:10.1177/0741932516646856

Saltapidas, H., & Ponsford, J. (2007). The influence of cultural background on motivation for and participation in rehabilitation and outcome following traumatic brain injury. *The Journal of Head Trauma Rehabilitation*, *22*(2), 132–139. doi:10.1097/01.HTR.0000265101.75177.8d PMID:17414315

Salter, K., Jutai, J., Foley, N., Hellings, C., & Teasell, R. (2006). Identification of aphasia post stroke: A review of screening assessment tools. *Brain Injury: [BI]*, *20*(6), 559–568. doi:10.1080/02699050600744087 PMID:16754281

Sander, A., Clark, A., & Pappadis, M. R. (2010). What is community integration anyway? Defining meaning following traumatic brain injury. *The Journal of Head Trauma Rehabilitation*, *25*(2), 121–127. doi:10.1097/HTR.0b013e3181cd1635 PMID:20134333

Sanger, B. D., & Bashir, A. S. (2018). Wait. What??? Guiding intervention principles for students with verbal working memory limitations. *Language, Speech, and Hearing Services in Schools*, *49*(3), 449–462. doi:10.1044/2018_LSHSS-17-0101 PMID:29978212

Santiago, C., Raviv, T., & Jaycox, L. (2018). *Creating healing school communities: School based interventions for students exposed to trauma*. Washington, DC: American Psychological Association. doi:10.1037/0000072-000

Sass-Lehrer, M. (2017). Early intervention for children birth-3: Families, communities, & communication. In L. R. Schmeltz (Ed.), *The NCHAM e-book: A resource guide for early hearing detection and intervention* (pp. 17-1–17-16). Logan, UT: National Center for Hearing Assessment and Management.

Schneider, B., Martinez, S., & Owens. (2007). Barriers to educational opportunities for Hispanics in the United States. In *Hispanics and the Future of America*. Washington, DC: National Academies Press. Available from https//:www.ncbi.nlm.nih.gov/books/NBK19909

Schopler, E., Van Bourgondien, M. E., Wellman, G. J., & Love, S. R. (2010). *Childhood Autism Rating Scale* (2nd ed.). Los Angeles, CA: Western Psychological Services.

Schroeder, M., Andrews, J. W., & Hines, Y. L. (2009). Cross-racial supervision: Critical issues in the supervisory relationship. *Canadian Journal of Counselling*, *43*(4), 295–310.

Schultz, E. K., Simpson, C. G., & Lynch, S. A. (2012). Specific learning disability identification: What constitutes a pattern of strengths and weaknesses? *Learning Disabilities*, *18*(2), 87–97.

Schyve, P. M. (2007). Language differences as a barrier to quality and safety in healthcare: The Joint Commission perspective. *Journal of General Internal Medicine*, *2*(S2), 360–361. doi:10.100711606-007-0365-3 PMID:17957426

Sciuchetti, M. B. (2017). Addressing inequity in special education: An integrated framework for culturally responsive social emotional practice. *Psychology in the Schools*, *54*(10), 1245–1251. doi:10.1002/pits.22073

Scott, A. N., Hauerwas, L. B., & Brown, R. D. (2014). State policy and guidance for identifying learning disabilities in culturally and linguistically diverse students. *Learning Disability Quarterly*, *37*(3), 172–185. doi:10.1177/0731948713507261

Segura, R. (2010). *Central Americans in Los Angeles*. Chicago, IL: Arcadia Publishing.

Semel, E., Wiig, E. H., & Secord, W. A. (2003). *Clinical Evaluation of Language Fundamentals* (4th ed.). Bloomington, MN: NCS Pearson, Inc.

Serjeant, G. R., Norman, W., & Todd, G. B. (1975). The internal auditory canal and sensorineural hearing loss in homozygous sickle cell disease. *The Journal of Laryngology and Otology*, *89*(4), 453–455. doi:10.1017/S0022215100080580 PMID:1127338

Serpa, J. A., & White, A. C. (2012). Neurocysticercosis in the United States. *Pathogens and Global Health*, *106*(5), 256–260. doi:10.1179/2047773212Y.0000000028 PMID:23265549

Shandera, W. X., White, A. C. Jr, Chen, J. C., Diaz, P., & Armstrong, R. (1994). Neurocysticercosis in Houston, TX: A report of 112 cases. *Medicine*, *73*(1), 37–52. doi:10.1097/00005792-199401000-00004 PMID:8309361

Sharfi, K., & Rosenblum, S. (2014). Activity and participation characteristics of adults with learning disabilities - a systematic review. *PLoS One*, *9*(9), e106657. doi:10.1371/journal.pone.0106657 PMID:25184315

Sheinart, K. F., Tuhrim, S., Horowitz, D. R., Weinberger, J., Godman, M., & Godbold, J. H. (1998). Stroke recurrence is more frequent in blacks and Hispanics. *Neuroepidemiology*, *17*(4), 188–198. doi:10.1159/000026172 PMID:9701833

Sherer, M., Nick, T. G., Sander, A. M., Hart, T., Hanks, R., Rosenthal, M., ... Yablon, S. A. (2003). Race and productivity outcome after traumatic brain injury: Influence of confounding factors. *The Journal of Head Trauma Rehabilitation*, *18*(5), 408–424. doi:10.1097/00001199-200309000-00003 PMID:12973271

Silliman, E. R., Bahr, R. H., Hnath-Chisolm, T., & Mahecha, N. R. (2002). Spanish and English proficiency in the linguistic encoding of mental states in narrative retellings. *Linguistics and Education*, *13*(2), 199–234. doi:10.1016/S0898-5898(01)00062-6

Silverstein, M. (2008). Getting home safe and sound: Occupational safety and health administration at 38. *American Journal of Public Health, 98*(3), 416–423. doi:10.2105/AJPH.2007.117382 PMID:18235060

Simms, M. C., Fortuny, K., & Henderson, E. (2009). *The urban institute fact sheet racial and ethnic disparities among low income families.* Retrieved from https://www.urban.org/sites/default/files/publication/32976/411936-racial-and-ethnic-disparities-among-low-income-families.pdf

Simms, L., Baker, S., & Clark, M. D. (2013). The standardized visual communication and sign language checklist for signing children. *Sign Language Studies, 14*(1), 101–124. doi:10.1353ls.2013.0029

Simon-Cereijido, G. (2015). Preschool language interventions for Latino dual language learners with language disorders: What, in what language, and how. *Seminars in Speech and Language, 36*(2), 154–164. doi:10.1055-0035-1549110 PMID:25923000

Simón-Cereijido, G., & Gutiérrez-Clellen, V. F. (2009). A cross-linguistic and bilingual evaluation of the interdependence between lexical and grammatical domains. *Applied Psycholinguistics, 30*(2), 315–337. doi:10.1017/S0142716409090134 PMID:19444336

Simon, K. B. (2018). Catalyzing the separation of Black families: A critique of foster care placements without prior judicial review. *Columbia Journal of Law and Social Problems, 51*(3), 347–385.

Simons, G. F., & Fennig, C. D. (Eds.). (2017), *Ethnologue: Language of the world* (12th ed.). Dallas, TX: SIL International. Retrieved from http://www.ethnologue.com

Simonsen, B., Freeman, J., Goodman, S., Mitchell, B., Swain-Bradway, J., Flannery, B., . . . Putman, B. (2015). *PBIS technical brief on classroom PBIS strategies.* Retrieved from https://www.pbis.org/common/ cms/files/pbisresources/ Supporting%20and%20Responding% 20to%20Behavior.pdf.

Simonsen, B., Fairbanks, S., Briesch, A., Myers, D., & Sugai, G. (2008). Evidence-based practices in classroom management: Considerations for research to practice. *Education & Treatment of Children, 31*(3), 351–380. doi:10.1353/etc.0.0007

Ski-Hi Institute. (2004). *Ski-hi language development scale* (2nd ed.). North Logan, UT: Hope, Inc.

Smith, A. (2000). *Ethnomed: Mexican cultural profile*. Retrieved from http://ethnomed.org/ethnomed/cultures/mexican/mexican_cp.html

Smith, D. P., & Bradshaw, B. S. (2006). Rethinking the Hispanic paradox: Death rates and life expectancy for US non-Hispanic White and Hispanic populations. *American Journal of Public Health, 96*(9), 1686–1692. doi:10.2105/AJPH.2003.035378 PMID:16380579

Smith, J. (2004). Unraveling the SES: Health connection. *Population and Development Review, 30*, 108–132.

Smith, J. H., Bottemiller, K. L., Flemming, K. D., Cutrer, F. M., & Strand, E. A. (2013). Inability to self-report pain after a stroke: A population-based study. *Pain, 154*(8), 1281–1286. doi:10.1016/j.pain.2013.04.006 PMID:23725781

Smith, L., & Thelen, E. (2003). Development as a dynamic system. *Trends in Cognitive Sciences, 7*(8), 343–34. doi:10.1016/S1364-6613(03)00156-6 PMID:12907229

Snow, C. E., Burns, M. S., & Griffin, P. (1998). *Preventing reading difficulties in young children.* Washington, DC: National Academies.

Sonderup, L. (2010). Hispanic marketing: A critical market segment. *Advertising & Marketing Review.* Retrieved from https://www.cdc.gov/healthcommunication/pdf/thisjustin/tji_1_201108.pdf

Spagat, E., & Galvan, A. (2019, July 31). Over 900 more children separated at the border since a judge halted the practice: ACLU. *Time*. Retrieved from https://time.com/5639549/900-children-separated-border-aclu/

Spann, M. N., Mayes, L. C., Kalmar, J. H., Guiney, J., Womer, F. Y., Pittman, B., ... Blumberg, H. P. (2012). Childhood abuse and neglect and cognitive flexibility in adolescents. *Child Neuropsychology*, *18*(2), 182–189. doi:10.1080/09297049.2011.595400 PMID:21942637

Sparrow, S. S., Cicchetti, D., & Saulnier, C. (2016). *Vineland Adaptive Behavior Scales* (3rd ed.). Bloomington, MN: Pearson.

Spaulding, S. A., Horner, R. H., May, S. L., & Vincent, C. G. (2008). *Evaluation brief: Implementation of school-wide PBS across the United States*. Retrieved from http://pbis.org/evaluation/evaluation_briefs/default.aspx

Spencer, P. E., & Marschark, M. (2010). *Evidence-based practice in educating deaf and hard-of hearing students*. New York, NY: Oxford University Press.

Spratt, E. G., Friedenberg, S. L., Swenson, C. C., LaRosa, A., De Bellis, M. D., Macias, M. M., & … . (2012). The effects of early neglect on cognitive, language and behavioral functioning n childhood. *Psychology (Irvine, Calif.)*, *3*(2), 175–182. doi:10.4236/psych.2012.32026 PMID:23678396

Steele, W., & Malchiodi, C. A. (2016). *Trauma-informed practices with children and adolescents*. New York: Routledge.

Stein, D. G. (2001). Brain damage, sex hormones recovery: A new role for progesterone and estrogen? *Trends in Neurosciences*, *24*(7), 386–391. doi:10.1016/S0166-2236(00)01821-X PMID:11410269

Stockman, I. (1996). Phonological development and disorders in African American children. In A. G. Kamhi, K. E. Pollock, & J. L. Harris (Eds.), *Communication development and disorders in African American children: Research, assessment, and intervention* (pp. 117–153). Baltimore, MD: Paul H. Brookes.

Stredler-Brown, A. (2010). Communication choices and outcomes during the early years: An assessment and evidence-based approach. In M. Marschark & P. E. Spencer (Eds.), *The Oxford handbook of deaf studies, language, and education* (Vol. 2, pp. 291–315). New York, NY: Oxford University Press.

Stuart, A. (2019). Hearing loss in children with homozygous sickle cell disease. *The Hearing Journal,72*(7), 16 & 18-19.

Stuart, A., Jones, S. M., & Walker, L. J. (2006). Insights into elevated distortion product otoacoustic emissions in sickle cell disease: Comparisons of hydroxyurea-treated and non-treated young children. *Hearing Research*, *212*(1-2), 83–89. doi:10.1016/j.heares.2005.10.014 PMID:16364581

Stuart, A., & Preast, J. L. (2012). Contralateral suppression of transient evoked otoacoustic emissions in children with sickle cell disease. *Ear and Hearing*, *33*(3), 421–429. doi:10.1097/AUD.0b013e31823effd9 PMID:22246207

Su, B. M., & Chan, D. K. (2017). Prevalence of hearing loss in US children and adolescents: Findings from NHANES 1988-2010. *JAMA Otolaryngology-Head & Neck Surgery*, *143*(9), 920–927. doi:10.1001/jamaoto.2017.0953 PMID:28750123

Substance Abuse and Mental Health Services Administration (SAMHSA). (2014). *Treatment improvement protocol (TIP) Series, No. 57. Trauma Informed Care in Behavioral Health Services*. Rockville, MD: Author.

Subtitle VII-B of the McKinney-Vento Homeless Assistance Act (42 u.S.C. 11431 et seq.).

Sullivan, K., & Tager-Flusberg, H. (1999). Second-order believe attribution in Williams Syndrome: Intact or impaired? *American Journal of Mental Retardation*, *104*(6), 523–532. doi:10.1352/0895-8017(1999)104<0523:SBAIWS>2.0.CO;2 PMID:10587733

Sylvestre, A., Bussieres, E. L., & Bouchard, C. (2016). Language problems among abused and neglected children: A meta-analytic review. *Child Maltreatment*, *2*(1), 47–58. doi:10.1177/1077559515616703 PMID:26620719

Tatemichi, T. K., Desmond, D. W., Stern, Y., Paik, M., Sano, M., & Bagiella, E. (1994). Cognitive impairment after stroke: Frequency, patterns, and relationship to functional abilities. *Journal of Neurology, Neurosurgery, and Psychiatry*, *57*(2), 202–207. doi:10.1136/jnnp.57.2.202 PMID:8126506

Taylor, C. (2012). *The Black Carib wars: Freedom, survival and the making of the Garifuna*. Jackson, MS: University Press of Mississippi. doi:10.14325/mississippi/9781617033100.001.0001

Teasdale, G., & Jennett, B. (1974). Assessment of coma and impaired consciousness. A practical scale. *Lancet*, *2*(7872), 81–84. doi:10.1016/S0140-6736(74)91639-0 PMID:4136544

Technical Assistance Center on Positive Behavioral Intervention and Supports. (2010). *SWPBIS implementation blueprint and self-assessment. Positive behavioral intervention and supports.* Retrieved from http://www.pbis.org/Common/Cms/files/pbisresources/SWPBS_ImplementationBlueprint_vSep_23_2010.pdf

Technical Assistance Center on Positive Behavioral Interventions and Supports. (2017). *Student-sample behavior expectations.* Retrieved from https://www.pbis.org/training/staff/student

Teicher, M. H., Andersen, S. L., Polcari, A., Anderson, C. M., Navalta, C. P., & Kim, D. M. (2003). The neurobiological consequences of early stress and childhood maltreatment. *Neuroscience and Biobehavioral Reviews*, *27*(1-2), 33–44. doi:10.1016/S0149-7634(03)00007-1 PMID:12732221

Telles, E. F., & Ortiz, V. (2008). *Generations of exclusion: Mexican American assimilation and race*. New York, NY: Russel Sage Foundation.

The Audiology Project. (2019). Our vision – The Audiology Project story. Retrieved from https://www.theaudiology-project.com/our-vision

The Hearing Review. (2012, January 30). More age-related hearing loss in female diabetics with poor glucose control. Retrieved from http://www.hearingreview.com/2012/01/more-age-related-hearing-loss-in-female-diabetics-with-poor-glucose-control/

Thelen, E., & Smith, L. (1994). *A dynamic systems approach to the development of cognition and action.* Cambridge, MA: MIT Press.

Thordardottir, E., & Brandeker, M. (2013). The effect of bilingual exposure versus language impairment on nonword repetition and sentence imitation scores. *Journal of Communication Disorders*, *46*(1), 1–16. doi:10.1016/j.jcomdis.2012.08.002 PMID:23021785

Thorndike, R. L., Hagan, E. P., & Sattler, J. M. (1986). *The Stanford-Binet Intelligence Scale* (4th ed.). Chicago, IL: Riverside Publishing.

Threats, T. (2010). The ICF and speech-language pathology: Aspiring to a fuller realization of ethical and moral issues. *International Journal of Speech-Language Pathology*, *12*(2), 87–93. doi:10.3109/17549500903568476 PMID:20420350

Throneburg, R., Calvert, L., Sturm, J., Paramboukas, A., & Paul, P. (2001). A comparison of service delivery models: Effects on curricular vocabulary skills in the school setting. *American Journal of Speech-Language Pathology*, *9*(1), 10–20. doi:10.1044/1058-0360.0901.10

Tomoeda, C. K., & Bayles, K. A. (2002). Cultivating cultural competence in the workplace, classroom, and clinic. *ASHA Leader*, *7*(6), 4–17. doi:10.1044/leader.FTR1.07062002.4

Toth, S. L., Stronach, E. P., Rogosch, F. A., Caplan, R., & Cicchitti, D. (2011). Illogical thinking and thought disorder in maltreated children. *Journal of the American Academy of Child and Adolescent Psychiatry, 50*(7), 659–668. doi:10.1016/j.jaac.2011.03.002 PMID:21703493

Turkstra, L. S., Coelho, C., & Ylvisaker, M. (2005). The use of standardized tests for individuals with cognitive-communication disorders. *Seminars in Speech and Language, 26*(4), 215–222. doi:10.1055-2005-922101 PMID:16278794

Turnbull, A., Turnbull, H. R., Erwin, E. J., & Shogren, K. A. (2015). *Families, professionals, and exceptionality: Positive outcomes through partnerships and trust* (7th ed.). Bloomington, MN: Pearson.

Turran, C. M., & Goldman, N. (2007). Socioeconomic differences in mortality among US adults: Insights into the Hispanic paradox. *The Journals of Gerontology. Series B, Psychological Sciences and Social Sciences, 63*(3), S184–S192. doi:10.1093/geronb/62.3.S184 PMID:17507594

U.S. Census Bureau. (2008). Washington, DC: Population Estimates – Hispanic or Latino.

U.S. Census Bureau. (2012). *U.S. Census Bureau projections show a slower growing, older, more diverse nation a half century from now.* Retrieved from https://www.census.gov/newsroom/releases/archives/population/cb12-243.html

U.S. Census Bureau. (2018a, June 17). *American Community Survey (ACS): Comparing 2012 American Community Survey Data.* Retrieved from https://www.census.gov/programs surveys/acs/guidance/comparing-acs-data/2012.html

U.S. Census Bureau. (2018b, June 17). *American Community Survey (ACS): Comparing 2015 American Community Survey Data.* Retrieved from https://www.census.gov/programs-surveys/acs/guidance/comparing-acs-data/2015.html

U.S. Centers for Disease Control and Prevention (CDC). (2014). Autism and Developmental Disabilities Monitoring Network surveillance year 2010 principal investigators. Prevalence of autism spectrum disorders–Autism and Developmental Disabilities Monitoring Network, 11 sites, United States, 2010. *Morbidity and Mortality Weekly Report, 63*(SS02), 1–18. PMID:24402465

U.S. Customs and Border Protection. (2019, August 13). *Central America-Dominican Republic Free Trade Agreement (CAFTA-DR).* Retrieved from https://www.cbp.gov/trade/free-trade-agreements/cafta-dr

U.S. Department of Education, Office of Special Education. (2019). Children and youth with disabilities. In National Center for Education Statistics. *The Condition of Education.* Retrieved from https://nces.ed.gov/programs/coe/pdf/coe_cgg.pdf

U.S. Department of Health & Human Services, Administration for Children and Families, Administration on Children Youth and Families, Children's Bureau (ACF). (2019). *Child Maltreatment 2017.* Available from https://www.acf.hhs.gov/cb/research-data-technology/statistics-research/child-maltreatment

U.S. Department of Health and Human Services, Office of Minority Health. (2016). *Profile: Hispanic/Latino Americans.* Retrieved from https://minorityhealth.hhs.gov/omh/browse.aspx?lvl=3&lvlid=64

U.S. Department of Health and Human Services, Office of the Assistant Secretary for Planning and Evaluation (USDHHS – ASPE). (2019). *Poverty guidelines.* Retrieved from https://aspe.hhs.gov/poverty-guidelines

U.S. Department of Labor. (2018). *TED: The Economics Daily.* Bureau of Labor Statistics. Retrieved from https://www.bls.gov/opub/ted/2018/76-point-9-percent-of-hispanic-men-employed-january-2018.htm?view_full

U.S. National Library of Medicine. (2019, Dec 10). *Your guide to understanding genetic conditions: Sickled cells.* National Library of Medicine (US). Genetics Home Reference. Retrieved from https://ghr.nlm.nih.gov/gallery?start=60

Uhry, J., & Clark, D. (1995). *Dyslexia: Theory & practice of instruction.* Austin, TX: Pro-ed.

United Nations Children's Fund (UNICEF). (1993). *The teacher's handbook: Teaching the UN Convention Rights of the Child*. Geneva, Switzerland: Author.

Uomoto, J. M., & Wong, T. M. (2000). Multicultural perspective on the neuropsychology of brain injury assessment and rehabilitation. In E. Fletcher-Janzen, T.L., Strickland, & C.R. Reynolds (Eds.), Handbook of cross-cultural neuropsychology (pp. 169-184). New York, NY: Kluwer Academics/Plenum Publishers. doi:10.1007/978-1-4615-4219-3_11

Valdes, G., & Figueroa, R. A. (1994). *Bilingualism and testing: A special case of bias*. Norwood, NJ: Ablex.

van der Kolk, B. (1994). The body keeps the score: Memory and the emerging psychobiology of post-traumatic stress. *Harvard Review of Psychiatry*, *1*(5), 253–265. doi:10.3109/10673229409017088 PMID:9384857

van der Kolk, B. (2015). *The body keeps the score: Brain, mind and body in the healing of trauma*. New York: Penguin Books.

Varona, J. F., Bermejo, F., Guerra, J. M., & Molina, J. A. (2004). Long-term prognosis of ischemic stroke in young adults. *Journal of Neurology*, *251*(12), 1507–1514. doi:10.100700415-004-0583-0 PMID:15645352

Vega, W. A., Rodriguez, M. A., & Gruskin, E. (2016). Health disparities in the Latino population. *Epidemiologic Reviews*, *31*(1), 99–112. doi:10.1093/epirev/mxp008 PMID:19713270

Vining, C., Edgarita, L., Inglebret, E., & Brendal, M. (2017). Speech-language assessment considerations for American Indian and Alaskan Native Children who are dual language learners. *Perspectives of the Special Interest Groups, 2*(Sig 14), 29–40.

Vis, J. C., Duffels, M. G., Winter, M. M., Weijerman, M. E., Cobben, J. M., Huisman, S. A., & Mulder, B. J. (2009). Down syndrome: A cardiovascular perspective. *Journal of Intellectual Disability Research*, *53*(5), 419–425. doi:10.1111/j.1365-2788.2009.01158.x PMID:19228275

Voulgarides, C. K. (2018). *Does compliance matter in special education? IDEA and the hidden inequities of practice. In Disability, Culture, and Equity Series* (pp. 31–49). New York, NY: Teachers College Press.

Vygotsky, L. S. (1978). *Mind in society: The development of higher psychological processes*. Cambridge, MA: Harvard University Press.

Vygotsky, L. S. (1986). *Thought and language*. Cambridge, MA: The MIT Press.

Walker, L. J., Stuart, A., & Green, W. B. (2004). Outer and middle ear status and distortion product otoacoustic emissions in children with sickle cell disease. *American Journal of Audiology*, *13*(2), 164–172. doi:10.1044/1059-0889(2004/021) PMID:15903142

Wallin, M. T., & Kurtze, J. F. (2004). Neurocysticercosis in the United States: Review of an important emerging infection. *Neurology*, *63*(9), 1559–1564. doi:10.1212/01.WNL.0000142979.98182.FF PMID:15534236

Wamser-Nanney, R., Sager, J. C., & Campbell, C. L. (2019). Maternal support as a predictor of children's sexualized behaviors following childhood sexual abuse. *Child Maltreatment*, *24*(1), 36–44. doi:10.1177/1077559518786821 PMID:30004257

Wardlaw, J. M., & Mielke, O. (2005). Early signs of brain infarction at CT: Observer reliability and outcome after thrombolytic treatment – systematic review. *Radiology*, *235*(2), 444–453. doi:10.1148/radiol.2352040262 PMID:15858087

Warner, E., Koomar, J., Lary, B., & Cook, A. (2013). Can the body change the score? Application of sensory modulation principles in the treatment of traumatized adolescents in residential settings. *Journal of Family Violence*, *28*(7), 729–738. doi:10.100710896-013-9535-8

Washington, K. (2007). Using the ICF within speech-language pathology: Application to developmental language impairment. *International Journal of Speech-Language Pathology*, *9*(3), 242–255. doi:10.1080/14417040701261525

Wechsler, D. (2014). *Wechsler Intelligence Scale for Children-V* (5th ed.). San Antonio, TX, US: Psychological Corporation.

Weimar, C., Konig, I., Kraywinkel, K., Ziegler, A., & Diener, H. (2004). Age and national institutes of health stroke scale score within 6 hours after onset are accurate predictors of outcome after cerebral ischemia - Development and external validation of prognostic models. *Stroke*, *35*(1), 158–162. doi:10.1161/01.STR.0000106761.94985.8B PMID:14684776

Westby, C.E., & Robinson, L. (2017, October). *Social communication and pragmatic language: Developmental perspective from infancy through adolescence.* Invited Keynote, Van Riper Lecture Series, Western Michigan University, Kalamazoo, MI.

Westby, C. E. (2007). Maltreatment: A global issue. *Language, Speech, and Hearing Services in Schools*, *38*(2), 140–148. doi:10.1044/0161-1461(2007/014) PMID:17428960

Westby, C., Burda, A., & Mehta, Z. (2003). Asking the right questions in the right ways. *ASHA Leader*, *8*(8), 4–17. doi:10.1044/leader.FTR3.08082003.4

Westby, C., & Washington, K. (2017). Using the International Classification of Functioning, Disability and Health in assessment and intervention of school-aged children with language impairments. *Language, Speech, and Hearing Services in Schools*, *48*(3), 137–152. doi:10.1044/2017_LSHSS-16-0037 PMID:28630972

White, A. C., & Atmar, R. L. (2002). Infections in Hispanic immigrants. *Clinical Infectious Diseases*, *34*, 1627–1632. doi:10.1086/340620 PMID:12032899

Whiteside-Mansell, L., Bradley, R., & McKelvey, L. (2009). Parenting and preschool child development: Examination of three low-income cultural groups. *Journal of Child and Family Studies*, *18*(1), 48–60. doi:10.100710826-008-9206-1

Wiggins, E. (2014). *History of the National Black Association for Speech-Language and Hearing (NBASLH): The first twenty years*. Norfolk, VA: Poetica Publishing Company.

Wiig, E. H., Semel, E., & Secord, W. A. (2013). Clinical Evaluation of Language Fundamentals –Fifth Edition (CELF-5). Bloomington, MN: NCS Pearson.

Wiig, E. H., Semel, E., & Secord, W. A. (2013). Clinical Evaluation of Language Fundamentals, Fifth edition (CELF-5). New York: Pearson.

Wild, A., Vorperian, H. K., Kent, R. D., Bolt, D. M., & Austin, D. (2018). Single-word speech intelligibility in children and adults with Down syndrome. *American Journal of Speech-Language Pathology*, *27*(1), 222–236. doi:10.1044/2017_AJSLP-17-0002 PMID:29214307

Williams, K. T. (2007). Expressive Vocabulary Test – Second Edition (EVT-2). Circle Pines, MN: American Guidance Service.

Williams, C. J., & McLeod, S. (2012). Speech-language pathologists' assessment and intervention practices with multilingual children. *International Journal of Speech-Language Pathology*, *14*(3), 292–305. doi:10.3109/17549507.2011.636071 PMID:22472031

Wolters, G., Stapert, S., Brands, I., & van Heugten, C. (2010). Coping styles in relation to cognitive rehabilitation and quality of life after brain injury. *Neuropsychological Rehabilitation*, *20*(4), 587–600. doi:10.1080/09602011003683836 PMID:20446171

Wood, C., Diehm, E. A., & Callender, M. E. (2016). An investigation of language environment analysis measures for Spanish-English bilingual preschoolers from migrant low-socioeconomic status backgrounds. *Language, Speech, and Hearing Services in Schools*, *47*(2), 123–124. doi:10.1044/2015_LSHSS-14-0115 PMID:27019230

Wood, C., Wolford, M. C., & Schatschneider, C. (2018). Relationship between performance on oral narrative retells and vocabulary assessments of Spanish-speaking children. *Communication Disorders Quarterly*, *39*(3), 402–414. doi:10.1177/1525740117722507

World Health Organization (WHO). (2019). Diabetes programme: About diabetes. Retrieved from https://www.who.int/diabetes/action_online/basics/en/index3.html

World Health Organization. (2001). *International Classification of Functioning, Disability, and Health*. Geneva, Switzerland: World Health Organization.

World Health Organization. (2007). *International Classification of Functioning, Disability, and Health, Children and Youth Version*. Geneva, Switzerland: WHO Press.

World Health Organization. (2013). *How to use the ICF: A practical manual for using the International Classification of Functioning, Disability and Health (ICF). Exposure draft for comment. October 2013*. Geneva, Switzerland: WHO Press.

Wu, S., Vega, W. A., Resendez, J., & Jin, H. (2016). *Latinos & Alzheimer's disease: New numbers behind the crisis*. Retrieved from: https://health.ucdavis.edu/latinoaging/news/pdf/Latinos_and_AD_USC_UsA2-Impact-Report.pdf

Würth, K., Langewitz, W., Reiter-Theil, S., & Schuster, S. (2018, July 4). Their view: Difficulties and challenges of patients and physicians in cross-cultural encounters and a medical ethics perspective. *BMC Medical Ethics*, *19*(70). Retrieved from https://bmcmedethics.biomedcentral.com/articles/10.1186/s12910-018-0311-4 PMID:29973220

Yanni, E., Grosse, S. D., Yang, Q., & Olney, R. S. (2009). Trends in pediatric sickle cell disease-related mortality in the United States, 1983-2002. *The Journal of Pediatrics*, *154*(4), 541–545. doi:10.1016/j.jpeds.2008.09.052 PMID:19028391

Yan, R. (2009). *Assessing English language proficiency in international aviation: Issues of reliability, validity, and aviation safety*. Saarbrucken, Germany: VDM.

Yan, R. (2013). Assessing the English language proficiency of international aviation staff. In A. J. Kunnan (Ed.), *The companion to language assessment (CLA)* (pp. 484–496). Chichester, UK: Wiley-Blackwell. doi:10.1002/9781118411360.wbcla050

Yan, R., & Oller, J. W. Jr. (2007). Processing-dependent measures as a failed solution to the assessment of individuals from language and dialect minorities. *Communicative Disorders Review*, *1*(3-4), 201–213.

Yawn, B. P., & John-Sowah, J. (2015, December 15). Management of sickle cell disease: Recommendations from the 2014 Expert Panel Report. *American Family Physician*, *92*(12), 1069–1076. PMID:26760593

Yehuda, N. (2016). *Communicating trauma: Clinical presentations and interventions with traumatized children*. New York: Routledge.

Yoo, S. H., Kim, J. S., Kwon, S. U., Yun, S. C., Koh, J. Y., & Kang, D. W. (2008). Undernutrition as a predictor of poor clinical outcomes in acute ischemic stroke patients. *Archives of Neurology*, *65*(1), 39–43. doi:10.1001/archneurol.2007.12 PMID:18195138

Yoshinaga-Itano, C. (2003). From screening to early identification and intervention: Discovering predictors to successful outcomes for children with significant hearing losses. *Journal of Deaf Studies and Deaf Education*, *8*(1), 11–30. doi:10.1093/deafed/8.1.11 PMID:15448044

Yoshinaga-Itano, C., Sedey, A. L., Coulter, D. K., & Mehl, A. L. (1998). Language of early- and later-identified children with hearing loss. *Pediatrics*, *102*(5), 1161–1171. doi:10.1542/peds.102.5.1161 PMID:9794949

Young, A., Carr, G., Hunt, R., McCracken, W., Skipp, A., & Tattersall, H. (2006). Informed choice and deaf children: Underpinning concepts and enduring challenges. *Journal of Deaf Studies and Deaf Education*, *11*(3), 322–336. doi:10.1093/deafed/enj041 PMID:16717258

Young, J. C., & Widom, C. S. (2014). Long-term effects of child abuse and neglect on emotion processing in adulthood. *Child Abuse & Neglect*, *38*(8), 1369–1381. doi:10.1016/j.chiabu.2014.03.008 PMID:24747007

Young, R. W., & Morgan, W. (1987). *The Navajo language: A grammar and colloquial dictionary*. Albuquerque, NM: University of New Mexico Press.

Younkins, E. (1998, Jan). *Individualism and freedom: Vital pillars of true communities*. Retrieved from http://fee.org/freeman/detail/individualism-and-freedom-vital-pillars-of-true-communities

Zentella, A. (1997). *Growing up bilingual*. Malden, MA: Blackwell.

Zheng, S., & Hu, X. (2018). Parents reporting adverse childhood experiences among young children with disabilities: Informing systems transformation. *Topics in Early Childhood Special Education*, *38*(3), 162–173. doi:10.1177/0271121418790674

Zimmerman, I. L., Steiner, V. G., & Pond, R. E. (2011). Preschool Language Scales 5th Edition: Administration and Scoring Manual. Bloomington, MN, Pearson.

Zimmerman, I. L., Steiner, V. G., & Pond, R. E. (2012). Preschool Language Scales (5th ed.). Bloomington, MN: Pearson. (in Spanish)

Zimmerman, I. L., Steiner, V. G., & Pond, R. E. (2012). Preschool Language Scales 5th Edition: Articulation Screener. Bloomington, MN, Pearson.

Zirkel, P. A. (2018). The legal meaning of special education eligibility: The latest case law. *Communique*, *46*(7), 14–16.

Zsembik, B. A., & Fennell, D. (2005). Ethnic variation in health and the determinants of health among Latinos. *Social Science & Medicine*, *61*(1), 53–63. doi:10.1016/j.socscimed.2004.11.040 PMID:15847961

About the Contributors

Diane M. Scott, PhD, CCC-A, has been working in the field of communication sciences and disorders for over 35 years. Her specific areas of interest include multicultural issues in communication disorders, pediatric audiology, and genetic issues in communication disorders. She has worked in academia for most of her professional career, serving as faculty at Hampton University, Michigan State University, and Howard University. Dr. Scott also served as director of the Office of Multicultural Affairs at the American Speech-Language-Hearing Association. Currently, she is a full professor at North Carolina Central University.

* * *

Sheila J. Bridges-Bond, Ph.D., CCC-SLP, is an associate professor in the Communication Disorders Department at North Carolina Central University (NCCU) in Durham, NC. With a specialization in augmentative and alternative communication, her clinical work, teaching, and research have focused on social justice, and global issues in service delivery to CLD families. A long-time member of the American Speech-Language-Hearing Association (ASHA) and the National Black Association for Speech-Language and Hearing (NBASLH), Dr. Bridges-Bond is an ASHA Fellow and has served on local and national boards and professional committees.

Karen Garrido-Nag, Ph.D., CCC-SLP, is an Associate Professor at Gallaudet University. Her main area of teaching is on pediatric child language development and disorders. She has also worked as a Speech-Language Pathologist in early intervention, school systems and private practice. Her areas of research are in typical and disordered neurophysiology of speech and language processing. She is the director of the Developmental Neurolinguistics and Cognition Lab

Kellyn Hall, Ph.D. CCC/SLP, is a clinician, researcher, teacher, and author with over 30 years' experience working in a variety of medical settings. She is currently an Associate Professor in the Communication Sciences and Disorders program at North Carolina Central University where she teaches medical speech-language pathology courses. Her clinical interests are in adult and pediatric feeding and swallowing disorders, voice disorders, and telepractice.

Davis E. Henderson, PhD, CCC - SLP, graduated from Arizona State University with his Doctor of Philosophy from the Department of Speech and Hearing Science, under the direction of Dr. Maria Adelaida Restrepo. He received my Masters from Central Michigan University, my Bachelor of Arts from the University of New Mexico. His expertise includes language development, language disorders, Navajo linguistics, and psychometrics. Dr. Henderson's research focuses on assessment of Native American children, specifically in the Navajo community. His research provides an in-depth knowledge in the area of speech and language development and disorders among Native American children. Prior to his PhD training, he worked on the Navajo Reservation as a speech-language pathologist for 5 years.

RaMonda Horton, Ph.D, CCC-SLP is an Associate Professor in the Speech-language Pathology program at Midwestern University in Downers Grove, IL. Her teaching, research, and clinical interests are in the area of early language development and disorders, school-based services, and multicultural issues in communication disorders.

Yvette D. Hyter, Ph.D., is Professor of Speech, Language, and Hearing Sciences at Western Michigan University in Kalamazoo, USA and a Fellow of the American Speech Language and Hearing Association. Her research and teaching focus on the influences of culture on communication development and disorders, with emphasis in the areas of (1) pragmatic language and social communication of speakers of African American English and (2) culturally responsive and globally sustainable practices. As a founding member of the Southwest Michigan Children's Trauma Assessment Center, Professor Hyter's clinical concentration is twofold: (1) the social pragmatic language of children with histories of maltreatment and prenatal alcohol exposure and (2) transdisciplinary assessments. She developed a social pragmatic communication assessment battery for young children that is currently being tested in Brazil, Cyprus, Greece, and the United States. As Co-Director of a nonprofit, Cultural Connections: Transnational Research and Education Laboratory, Professor Hyter co-teaches study-abroad courses in West Africa and in the U.S. Midwest about the causes and consequences of globalization on systems, policies, and practices. She has published articles underscoring the need for conceptual frameworks guiding practice in globally sustainable ways, a co-authored book on culturally responsive practices, and served in leadership positions regarding global practice, diversity, inclusion, and equity.

Leslie Johnson is a native of North Carolina and enjoys giving back to the state she loves by serving at a state-supported institution. She is dedicated to her family, students, and School of Education faculty team. Her teaching and research is driven by her clinical experiences as a Speech Language Pathologist and she hopes that her students and research will drive future clinical practice.

Yolanda Keller-Bell is an Associate Professor at North Carolina Central University. Her research focuses on language and literacy development in children with developmental disabilities and individuals from diverse populations.

James McCann, EdD, CCC-SLP received his EdD from the GWU Graduate School of Education and Human Development's Special Education and Disabilities Studies Program in 2018. His dissertation research examined the relationship between visual language and early literacy development in deaf and hard-of-hearing children. He received his MS in Speech-Language Pathology from Gallaudet University in 2001, and his BS in Communication Sciences and Disorders with a minor in Spanish in 1999 from Penn State University. Dr. McCann's research interests are identifying language disorders separate from language delay due to lack of accessible language in deaf and hard-of-hearing children acquiring visual language; identifying evidence based practice for language instruction and intervention with D/HOH children; investigating eye gaze and its relationship to language and literacy development and its relationship to instructional practice; acquisition and preservation of heritage language in bilingual children with language impairment; and the communication development of deaf and hard-of-hearing children with complex communication needs who require augmentative and alternative communication (AAC) strategies due to significant additional motor, intellectual, and/or sensory needs.

Katrina Miller's 25 plus years' commitment to the communication disorders profession has improved the lives of her clients and over 300 speech-language pathology students. As a Clinical Associate Professor at North Carolina Central University she founded the Neurogenic Aphasia Group. As a clinical educator, Dr. Miller has traveled to China to train BLCU and NCCU students in the field of speech-language pathology. Her area of interest includes clinical education/supervision, adult neurogenics and adult group therapy.

Celeste Roseberry-McKibbin received her Ph.D. from Northwestern University. She is a Professor of Communication Sciences and Disorders at California State University, Sacramento. Dr. Roseberry is also currently a part-time itinerant speech pathologist in San Juan Unified School District where she provides direct services to students from preschool through high school. She has worked in educational and medical settings with a wide variety of clients ranging from preschoolers through geriatric patients. Dr. Roseberry's primary research interests are in the areas of assessment and treatment of culturally and linguistically diverse students with communication disorders as well as service delivery to students from low-income backgrounds. She has over 70 publications, including 16 books, and has made over 370 presentations at the local, state, national, and international levels. Dr. Roseberry is a Fellow of ASHA, and winner of the American Speech and Hearing Association's Certificate of Recognition for Special Contributions in Multicultural Affairs. She received the national presidential Daily Point of Light Award for her volunteer work in building literacy skills of children in poverty. She lived in the Philippines as the daughter of Baptist missionaries from ages 6 to 17.

Christine Begay Vining, PhD., CCC-SLP, is a bilingual Navajo Speech-Language Pathologist at the Center for Development & Disability, Department of Pediatrics, Health Sciences Center, University of New Mexico in Albuquerque, NM. She received her bachelor and master's degrees from the University of Arizona and doctorate from the University of New Mexico. Chris has worked with children, youth and young adults with neurodevelopmental disabilities, their families, and communities throughout New Mexico in many settings including therapeutic, early intervention, public school and university clinics. As program manager of several clinical and community based programs, she has worked to improve systems of care and education through collaboration at various systemic levels (i.e., family, community, university and state) with emphasis on rural, underserved areas including Native American communities. Currently, she provides clinical services, and helps to build capacity and resources across the state through training and technical assistance and information dissemination. In the Autism and Other Developmental Disabilities Division, she serves individuals referred for autism services in the Autism Spectrum Evaluation Clinic and Parent Home Training. She provides consultative and direct services to Navajo

Nation Growing in Beauty Program to build capacity in services related to autism spectrum disorders and other developmental delays. In addition, she represents the speech-language pathology discipline on the faculty team for the NM Leadership Education in Neurodevelopmental and Related Disabilities (LEND) program and facilitates opportunities for infusing cultural and linguistic competence with the LEND curriculum. She collaborates with faculty to provide an interdisciplinary training program that strives to improve the health of infants, children, and adolescents with or at risk for neurodevelopmental and related disabilities and their families. With their expertise, faculty members mentor, research, and teach as they support leadership development, team building, public policy & advocacy, research, and problem based and experiential learning. Her interest and work has also including improving cultural competency and advancing diversity, equity and inclusion efforts. She is Fellow of the Association. American Speech-Language-Hearing Association (ASHA). She has served as president for the New Mexico Speech-Language Association ((NMSHA) and has been a member of the Executive Board of Council of State Association Presidents (CSAP) and the Multicultural Issues Board of ASHA. She is a member of Native American Leadership Council for Speech-Language Pathologists and Audiologists, a constituency of ASHA. She has also served as co-chair for the Association of University Centers on Disabilities (AUCD) Multicultural Council and served on the AUCD Board of Directors.

Ruixia Yan is an Associate Professor, CCC-SLP in the Program of Communication Disorders, North Carolina Central University. Dr. Yan's areas of research include but not limited to child language disorders, speech sound disorders, multilingualism in communication disorders, etc.

Index

F

H

I

L

M

N

O

P

R

S

T

V

W

www.ingramcontent.com/pod-product-compliance
Lightning Source LLC
LaVergne TN
LVHW060409300926
849162LV00006B/1384